# CONSCIOUS HEALTH

*Choosing Natural Solutions for*
*Optimum Health and Lifelong Vitality*

## Ron Garner

NAMASTE PUBLISHING

BEAUFORT BOOKS

### DISCLAIMER

Although the author has extensively researched sources to ensure the accuracy and completeness of the information contained in this book, no responsibility is assumed for errors, inaccuracies, omissions, or inconsistencies herein. Any slights of people or organizations are unintentional. Neither the author nor the publisher is engaged in rendering professional advice or services to the individual reader. This book is not intended to be and should not be considered as a replacement for consultation, diagnosis, or treatment by a doctor or licensed healthcare practitioner. Please consult your personal physician or healthcare practitioner before starting any diet, taking nonprescription supplements, or beginning any new health treatment. The intent of this book is only to offer information to help you cooperate with your healthcare practitioner in your mutual search for health. Neither the author nor the publisher shall be liable or responsible for any loss or damage allegedly arising from any information or suggestion in this book.

While the author has made every effort to provide accurate Internet addresses at the time of publication, neither the publisher nor author assumes any responsibility for errors or for changes that occur after publication. Further, the publisher does not have control over and does not assume responsibility for author or third-party websites and their content.

#### LIBRARY OF CONGRESS CATALOGING-IN-PUBLICATION DATA

Garner, Ron (Ronald A.)
Conscious health : choosing natural solutions for optimum health and lifelong vitality /
Ron Garner.

p. cm.
Includes bibliographical references.
ISBN 0-8253-0540-3  (978-0-8253-0540-5 : alk. paper)

1. Naturopathy—Popular works. 2. Health—Popular works.
3. Self-care, Health—Popular works. I. Title

RZ440.G338
615.5'35—dc22     2006005017

#### CO-PUBLISHED BY

NAMASTE PUBLISHING
4563 West 3rd Avenue
Vancouver, BC  Canada  V6R 1N3
www.namastepublishing.com
namaste@telus.net

BEAUFORT BOOKS
27 West 20th Street, Suite 1102
New York, NY  10011
www.beaufortbooks.com
service@beaufortbooks.com

#### DISTRIBUTED IN NORTH AMERICA BY

MIDPOINT TRADE

Printed in Canada

*To all those who have a vision of creating*
*optimal health for themselves;*

*who dare to depart from conditioned thinking and*
*believe that health is there for them instead of a life*
*with inevitable disease;*

*who are willing to learn and to cooperate with their*
*bodies to achieve vibrant health;*

*and who want to live their lives responsibly*
*through conscious choice.*

# CONTENTS

## 4   WHAT IS DISEASE? / 53

## 5   HEALTH AND DISEASE / 73

SECOND KEY: **CLEANSING**

# 13 DETOXIFYING AND HEALING / 235

# 16 SUPPLEMENTS / 311

## FOURTH KEY: BELIEVING

# 17 AWARENESS / 327

# 18 ATTITUDES AND EMOTIONS / 337

## 19 THE POWER OF BELIEF / 349

# LIST OF ILLUSTRATIONS

*(Illustration credits: see page 482)*

## Tables

## Figures

## ACKNOWLEDGEMENTS

I ACKNOWLEDGE with deep gratitude Drs. Joel Robbins, Leo Roy, and Michael O'Brien who provided the foundational education that enabled me to understand how the human body always strives to be healthy.

With reverence, I recognize the many early pioneers and heroes in health research such as Drs. Francis Pottenger and Weston Price, whose works were ignored and even denigrated by the commercially motivated establishments of their time. In addition, the teaching of Dr. M. T. Morter Jr. has given me clear understanding of the paramount importance of the body's acid/alkaline balance and how to monitor it. Most recently, I acknowledge the current pioneer Victoria Boutenko for her studies of the chimpanzee diet and its vital significance to humans.

I am grateful to the many friends, relatives, and health practitioners who encouraged me to bring this practical message of health forward. I thank and acknowledge the many readers who have already expressed sincere gratitude to me for presenting this information in a form which explains the causes of disease and takes the confusion out of health.

It has been a distinct pleasure to work with the caring, professional team at Namaste Publishing. I am very grateful to Pat Brand, Chris Dube, and Dalyce Epp for their editing excellence in helping me to improve this work, while still respecting my vision and writing style throughout the process.

With profound thanks I acknowledge Connie Kellough, President of Namaste Publishing, for her guidance, support, encouragement, and example of unconditional love. It was Connie who recognized the greater vision for this book, marshaled the editorial resources, and forged the distribution contacts necessary to bring it to a world audience.

Finally, I am eternally grateful for my developing awareness of the oneness of everything and the special role each of us plays as part of the greater whole.

*Conscious health means choosing health. It means choosing health with understanding, awareness, intention, and vision. Conscious health is the active and deliberate creation of a vital body, mind, and spirit, with full knowledge, understanding, and belief. We create our lives, and we have the power to re-create them. When we are fully conscious, we can take responsibility for our own health. We can make the necessary choices and decisions. We can determine our health destiny.*

## WHY I WROTE THIS BOOK

FOR MOST OF my life, as I suffered with eczema, asthma, and various allergies, I intuitively felt there had to be answers for true healing. I couldn't believe that life had to be a continuous one-way slide toward more illness, pain, and deteriorating physical condition. Drugs and skin ointments, which only treat symptoms, not causes, didn't make any long-term or curative sense to me. I read everything I came across in my search for information and answers about bodily afflictions and healing. In this process, I learned a great deal. However, the information was like pieces of a jigsaw puzzle spread out on a table. I had parts of the picture, but couldn't find the form, plan, missing pieces, and an explanation to bring it all together. I needed a vision.

1

This book is the result of ten years of study, thought, and experience. It brings together the practical proceeds of extensive research and personal application of the principles it sets down. I have tried to make it clear and easily understandable, yet comprehensive. It was my goal to sort out and make sense of the plethora of information available on the subject of health, and to distill it into one easy-to-understand volume for the average reader. I wanted to present a complete picture, and the *truth* concerning the health of the human body, not just theories. And in arriving at conclusions, I applied a simple test, "Does it work?"

The content in this book does not include much medical and health industry terminology: both can be confusing. Nor does it go into deep or detailed background explanations. Some concepts are mentioned in more than one place and may appear to be repetitious to the reader. There are two reasons for this. First, repeating basic principles helps with learning and understanding. Second, this book is written to be both a practical reference that can be read and understood on a topical basis and a complete work. It is intended to be a presentation of the "natural facts" about how and why the health of the body degenerates, and how that process can be reversed. I write in large part from my own experience.

I would like to encourage particularly those people who may be suffering from serious or long-standing health challenges to read this book, or at least the most pertinent sections, several times. When we understand the principles of health well enough to be able to explain them to others, we also gain the mindset to do what is necessary to change our own situation for the better.

It is my hope that you will find the information here to be enlightening and practical. May it help to create a new vision of hope for you on your own exciting personal journey to conscious health.

## WE CREATE OUR OWN HEALTH

"A journey of a thousand miles begins with a single step." This old adage speaks a powerful truth, and its meaning implies that before anything can be accomplished, one must first initiate some kind of action. But if it is to lead to success, what gives an action its power? How can we know that our first step will lead to success?

To walk a thousand miles we must *intend* to do it, *believe* that we can accomplish it, make the determined *decision* to do it, and then take action to *implement* our decision. Only the person who is doing it can create the desired outcome for his or her own benefit. Someone else can't do it for them. This is how the universe operates.

We live in a universe of creation that has nothing to do with religion, but everything to do with the spirit of belief. And that is what is exciting about it. When we think we can, to the point of believing it, we create the life we want, which includes a healthy body, mind, and spirit. We are mini-creators. We create our own lives. We create our bodies. The thoughts that constantly circulate in our heads are reflections of our beliefs, and our beliefs do the creating.

Cellular biologist Dr. Bruce Lipton discovered through his research with living cells that belief or perception creates our reality. What we believe at the subconscious level actually instructs our cells how, and in what form, to reproduce.[1]

You've heard it said when someone finds themselves in an uncomfortable situation in their life, "You made your own bed, now lie in it!" In other words, you took certain actions that got you to where you are now; you made decisions that led to your situation; you produced it yourself.

Whether we realize it or not, we are doing it! Every moment, we are creating our own reality, including our state of health or disease. We create one or the other by how conscious and honoring we are of our bodies. Our bodies reflect our subconscious or core beliefs. They reflect our knowledge of how they build themselves and how we choose to act on that knowledge. They reflect our wisdom or our ignorance. They reflect our caring or our apathy.

The self-creating process works from our subconscious core beliefs. We are *unconscious* of this process to the extent that we are unaware of our core beliefs. The creation and self-direction of our life becomes magic when we are *conscious* of the underlying beliefs that generate our reality.

There is a legal maxim that states, "Ignorance is not a defense of the law," meaning that lack of knowledge is not a valid excuse for breaking the law and will not save us from the consequences. So it is with our bodies. They were created to function under natural law. They have requirements that must be met to be healthy. Ignorance of any of these needs, be they nutritional, energetic, or attitudinal, does not nullify the natural consequence of degenerating health as we grow older.

The purpose of this book is to help you become consciously aware that you have the power to create the health and happiness you choose. Five transformational tools are presented to empower you to take responsibility for your own health. Healthcare practitioners and caregivers are encouraged to use the information they find here, which may not have been part of their own training.

This book presents a *complementary* and *evolutionary* paradigm of healthcare. It brings together knowledge and understanding that can become shared and applied. Although the information is not new, the widespread application of it and the approach to "self-health" is.

Presently, diseases of all description appear to be beyond our control, and they are increasing. While medical science has made advances, "natural" approaches are achieving cures in areas previously thought to be incurable. Energy or vibrational medicine, practiced in the East for hundreds of years, is now being embraced in the West and advanced by discoveries in technology. But almost totally ignored is the potential of the creative or spiritual aspect within all of us to be our most powerful ally for health.

It is time for a marriage of everything that *works* for health, in a spirit of open-mindedness and love. It is time to consciously incorporate the best of science, nature, and spirit to build the bodies and lives we were designed to create from the very beginning.

## GAINING A VISION FOR HEALTH

Vitality. Even the word has a nice ring to it. It means, "full of life and energy," or "the overall energy of the body." Vitality is the feeling of life within us. Wouldn't it be wonderful not to have our bodies break down, become more painful, and develop diseases as we grow older? This is possible! That is the way the human body was designed to operate. And it will, if we do our part to help it.

What happened to the vitality we used to enjoy? What about others, our age or older, who seem to be in good health? Is it possible that we can regain this quality of life? When we look back on our lives and see the progression of our worsening conditions and the loss of energy, do we wonder about it? Do we just accept our substandard or deteriorating health as an inevitable part of life? Is this what life is all about: loss of energy with more pain and suffering as we grow older? Is it inevitable, as statistics tell us, that we can probably expect to contract a disease such as diabetes, arthritis, heart disease, or cancer? What can we do?

What you are about to read attempts to take the mystery out of health and disease. It will provide the understanding that many people, even some health professionals, do not have. When you finish reading this book you will know:

- What marvelous, naturally intelligent creations our bodies are.
- What the purpose of a cold or flu is, and why we get them.
- That diseases such as arthritis, heart disease, and even cancer are actually the body's effort to keep us alive longer.
- What drugs are and what they do to our bodies.
- Where energy actually originates from.
- What real food for our bodies is.
- What the best kind of water for our bodies is.
- What the "workers" inside our bodies are.
- The difference between real food and junk food.
- What our bodies need to stay healthy, or to regain health.
- That the human body actually runs on electricity, not tiny particles of digested matter.
- That anything that interferes with the electrical nature and functions of our bodies undermines our health.
- That everything we eat and drink must be electrically compatible with

the body or it cannot be used for health.

- What the natural chemistry of our bodies needs to be to keep us healthy, and how when it gets out of balance, it leads to disease.
- What we must do to reverse the disease process and become healthy.
- Which supplements can help the body and which ones place extra burdens on it.
- That our attitudes and beliefs are the basis for everything in our lives.
- That our health depends on the nutritional and lifestyle choices we make.

## AN OWNER'S MANUAL

Every new car comes with an owner's manual to inform the driver of its maintenance requirements and to explain its various features. In order to perform reliably and optimally, the car requires quality fuel and lubrication materials, and needs to be cleaned and have its oil changed regularly. If a car is not maintained properly it will eventually develop problems and stop operating. The owner of a newer vehicle needs to become familiar with technical features such as interior climate controls and onboard navigation systems in order to make full use of features the car has to offer.

Caring for the human body can be likened to maintaining an automobile. The difference is that we do not come equipped with an owner's manual. Nonetheless, our needs are similar. Our bodies need to be supplied with a full range of nutrients that promote life, and need to be able to regularly eliminate digestive, metabolic, and toxic wastes. If these requirements are not met, problems develop and diseases start to appear. For optimum performance, the human body needs its owner to understand the energy healing features that are built into it that create physical and emotional health. We need understanding.

When people ask me what this book is about, I tell them that it explains: how the human body was designed to operate, what its requirements for healthy operation are, why it develops disease symptoms, how the disease process can be reversed, and how one can enjoy health and vitality well into old age. This book was written to give the understanding people require to be able to monitor and maintain their own health programs. It is a human body owner's manual for self-empowerment.

## STARTING TO QUESTION

Food is the basis of most of our disease problems. We have been conditioned to think that we can eat and drink anything we like, and when things start to go wrong in our bodies, to go to the doctor. But is that working? Is there less heart disease, diabetes, allergies, and cancer now than there used be? Something is missing!

After we've been to all the doctors in search of help for our physical ailments and are still no better, where do we turn? After the doctors say, "I'm sorry, there's nothing more we can do," or worse yet, "You only have two to six months to live. We've done all we can," you don't want to give up, but what can you do? Could there be another route besides the usual doctors and prescription drugs? Health is the most precious thing we have, so why do we turn control of it over to someone else? Putting our trust in conventional healthcare systems alone, and letting someone else make health decisions for us, isn't bringing the results we need and want. Are these systems really focused on health care, or are they focused on disease care? Is there an alternative to conventional medicine? Is there any hope in so-called "natural health," or the ways of Mother Nature?

If these thoughts have gone through your mind, you are beginning to think for yourself. Something inside you doesn't want to give up or give in. We shouldn't give up. We can educate ourselves about how the human body was designed to work. We can start making decisions for ourselves about the treatment of our conditions. We can start working in a caring way *with* the body. A better degree of health with more vitality is possible. It is there, because that's the way the body was meant to be. The truth of the matter is that health is a conscious choice when we have become aware of how it is created.

## IT'S UP TO US

We have to become knowledgeable about what the body requires for health, and supply those needs to it. There is an alternative to the conventional *healthcare* that is provided by someone else. *Selfcare* implies making informed choices for ourselves according to the natural principles our bodies are based on. The earlier we start on this path, the better our chances of success will be. Many people have made the decision to apply the recommendations in this book to their lives, and an increasing number are enjoying improved health by using the approach that nature intended for the nurture of our bodies. Health is a matter of choice, not a matter of chance.

How do we take back our health power? We get back to the basics that our bodies need to be healthy. We need to apply the *5 Keys*.

1 Learning—Gain health knowledge.
2 Cleansing—Detoxify your body.
3 Feeding—Give your body the nutrition it needs.
4 Believing—Think positive creative thoughts.
5 Implementing—Take action.

Let's start the process of building understanding about how health and disease really work, so we can be empowered to make the right choices to change our health and our lives.

~ FIRST KEY

# LEARNING

# 1 | GAINING PERPSECTIVE

∾

*Wonder is the beginning of wisdom.*
GREEK PROVERB

∾

## A BRIEF PERSONAL HISTORY

SOON AFTER I was born, I had eczema over most of my body. As a child, I had brief periods of asthma, and the eczema was intense every spring and summer until I was about 16. From age 17 to 21, I enjoyed good health—the best of my life. However, by age 22, hay fever started with each spring and lasted into the summer. By age 25, the asthma returned, and I had to carry a bronchial dilator with me at all times. After living on a farm for a year, I became allergic to most grass and tree pollens, dust, dogs, cats, horses, and cows, as well as eggs and bee pollen. When my doctor put me on prednisone, I began reading about the dangers of this strong form of cortisone, and I weaned myself off it with great difficulty. For most of my adult life, until I began to change my lifestyle, I suffered with all these afflictions, plus indigestion and chronic diarrhea. In later years, food allergies began to be more of a problem as well.

All my life, I felt there had to be answers as to why we become sick and diseased, and how we can return to health. I asked my physicians, "Why do doctors only treat symptoms? Why don't they talk about the causes of illnesses?" I received no answers from them, so I asked myself, "What can *I* do? Do I have any power to change my health?"

In my search I continued reading material from the natural health field, feeling that the answers had to be somewhere. In this process, I found wisdom in the writings of some great practitioners and teachers: people like Doctors Arnold Ehret, Bernard Jensen, Norman Walker, and Paul Bragg. These men practiced what they preached. Dr. Walker worked until the day he died at the age of 109 while having an afternoon nap. Dr. Bragg opened the first health food store in the U.S. and wrote many books on health, and died at 95 by drowning while surfing off a California beach.

However, it was not until I came upon the teaching, research, and practice of Dr. Joel Robbins that the puzzle came together for me. Dr. Robbins explained clearly the truths about health and the disease process. Subsequently, I studied under him via the College of Natural Health, which he founded. I was awarded a Doctorate diploma, which entitles the holder to practice as a nutritional counselor in the United States of America.

During those studies, I was introduced to the writings of Dr. Henry Bieler, who wrote *Food is Your Best Medicine*. He treated patients for over 50 years without prescribing a drug. I also encountered the pioneering work of Dr. Royal Lee. In the 1940s, he invented machinery to produce whole food supplements that retain their life forces, using combinations of various foods. I also met Dr. Leo Roy, who spent most of his life helping people with their health and researching and writing about how the body heals itself. More recently, I became acquainted with Dr. Michael O'Brien's work and his belief that it is never too late for a body to return to health.

Through these mentors, I came to understand how our body functions. I also learned that mainstream conventional medicine does not understand what causes most diseases. For the most part, modern medicine practices disease treatment, and subscribes to the belief that the symptom is the problem. That is, if you can eliminate the symptom, you have conquered the disease. But that is not true. I am not saying that modern medical care has no place. On the contrary, when we are in a crisis such as a traumatic injury, heart attack, or severe allergic reaction, we have some of the finest lifesaving care, procedures, technology, and medicine in the world available to us. My own life was saved by penicillin when I had blood poisoning at the age of 13. However, for our general health and to avoid developing diseases, we need to become informed and accept personal responsibility for our own health. We need to understand that disease is a process and not a "happening." It is our lifestyle choices that determine whether a health process or a disease process takes hold in our bodies.

In 1994, I began in earnest to change my own nutritional program under the initial guidance of Dr. Robbins. It required hard work and determination to get to where I am now, but it was worth it. Since that time, the dry skin, indigestion, diarrhea, hay fever, asthma, getting up three or four times in the night, and lack of energy have been corrected. I have an energetic feeling of well-being, and now need less sleep each night. In retrospect, I realize I made a lot of mistakes because I didn't fully understand the health-rebuilding process. Now, I have energy that I haven't enjoyed for many years. It feels wonderful to wake up feeling refreshed after a night's sleep, able to think clearly without mental fog.

In the year 2000, when I added a group of electrically synergistic supplements to my diet, the rate of improvement in my health and vitality increased even further. Then, in 2004, I made a sustained effort to bring my acid-alkaline values into healthy alignment. Finally, I began to see the overall results I had been seeking and my health made great strides. But there was one more nutritional component to learn: the importance of significantly increasing the proportion of whole raw greens to my diet.

It is exciting to see and feel good health return again. It takes self-discipline and perseverance to change a lifestyle and to reverse the effects of many years of living contrary to nature's laws. If you are prepared to take responsibility for your own health, then, as Dr. Joel Robbins says, "Ten years from now you can feel better, and be healthier, than you were ten years ago."[2] I am happy to say I can testify to that statement! This process took me twelve years of learning and experimentation, but because of the information in this book you can make great health gains in much less time—without the mistakes I made.

I would love to have known the information in this book earlier in my life. What a difference it would have made to my own health program. That's the whole point. The earlier that we convert to a health-building lifestyle, the younger our bodies will look and be for a longer time. When supplied with its needs, the body naturally responds with vitality. It's an interesting and exciting adventure. And, in the process of learning and applying these principles, we can also help our loved ones and friends experience positive changes in their own health and lives.

First, let's walk through some basic information. Understanding is necessary for us to persist in carrying through with our new health objectives. As we educate ourselves about how to be healthy, we become empowered to take the necessary steps toward achieving our own vitality for life!

## CREATING HEALTH OR IDENTIFYING DISEASES?

This book is about how to create health. It is not about diseases. Some degenerative disease conditions are discussed, but only for the purpose of showing that they develop when the body has lost its natural balance, or homeostasis, through being deprived of its basic needs. Disease develops when the natural laws of health are broken. We need a thorough understanding and appreciation of those laws.

The human body knows how to be healthy. Our job is to supply what it needs to do its job, and not to dictate which conditions it must work on. This concept is contrary to our western way of looking at health, which focuses on trying to cure diseases. Conventional western medicine treats disease conditions or symptoms. It does not treat the basic causes of disease, the reasons why health begins to degenerate in the first place.

The "chasing the disease" approach simply doesn't work in the long run because it can't! If you don't address the *cause* of a problem, it will just surface again later. It may arise in a different form, or it may come back in the same form but be much more serious.

When natural laws of caring for the body are ignored, aging and deterioration take place in a manner that, sooner or later, results in serious loss of quality of life. As some older friends have said to me, "It's no fun growing old." And, with skyrocketing healthcare expenses plus reduced services, how cost-effective is the standard medical route? And how reliable is it? How long are the waiting lists for surgery, or even to get an appointment with a specialist? What are the costs for heart operations or cancer treatments? And, in the end, are they curative?

The fact is, we do not have to concentrate on any one specific disease condition. We need to focus on *health* because that's the way our body naturally operates.

## HOW TO START GETTING HEALTHIER

On our road to renewed health, we must *decide* that we are going to be healthy. This is our *active intent*. We must take responsibility for our own health. We must take control of our own lives. It begins with this first determined thought. Next, we must become fully *aware* of how our health is gained and maintained. This where the 5 KEYS OF CONSCIOUS HEALTH come in.

## THE 5 KEYS

### Key # 1: Learning—Gain Health Knowledge

The first step is education about how health is gained and maintained. We need knowledge; it is the beginning of power. Understanding is the primary key to correcting the *wrongs* in our lives and consistently doing the *rights*. Education brings understanding that enables us to put the learned principles to work in our lives so we can start to see positive results.

Many people die from lack of knowledge. Always be searching for the truth. And, just because something is accepted practice doesn't mean it is the truth. False knowledge is more dangerous than ignorance. Accepting one false principle about health and nutrition erodes the benefits of our gained wisdom.

### Key # 2: Cleansing—Detoxify Your Body

Over years of not living in accordance with the way nature intended, our bodies become burdened with stored wastes that shouldn't be there.

15

Toxins are the cause of reduced function and premature aging. Just like the engine or radiator of our car, if they aren't cleaned on a regular basis, they overheat and wear out. Before we can return to vibrant health, we have to do some housecleaning for our bodies too. This is called detoxification.

### Key # 3: Feeding—Give Your Body the Nutrition it Needs

You need to feed your body what it can use to rejuvenate itself. As we have already learned, the human body is very wise; given the proper tools, it knows what to do to achieve health. Our job is not to try to "fix" a disease—that's the body's job. Our job is to give the body what it needs and let it do the rest.

### Key # 4: Believing—Think Positive Creative Thoughts

Our thoughts stem from our beliefs, and our beliefs create what happens in our lives. A habit of negative thinking creates situations of unhappiness or lack. Positive thoughts, based on positive subconscious beliefs, create happiness and abundance. We need to think carefully about what we think!

### Key # 5: Implementing—Take Action

Once we have made the decision to be healthy and have started to educate ourselves about what helps our bodies to cleanse, heal, and stay healthy, we must then be determined to put healthy lifestyle principles into practice. We must take consistent action.

As we gain experience by applying healthy principles to our diet and lifestyle, we can learn to read the various signals our bodies send us when they are stressed and when they are healing. We become detectives, figuring out from the clues our bodies give what they need us to do to make and keep ourselves healthy.

The only way to true health is by taking full responsibility for it. Every "body" is different, with different deficiencies and weaknesses. No one knows you and your body like you do. Individual health is a very personal thing, and no doctor or therapist can know enough about you to "fix" your problems. It is only you, with your intimate knowledge of your self, your growing knowledge about what a body needs for health, and your continuous attention to your bodily signals, who can make the adjustments and changes that are required. Only then can it serve you with real and lasting health. It is a symbiotic relationship: we supply the body with its needs, and it serves us with good health.

For those who are just beginning, this book is an important first step. It provides education about what the body requires in order to be healthy. The ensuing steps, of making positive changes in our lives and continuing with our health education, are up to us. This venture is the most interesting, exciting, and rewarding discovery I have made in my life. I hope it will be for you as well.

## BREAKING THROUGH OUR CONDITIONING

Ignorance is defined as "not knowing." As we break into knowledge or "knowing," the first step is realizing that "we don't know that we don't know." For most of our lives, we have been taught by our parents, peers, culture, church, and government to look to others for direction, and to do what we are told. In other words, we have been conditioned not to think for ourselves. This has had a disempowering effect on us. For the most part, we have come to think that we don't or can't know enough, and that others are more capable than we are. This, inevitably, has led to a lack of confidence in our ability to make decisions for ourselves.

A little book that I recommend in the highest terms is *The Four Agreements* by Don Miguel Ruiz. In this book, Ruiz shares wisdom from thousands of years ago handed down by Toltec men and women of knowledge in southern Mexico. It cleverly explains how, as small children, we make "agreements" in our minds based on what we encounter in our external, parental, and cultural environments about what must be "true"; then, we accept them and they become our beliefs. But, the vast majority of them are not true. When we read and practice "the four agreements," they will revolutionize how we understand ourselves and act in our relationships, and we will gain personal freedom.

When we were born, of necessity we depended on our parents for survival, protection, and direction. We accepted their rules and ways of thinking. As we grew older, we went to school and took direction from our teachers. Then, when we got a job, we took direction from the boss; we had to if we wanted to stay in the job. In matters of spirituality and religion, we were taught to listen to the minister, pastor, priest, rabbi, or sheikh. In matters of our health, we have been conditioned by our upbringing, the media, and the pharmaceutical industry to go to the doctor because "The doctor knows best." But is this always the case?

We think we are free, in control, and well taken care of, but are we *really*? The answer in health, as in all other parts of our lives, is to *think for ourselves*. One of the most important truths I have learned in my life is: "It is not so much who we know, or what we think we know that is most important, but the questions we ask." Always be thinking for yourself, and be open to learning something new. Think like a little child again, and ask the "why" questions.

## HEALTH IS A CHOICE

Once we overcome our ignorance of what the body requires to be healthy, the state of our health becomes our choice. The lifestyle we choose to live determines our health. Every day we make decisions about what to eat and drink, how much exercise, rest, and fresh air to get, how to take care of our personal hygiene, and whether our attitudes will be positive or negative. We create our own health; it is our responsibility.

## UNDERSTANDING YOUR BODY

The human body is programmed to be healthy. It is not programmed for disease. It will reward us with health when its requirements are met because it has a remarkable ability to bounce back. This will happen automatically. That's great news. However, as we take responsibility for our own health with "self-care," it really helps to have a basic understanding of how the body operates.

The next two chapters will focus on how the human body was created to function. Chapter 2 discusses how the wonderful human body works to build health and fight disease, and how it sets priorities to always work in our best interest. Chapter 3 provides a basic physiological explanation of the body's main operating systems.

# 2 | THE WONDERFUL HUMAN BODY

~

*… this consummation of the design of nature,*
*which is able to bear and house a spiritual being.*
Sir George Trevelyan

~

## WHAT OUR BODIES NEED

As we begin to understand how it works, we realize what a perfectly designed and amazing body we have. If it is given the proper nutrition, exercise, and rest, and is supported by positive attitudes and freedom from serious emotional stress, the human body is fully capable of staying healthy for 120 years or more. It has innate intelligence, a built-in *knowing*. It is designed to self-correct by instinct. All we have to do is work *with* it, not *against* it. Even in the face of all the wrongs we inflict on the body, it still strives valiantly to keep us healthy for as long as it can. It struggles in the face of deficiencies and hardships. It truly is a faithful servant.

The body's efficiency weakens only when we neglect its needs, or ignore the complaints it sends us in the form of symptoms. Of course the longer this continues, the less vitality it has until finally it begins to break down and succumbs to disease. What else can we expect?

It is an odd characteristic of human nature that we usually take better care of our cars and other machines, servicing them with proper parts and materials. We wouldn't think of putting diesel fuel in a gasoline engine or dirty oil in the crankcase. Similarly, we try to take care of our household plants and gardens so they will yield good blossoms, fruit, and vegetables. We wouldn't use salted water, soft drinks, or alcoholic beverages on the potted plants in our houses, or feed them grease from cooking. If we want them to be healthy, we cultivate and nourish the soil. We know that they need clean water, air, sunshine, and agreeable temperatures.

Yet, when it comes to our bodies, we typically ignore common sense. We treat them as if they were super "garbage digesters" with stainless steel parts. We don't question whether the food we consume helps or hinders the body. We dump greasy foods, sugar, salt, alcohol, harmful food additives, drugs, and more into our stomachs. Some of us smoke. We deprive our bodies of regular rest. Some of us worry ourselves half to death on a regular basis. Yet, we expect to be healthy. When we do become diseased, we think it is bad luck, or that some germ or virus zapped us. But the germ or virus would not have gained a foothold in the body if our immune system, with its specialized cells to resist disease-producing organisms, had remained strong. And, the body will be strong if we give it what it needs to be healthy, and if we keep it relatively free of toxic wastes.

The human body has a tremendous innate ability and corrective capability, but it has limits. We know it cannot go on indefinitely without sleep, but it cannot go on indefinitely without having its other needs met either. If deficiencies are not corrected, and abuses are not stopped, sooner or later it will begin to break down and health disturbances will begin to manifest in some area of the body. The location is often related to genetic weaknesses passed on from our parents and grandparents. Under stress, these areas tend to be the first to show signs of disease such as allergy, asthma, high blood pressure, heart disease, arthritis, diabetes, and emotional disorders.

We can be the body's greatest friend or its worst enemy. Our choices of food, rest, exercise, fresh air, sunshine and attitudes have the greatest impact on our health. We need to know what our bodies require to be healthy. But, before that, we need to understand how our bodies function.

## OUR BODIES ARE ELECTRIC

Our bodies run on electricity. Everything in the universe is an expression of energy. While we have been taught that the atom is "the smallest particle of an element," leading scientists now reason this is not so. There are tremendous spaces even within an atom. Consider two models: one of the sun and the orbiting earth, and the other of an atom with its nucleus and electrons. The distance between the nucleus of an atom and its orbiting electrons is *proportionately* forty-seven times greater than the distance between the sun and our orbiting earth.[1] Even the central components of an atom, the proton and neutron, are not the smallest parts. In fact, there are spaces within them. Scientists have found even smaller particles called quarks that also have great spaces between them. And on it goes. Nothing is solid. What we consider to be "matter" is actually energy in various forms.[2] By arranging clusters of atoms in different patterns, we get different matter. Each "particle" of that matter is actually a matrix of energy configured in a certain pattern.

So what does this mean to our health? All atoms are polarized, with positively charged protons that attract, and negatively charged electrons that repel. This "polarized energy" is electricity. Each one of our cells is a little electric battery capable of being recharged by a properly shaped charge of energy. Just as a DC (direct current) battery cannot operate on AC (alternating current), our bodies, which are "natural," cannot operate on foods that are "unnatural" or synthetic, because their electrical configurations are not compatible with our body requirements. Such foods contain no life force energy, just as dead batteries have no electricity or life. The human body can only be recharged from food sources that are electrically alive.

The electrical energy or vibratory frequency of a healthy human body is in the range of 62–78 megahertz (MHz).[3] As the body frequency is lowered, disease states begin to set in. Dead food, including cooked food that has no electrical vibrancy, plays a significant role in lowering the body's electrical reserve. The electrical configurations for our cells come from the food we eat, as the processes within the bodies break it down into its atomic parts. Food is transformed by digestive processes for use in our bodies as electricity.[4] Food properties change form depending on what is done to it. How food was grown, what kind of soil it was grown in, what sprays or chemicals were used, how and when it was harvested, how it was processed, and how it was cooked before it was consumed will determine the energy configurations of the food atoms. All these factors have a bearing on whether it can be used by the body for health. Each vitamin or mineral has a unique electrical configuration, and body cells select the matrices that fit its requirements. Only energy with a properly configured matrix can enter and charge cells. An analogy is of a key that must have a proper shape, or configuration, to enter a lock and open it. Our bodies require a full array of naturally formed vitamins, minerals, amino acids, and live enzymes. Synthetic matrices just don't fit. Anything unnatural has wrongly-configured matrices, and therefore cannot nourish and energize cells.

Most food is grown in soils that have been depleted of minerals, and treated with chemical pesticides and fertilizers. It is picked before it has ripened and assembled all its nutrients. Next, it is processed and denatured of all its enzymes by being cooked in various ways. Once again, we end up with electrical matrices that are unnatural, distorted, incomplete, and toxic. Everything done to food changes its electrical matrix. Such food, when broken down by our bodies and processed for energy, lacks the correct configurations our cells require for energy and tissue construction. This causes two things to happen. First, this unnatural energy must be eliminated from the body because it is toxic, and, if that is not possible, it must be stored in the tissues. Second, the body must rob the required vitamins, minerals, amino acids, and enzymes from its own tissues—cannibalizing itself—to manufacture energy for its cellular requirements. As this continues over time, the body's energy reserves become depleted, and its electromagnetic composition becomes distorted, which allows disease to develop. Health returns when the body's electrical balance is restored.

## THE BODY AS A CONSTRUCTION SITE

Caring for the human body can be compared to building a house. Once a building lot is obtained, two things are needed: construction materials and workers. In our bodies, the construction materials are the components of the food we eat. To build our house we wouldn't use board scraps, burned pieces of plywood, wiring that has been soaked in acid or oil, or weak cement that has been mixed with one measure of cement to fifty measures of sand or gravel. We would use quality materials to build a quality house that will be strong, look good, and serve us well. And, as we build our house, we would remove waste materials from the construction site and take them to the dump so our site is clean and the working environment efficient. To build strong bodies, we also need quality materials in the form of quality food, and we need an efficient elimination of waste materials from the body.

We can have all the very best materials to build our house in a pile at the construction site, but if we have no workers to assemble the materials they will sit there and eventually rot. It's the same with our bodies. There are only two things that do "construction" work in our bodies: *enzymes* and *bowel bacteria*. If enzymes are not available or are in short supply at each stage of the digestion process, the body cannot do its job of building a good house for us. Poisons are created, and weaknesses and problems develop. If a sufficient quantity of friendly bacteria is not present in the bowel, the body cannot manufacture certain enzymes, vitamins, and antibiotics. Putrefaction, or rot and stagnation, then occurs in the colon. All disease symptoms can be traced to these problems.

## A BRIEF OVERVIEW OF DIGESTION AND ELIMINATION

*Absorption* takes place mostly in the small intestine where the broken-down food substances are absorbed through the intestinal wall and sent to the liver to be processed. The liver metabolizes these food substances by combining them with enzymes and converting them into energy and nutrient components. It then sends these out to the cells of the body via the bloodstream.

*Assimilation* happens when nutrients carried in the blood are incorporated into the cells as energy and transformed into tissue.

*Elimination* is the removal of the normal waste products of digestion and cellular function.

## UNDERSTANDING DIGESTION

Digestion is the major starting point of health. All building materials for creating cells and tissues are transformed into molecular structures by digestive enzymes so the body can utilize them. Without these, every organ, tissue, and cell of our bodies degenerates. Almost all people who are victims of degenerative diseases have problems with their digestion, and most of these can be attributed to a lack of digestive enzymes.

Digestion begins in the mouth when food is chewed and mixed with saliva, which contains essential enzymes for digesting sugars. This is why it is very important to chew your food thoroughly.

As food enters the stomach, hydrochloric acid and enzymes are secreted to combine with enzymes already supplied in raw foods, beginning the digestion process. Efficient digestion in the stomach is very important. The environment in the stomach is acidic. Enzymes and pepsin in the stomach react on protein to form amino acids, which then pass into the small intestine as nutrients for the liver.

Partially digested food leaves the stomach and enters the small intestine for the final stage of digestion. The inner lining of the small intestine produces a secretion that creates an alkaline environment for this stage of digestion. Here, enzymes produced by the pancreas are secreted through the pancreatic duct into the small intestine. These digestive enzymes only work in an alkaline medium. Bile, secreted by the liver and stored in the gall bladder, is added to the mixture via the common bile duct as needed to break down fat molecules into smaller particles. Digested food particles that have now been broken down into molecular size nutrients are absorbed through the villi in the small intestine and transported through capillaries into the portal vein and moved directly to the liver.

Using more enzymes, the liver converts the nutrients into usable energy and fuel for all cells of the body. Purified and replenished with usable nutrients, blood from the liver is then pumped by the heart to the lungs to receive oxygen, and sent on to the cells in all parts of the body through blood vessels and capillaries.

Our stomachs, intestines, pancreases, and livers are the most excessively used and abused of all organs. If we continue our intake of wrong foods, drugs, and chemicals, our digestive systems fight a losing battle trying to keep us healthy. When we change to healthy lifestyle practices, our digestive systems can regain their efficiency.

Everything we put into our mouths must be completely available and usable by all the organs and cells of our bodies; otherwise, the potential health benefits pass right through us. Our digestive systems must have their requirements met at every station along the way: mouth, stomach, small intestine, and large intestine. It is the same as a production line for assembling cars, if the workers or correct materials are not available at each station along the way, the car is not built properly.

## UNDERSTANDING ELIMINATION

Elimination is the removal of waste products from the body. In addition to the processing of metabolic waste by the liver and kidneys, the body utilizes several other modes of elimination such as the lymphatic system, bowels, lungs, skin, and the mucus membranes of the nose, throat, ears, and eyes. The main portal for the removal of wastes, however, is via bowel movements through the colon.

When the colon becomes overburdened with excess wastes, it becomes congested, and the body resorts to using additional channels to eliminate toxins as long as it has sufficient energy to do this. When the body's vitality is high, mucus membranes and skin are also used as avenues of elimination. As a result, symptoms such as colds, sinusitis, ear infections, measles, chicken pox, and eczema arise. As vitality lowers, the body cannot afford the expenditure of energy required for the alternate elimination, and is forced to store toxins in its tissues. As this continues, toxins are stored in the deeper layers of the tissues where they eventually cause diseases such as arthritis, heart disease, senility, and cancer.

After food has been processed in the small intestine and nutrients extracted for use by the body, the remaining wastes are moved to the large intestine, or colon, before being expelled from the body as feces. Fecal matter in bowel movements contains fiber and wastes from the digestion of food. It also contains waste products from cellular metabolism.

We should have as many bowel movements each day as the number of substantial meals we eat. When the number of movements is less than this, a condition of stagnation exists. Wherever there is stagnant food matter, there is fermentation and rotting. Where there is rotting, toxins are formed. When fecal matter sits in the colon for longer than normal, toxins are absorbed back into the body causing autointoxication or poisoning. Poisoning leads to disease. From this progression, we can understand the phrase, "Disease begins in the colon." That is why it is so important to have regular and good elimination. V. E. Irons, a pioneer in promoting colon cleansing, maintained that 95% of people's health problems start in the colon with self-created conditions of intestinal toxemia.[5] Michael O'Brien, noted lecturer, product formulator in the nutritional industry, and former medical doctor, puts this figure even higher, at 99.99%. Dr. Bernard Jensen explained an example of this disease process in his book *Breathe Again Naturally*:

> The primary cause of asthma and all other respiratory conditions may be found in the eliminative system. … Chronic lung congestion indicates that the other eliminative channels are not doing their job. … Either wastes are being produced faster than the normal capacity of all eliminative channels to get rid of them, or one or more of the eliminative channels is under-active. We need to ask why the lungs and

bronchials are congested. We need to know what is going on in the other eliminative channels. To clean out the lungs and bronchial tubes, we need to develop a clean bloodstream and lymphatic system. To clean up the blood and lymph, we will have to take care of the bowel.[6]

Good elimination depends on the many digestive processes that happen in the alimentary tract above the colon. It is affected by the quality of food eaten, the digestive enzymes present, and how adequately food is chewed to break it down and mix it with saliva.

While we are working to improve our digestion, it is necessary to keep our bowels moving, which may require the use of enemas, colonics, or even a gentle herbal laxative. This is to avoid the reabsorption of toxins back into the body and to "re-educate" the bowel to induce its own contractions on a more regular basis. Supplements of friendly bacteria, also known as friendly flora and probiotics, should be taken to increase their population in the colon.

Without regular and healthy bowel movements, a body cannot be truly healthy. We need to observe our bowel movements regularly, and work with the principles and suggestions in this and other books to achieve the elimination of normal, healthy stools.

## THE IMMUNE SYSTEM

The immune system is a complex and delicately balanced system whose function is to defend the body against invaders and to fight disease. The components of this system work to eliminate potential antigens such as drugs, pollens, insect venom, chemicals in foods, malignant cells, and foreign tissue such as transplanted organs or transfused blood. It can deal with a wide range of pathogens such as viruses, fungi, bacteria, and parasites. The immune system maintains its own system of circulation via the lymphatic vessels, which permeate every organ in the body except the brain. The lymphatic system is sometimes referred to as the body's other circulation and elimination system. These vessels contain lymph, which is a pale, thick fluid consisting of fat-laden liquid and white blood cells. Lymph nodes, tonsils, bone marrow, spleen, liver, pancreas, lungs, and the intestines are also part of the immune system. As part of an immune response, white blood cells are mobilized and deployed to areas of the body requiring their assistance. Lymph nodes, which contain filters, swell because the lymphatic vessels drain infection by carrying it to the nearest area where an immune response can be organized. The lymph nodes most commonly recognized are in the neck and groin areas.

Our bodies possess two kinds of immunity. Everyone is born with innate immunity, or the ability to react to foreign substances. Our bodies also have learned immunity, which is the ability to learn, adapt, and remember. This explains why people do not contract chickenpox or measles more than once.

Immunity involves the production of a specific protein called an antibody, which is designed to destroy a particular invader called an antigen—a foreign, unusable protein molecule. The immune system is constantly searching for antigens that don't belong to the body. Its basic strategy is to recognize the enemy, mobilize forces, and attack.

As great as the immune system is, it can only work if it is cared for properly. This means getting all the right nutrients and enzymes, having the right environment, and avoiding those things that tend to depress immunity such as: household cleaners, the overuse of antibiotics and drugs, pesticides, chemical additives present in the foods we eat, exposure to environmental pollutants, and stress. Lowered immunity results in impaired healing ability and lowered defense against infection.

Symptoms of lowered immunity in our bodies can be: frequent colds and flu, herpes (cold sores), allergies, continual fatigue, candida yeast overgrowth, painful joints and muscles, parasite infections, psoriasis, eczema, and inflammatory disorders.

Healthy immunity is dependent on a healthy ecology in the gastrointestinal tract. This includes having the right food and all necessary enzymes to completely break it down into its component molecules so the body can process it for its needs. It depends on a healthy stock of bowel bacteria in the intestines. When the gastrointestinal tract is healthy, the body can manufacture the other enzymes, vitamins, and antibiotics it needs to be in top-notch health and to maintain a fully functional immune system.

## THE BODY'S NATURAL 24-HOUR CYCLE

This concept is very important and should be completely understood, appreciated, and incorporated into one's lifestyle to promote optimum health. The body must be given adequate time to be able to properly complete digestion, absorption, assimilation, and elimination each day.

In simple terms, we could think of the 24-hour day divided into three approximately equal sections. Although they do not happen completely consecutively, each function of digestion, absorption, assimilation, and elimination must be allowed sufficient time to complete. This is required in order to efficiently deliver nutrition to the cells and to eliminate metabolic wastes from them. In almost everyone's lifestyle, it is the elimination segment of time that gets shortchanged. Most people eat too much, too often; they overload their systems. When metabolic waste products are not completely eliminated from the body, they remain stored in the cells. The storage of waste products results in congestion, which sets the stage for degenerative diseases.

To help the body maintain its efficiency, our major time for eating and digesting mostly solid food should be roughly between noon and 8 p.m. Absorption and assimilation takes place over the next few hours. Complete elimination of cellular wastes requires the remaining hours until late morning to complete.

When we eat breakfast we are "breaking-the-fast"—the overnight time of no food intake. It is during fasts, when the body is able to rest from digesting, absorbing, and assimilating food nutrients, that clean-out and elimination functions are performed.

The body works best with a light digestive load. The typical practice of eating a large breakfast, lunch, and dinner, plus snacking throughout the day and eating before going to bed, significantly increases the digestive load. As well as rapidly depleting our enzyme reserves, the eliminative function is seriously restricted. We can let garbage accumulate in our kitchen for only so long before it causes a problem in our living environment. It is the same with our bodies.

When we learn to have mainly fresh squeezed juice or fruit for breakfast, and/or maybe a piece of fruit mid-morning, as well as not eating anything more after dinner at the end of the day, we cooperate with the body's 24-hour cycle. Reducing the amount of food we eat, and the number of times we eat it, increases the efficiency and health of the body.

## WHAT ARE THE BODY'S PRIORITIES?

As a faithful servant, the body always strives first to survive, and second, to maintain or restore health. Survival is paramount. If there are energy and nutritional reserves left over at the end of the day, only then can the body direct its focus to healing. In the absence of adequate nutrition and rest, all the body can and will do is work to survive.

With this overriding priority of survival, the body will work to protect the most vital organs even at the expense of other areas that are less essential to living. Fortunately, they are able to function at a reduced capacity and still allow us to live.

The body works hard to maintain a functioning blood system, heart, liver, kidneys, and lungs because of their importance to its survival. Its second priority of working on the health of the body becomes difficult in the context of a harmful and unhealthy lifestyle. Only when there are sufficient nutrients, good water, fresh air, rest, exercise, proper elimination of wastes, and relative freedom from the stress of harmful attitudes does the body have a surplus of energy which it can, and will, direct toward improving health and raising its overall level of vitality.

## HOW DOES THE BODY HEAL?

The body heals naturally, and in definite stages, *when* it has accumulated sufficient nutrition and energy above and beyond basic living requirements.[7] Healing consists of a resting phase and a healing phase. During the resting phase, our bodies store nutrients and energy in response to an improved diet and lifestyle; we notice that we are feeling better, and are encouraged by the changes we have made. The healing phase consists of detoxification, destruction of diseased cells, and rebuilding of cells. During this phase, the part of the body to be healed is brought into priority, and symptoms are reactivated.

### As Healing Begins

When the body is being supplied with quality nutrition so it can meet all of its daily requirements without borrowing nutrients from its own tissues for metabolic and eliminative processes, it can then turn its attention toward healing. The body must have nutrition left over in order to build a reserve for healing. Complete healing can only happen when all the requirements for glucose, protein, fatty acids, minerals, enzymes, and water are being met *and* there are some leftovers that can be stored.

As our lifestyles begin to improve, our energy levels also improve. When our nutrition, exercise, rest, and attitudes all begin to work with the body, we build up reserves of nutrients and energy in preparation for healing and corrective action. When the body is ready, not necessarily when it's convenient for us, it will start to do some active and intense detoxifying and healing. This is known as a healing crisis. The reactions may be mild or they may be severe. One should expect this and work toward it. The body's inherent desire is perfect health.

The most common detoxifying process utilized by the body in preparation for healing is a cold. During a cold, the body starts eliminating toxic wastes that have been held in storage throughout the body. Toxins are transported to the mucus membranes where they are combined with mucus for elimination from the body. As the body begins to make gains via detoxification, it then turns its attention to breaking down and removing diseased cells, replacing them with healthy ones.

## In Order of Priority

Considering that the body's first priority is to survive, its first healing efforts will be directed to the parts of the body most vital for survival. For example, there could be a life-threatening disease such as cancer or a heart problem in process within the body. In its wisdom, the body will want to correct this first to ensure survival.

During this time, it is essential that we not try to dictate, by physical, herbal, drug, or other stimulants, which part the body must work on. The fact that we may want to be ten or twenty pounds lighter, when the body's first concern may be to heal a disease condition in our pancreas, liver, or kidney, must be considered. Looking thinner, when a developing cancer may be threatening our life, quickly loses its importance. Even though we may not be aware of a disease condition, and medical doctors may not be able to diagnose it, our body knows. It has a built-in, innate intelligence. And it will take the necessary corrective action, as a matter of course, if we work with it.

## In Cycles

The body works on each priority area until it is no longer the highest priority, moving on to the next worst condition after that. Little by little, vitality is raised and overall health is improved. As conditions improve in each area, the body will cycle back again to work on areas that are partially healed, to increase health levels further. This way, it gradually works toward complete health. We need to be patient with this process, and realize how long it took for disease or poor health conditions to develop. They cannot be reversed and corrected in only one or two singular efforts by the body. Given our cooperation, however, the body will continue to work on healing until health is restored.

## It Depends On Us

In order to do a proper job of keeping us healthy and disease-free, the body depends on us. Just like our car, if we misuse and abuse it, it will break down. If we don't supply it with nutritious food, how can it produce long-term health for us? Our job is to understand what the body requires in order to do its job properly. It depends on us to supply those needs. Given the right tools, it will be able to perform the way it wants to and was meant to.

## It Always Seeks Balance

Health is balance. The body always works to maintain a condition of homeostasis, that is, biochemical and electrical balance. It tries to keep energy levels and vital functions as stable and even as possible. It is like water inside a U-shaped tube. When we are in a state of optimum health, the water levels are balanced and are at the top of both tube columns. But, as trauma, disease, or continued lack of good nutrition stress the body, it is as if the U-tube is tilted over and some of the water spilled. The body eventually returns to a balance, but with a little less vitality than it had before, just like the U-tube with a lower level of water in the two columns. As this process is repeated over time, the body still seeks to be stable, but no longer has the energy or clear functioning ability to effectively fight disease processes and bring about the desired return to full health.

## HOW WERE WE MEANT TO LIVE?

Cancer is virtually unknown among people such as the Hunzas of northern Pakistan, the Georgians of western Russia, and the Titikaka Indians of southeastern Peru. They do not have access to the kinds of healthcare resources we have, yet they live to very old ages virtually free of our debilitating diseases. They carry on working until they die or shortly before they die. They do not suffer, nor do they live with pain. Drs. Walker and Bragg, mentioned at the beginning of this book, experienced a similar pattern of healthy longevity.

What are these people doing that is different? The answers are found in their lifestyles of eating raw and unprocessed foods, drinking good water, getting regular exercise through their work, living in a clean air environment, being exposed to moderate amounts of sunshine, getting adequate rest, and maintaining positive life attitudes.

### What Is a Long Life?

Humans are capable of living to between 120 and 170 years. This reasoning is based on the fact that all animals usually live six to eight times their age of maturation. A horse generally matures around three years of age and often lives to twenty-four. So, if humans physically mature at twenty or twenty-one, we should be living much longer, and without all the diseases that are so prevalent now.[8]

## WHAT ARE HUMANS DESIGNED TO EAT?

Are humans designed to be frugivores (fruit eaters), herbivores (vegetation eaters), carnivores (meat eaters) or omnivores (combination eaters)? Consider the comparisons in Figure 2.1.

Given the physical differences in design between carnivores and humans, it soon becomes obvious what kinds of food we are best suited to gether and eat.

|  | CARNIVORE | HUMAN |
|---|---|---|
| TEETH | Long, sharp, pointed. No flat molars. Sharp canines. | All flat. Dullest of the primates. |
| JAW | Moves up and down. | Moves up and down plus sideways for grinding. |
| TONGUE | Rough and thin. | Smooth and thick to move food onto molars for grinding. |
| INTESTINES | 3 times length of body to facilitate quick elimination of toxic protein wastes. | 12 times length of body to extract maximum amount juice and nutrition. (Herbivores are similar) |
| LIVER | Contains the enzyme uricase to break down uric acid from meat. | Low tolerance for uric acid. |
| BLOOD AND SALIVA | Acidic. | Alkaline in health. |
| FEET OR HANDS | Clawed to catch and rip flesh. | Individual fingers with nails and opposable thumbs. Hands perfect for picking and peeling fruit. |

Table 2.1  Carnivore versus human physical characteristics

Now that we have had an overview of how the body is designed to set priorities and how it always works for health, let us take a quick look at its main physical operating systems.

# 3 | THE BODY'S OPERATING SYSTEMS

*I kept thinking how wonderful the human body is, and how, through our ignorance, we work to destroy it.*
HARVEY MILSTEIN

THIS CHAPTER IS a brief outline of the human body's main systems. It is presented on the premise that basic self-knowledge is fundamental to effective self-care.

Learning the basics is always a good place to start in any endeavor. When we have an understanding of the body's internal parts and where they are located, and can appreciate the important functions they perform, we are better able to work *with* the body to co-create health. With this knowledge, we are aware of the reasons why we need to adopt lifestyle changes, and can be motivated to make consistently wise choices.

## NERVOUS SYSTEM

The nervous system is the body's main communication network. Its purpose is to control and coordinate all systems of the body by means of nerve impulses from the brain. Critical to a properly functioning nervous system is a healthy spinal column.

### Central Nervous System

All voluntary motor activity, such as muscular movement, is directed through the central nervous system. Its components are the brain and the spinal cord through which all nerve impulses travel.

### Peripheral Nervous System

Peripheral nerves branch off the spinal cord on both sides of each vertebra to connect with various parts of the body. Impulses are received from the brain and sent to the brain via these pathways.

### Autonomic Nervous System

Involuntary functions such as digestion, bowel contractions, and heartbeats are directed through the autonomic nervous system. Impulses to speed up or slow down various body functions are directed through this system.

## DIGESTIVE SYSTEM

The purpose of the digestive system is to convert food into simple, usable components that the body can use to build and maintain health. The digestive tract is actually considered to be an external tube extending from the mouth to the anus because there are no direct openings from it into the body.

### Mouth and Salivary Glands

The mouth is the initial holding area for food, and is where the breakdown process begins through chewing and the mixing in of digestive enzymes produced by the salivary glands. The teeth, with the aid of the tongue, perform the chewing process. The tongue's taste buds alert us to both good foods and harmful or toxic substances. This is easily observable in babies and infants before they have been conditioned to eat unhealthy food. They simply spit it out.

**Esophagus**

The esophagus is a tube connecting the mouth and throat with the stomach. It transports food and liquid to the stomach via muscular activity known as peristalsis, not by gravity.

**Stomach**

The stomach is a muscular reservoir located mostly on the left side of the body just below the diaphragm. The muscles of the stomach are in three layers, each running in a different direction. They mix food with hydrochloric acid and various enzymes produced in the stomach, and empty the resulting contents of the stomach, known as chyme, into the small intestine.

The inner lining of the stomach is a mucus membrane that secretes protective mucus and digestive enzymes. The types and quantities of enzymes produced depend on the type and quantity of food put into the stomach. Two valves, called sphincters, are located at either end of the stomach to regulate the inflow and exit of food. The digestive medium in the stomach is acidic.

**Small Intestine**

The breakdown of food that begins in the mouth is intensified in the stomach, and is completed in the small intestine where more digestive enzymes are added to the digestive process. The inner lining of the small intestine contains thousands of finger-like projections called villi, which absorb nutrients from digested food. These nutrients pass through the mucus membrane and on to the liver for processing and distribution to the body. The digestive medium of the small intestine is alkaline. Wastes and undigested food from the small intestine are passed into the large intestine.

**Large Intestine**

The large intestine is called the colon. It is larger in diameter than the small intestine, and is approximately 4 to 6 feet in length. It performs two functions: absorbs fluids and minerals, and stores fecal matter until it is evacuated from the body via the rectum and anus. Between the small and large intestines is a sphincter valve called the ileocecal valve, which regulates the outflow of material from the small intestine and prevents backflow. The appendix is located at the beginning of the colon. It is a tubular protrusion, about 3 inches long, which opens into the large intestine and produces lubricating mucus to aid in the movement of fecal matter through the bowel.[1] When toxic overload conditions exist in the lower end of the small intestine and the colon, the appendix can become blocked and may abscess, requiring emergency detoxification measures or removal.

Regular bowel movements are very important for health. When strong body signals to empty the colon are ignored until the urges pass, sacs in the colon wall, called diverticula, can occur in order to create room for the buildup of feces. A diverticulum is a protrusion of the inner lining of a membrane through the outer muscular coat of a tubular organ to form a small pouch with a narrow neck. If bowel habits are not changed to allow these sacs to release their toxic load, diverticulitis or inflammation can develop due to irritation from stagnant feces. Prolonged fecal storage in diverticula pockets can lead to serious problems such as colon cancer. Toxic overload must be avoided.

### Liver

The liver is both a gland and an organ. It is located mostly on the right side of the body, under the diaphragm, nearly hidden and protected by the ribs. In an adult, it weighs about 3–5 pounds (1.4–2.3 kg). It secretes bile to break down oil and fat molecules into smaller particles, making the digestive enzymes in the small intestine more efficient. Bile alkalizes the acid chyme that enters the small intestine from the stomach. The free flow of healthy alkaline bile is critical to the overall health of the body.

Thousands of different types of enzymes are manufactured by the liver. Some of these transform the nutrients that come from the intestines via the portal vein into biochemical substances needed by the body. These are fed into the bloodstream and to the heart for transport to all areas and cells of the body. Other liver enzymes detoxify and render harmless: wastes

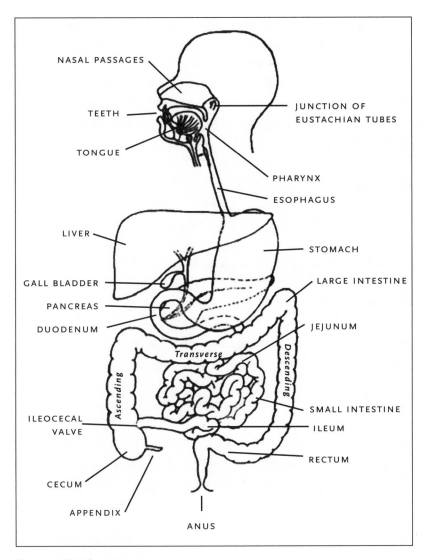

**Figure 3.1 Digestive system**

from dying cells, chemical pollutants, and non-foods that may have been taken into the body. These are filtered out of the bloodstream by the liver and sent to the colon for elimination from the body. Chlorine and alcohol are particularly harmful to the liver's health.

The basic building blocks, or starter hormones, for the endocrine system are also manufactured in the liver from complete amino acids, which are only supplied from raw protein in the diet.

The liver is truly magnificent and definitely one of the master organs of the body. It is impossible to have a healthy body without a healthy liver. Restoring and maintaining the health of the liver must always be a high priority because a free and healthy flow of bile is central to our health.

### Gall Bladder

The gall bladder is a muscular sac about three inches long located on the under surface of the liver. Its purpose is storing bile which is ready for use. When bile is needed, the gall bladder contracts, forcing the bile into the common bile duct, which carries it to the small intestine to aid in digestion. People who have had their gall bladders removed are at a distinct digestive disadvantage.

### Pancreas

The pancreas is a relatively flat organ about 7 inches (18 cm) long and 1½ inches (4 cm) wide. It is situated across the middle of the abdomen just behind the stomach. It produces pancreatic enzymes that break down carbohydrates, fats, and proteins. Pancreatic juice is carried to the small intestine via the pancreatic duct, which joins with the common bile duct. The pancreas also manufactures insulin, which passes directly into the bloodstream from the pancreas. Insulin is responsible for helping the body regulate the use of sugar and other carbohydrates.

## LYMPHATIC SYSTEM

### Lymph

Lymph is blood plasma that has left the blood stream to carry nutrients to cells of the body, and to carry wastes from the cells back to the blood stream via lymph vessels for removal from the body.

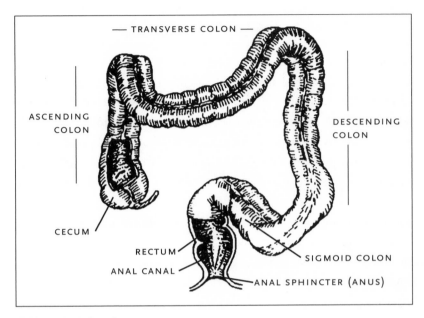

**Figure 3.2  Large intestine**

## Lymph Nodes

Lymph nodes are located within the lymph vessels to filter lymph fluid of toxins and bacteria so that the bloodstream is not overloaded. They also make new lymphocytes to help the body defend itself against infection. The most commonly known lymph nodes are found in the neck and groin areas.

## Spleen

The spleen is the largest mass of lymphatic tissue in the body and acts as a powerful blood waste filter. It is an organ about the size of a person's fist, and is located in the upper part of the abdominal cavity, just under the rib cage on the left side. It produces lymphocytes (white blood cells), destroys defective red blood cells, and serves as a blood reservoir. It recycles whatever molecules our bodies need to retain and reuse. During times of great stress or hemorrhage, the spleen can release stored blood to prevent shock.

## URINARY SYSTEM

### Kidneys

The kidneys are bean-shaped organs about 4 inches long, 2 inches wide, and 1 inch (2.5 cm) thick, located against the back wall of the abdomen at the lower rib cage portion. The body usually has two kidneys; their function is to maintain the pH balance of the blood in the body. After blood has circulated through the liver and heart, it then enters the kidneys for purification. The kidneys work to maintain proper pH balance in the blood by eliminating excess water, salts, and other elements in the form of urine. Depending on the body's needs at the time, most of the useful materials in urine are reabsorbed back into the blood stream. Urine trickles out of the kidneys on a continual basis, draining into the bladder, where amounts in excess of bodily needs are stored in preparation for expulsion from the body.

Kidneys that are stressed and under-functioning become that way due to an overstressed and congested liver. Therefore, the key to improving kidney function is to work on improving the health of the liver.

### Bladder

The bladder is an expandable muscular sac for the temporary storage of urine. It is located in the front lower part of the pelvic area and can hold between 7 and 10 ounces (200 and 300 ml) of urine. As it fills, a nerve reflex initiates the contraction of the muscles of the bladder impelling a need to expel its contents via the urethra.

## RESPIRATORY SYSTEM

The main function of the respiratory system is to supply oxygen to the bloodstream from the air we breathe, and to remove carbon dioxide, some water, and other gaseous waste products from the blood. Its main components are the nasal passages, the trachea or windpipe, and the lungs. The lungs are two cone-shaped organs occupying the greater part of the

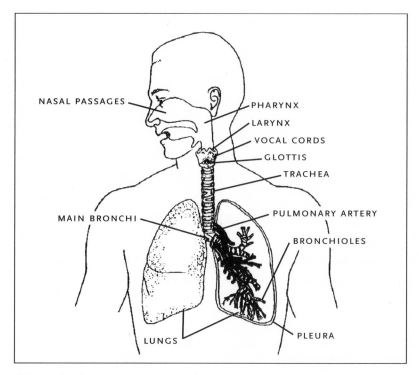

**Figure 3.3  Respiratory system**

chest cavity above the diaphragm. The respiratory system also plays a major role in working to maintain the acid/alkaline balance of the body.

## CIRCULATORY SYSTEM

### Heart

The circulatory system is made up of the heart and blood vessels. The heart is the pump for the blood in our body. It consists of four muscular chambers. Each chamber opening has a one-way valve to regulate the flow of blood in and out of the heart. Blood comes from the body into the right upper chamber known as the right atrium. From here it is pumped into the right lower chamber, known as the right ventricle. Then it is pumped to the lungs where carbon dioxide is exchanged for oxygen. The oxygenated blood flows back to the heart to the upper left chamber, called the left atrium. Blood is pumped from here into the lower left chamber, the left ventricle, and from this chamber it is pumped back out into the general circulation of the body via blood vessels.

### Blood Vessels

Blood vessels can be divided into three categories: 1. Arteries, which convey oxygenated blood away from the heart. 2. Capillaries, which are the smallest blood vessels of the body—so small in diameter that blood cells can only pass through them single file. Their cell walls are thin enough to allow nutrients and oxygen to pass through to the cells of the body, and to pick up carbon dioxide along with a certain amount of waste products from the cells. 3. Veins, which convey blood toward the heart, carry deoxygenated blood primarily loaded with carbon dioxide.

## ENDOCRINE SYSTEM

The endocrine, or hormonal system, helps to regulate a variety of metabolic functions in the body such as: controlling the rate of chemical reactions in cells, transporting substances through cell membranes, regulating the rate of cell growth, and initiating secretions of various glands or cells. Hormones are chemical substances secreted into the body fluids by glands, and which initiate a physiological effect on other cells of the body. Hormones can be viewed as chemical messengers that work to maintain functional balance in the body.

### Pituitary

The pituitary gland is about the size of a pea, and is located on the underside of the brain at approximately eye-level, and just in front of the ears, vertically. The pituitary gland is often called the master gland because it has influence over the rest of the hormonal system, as well as over many functions of the body.

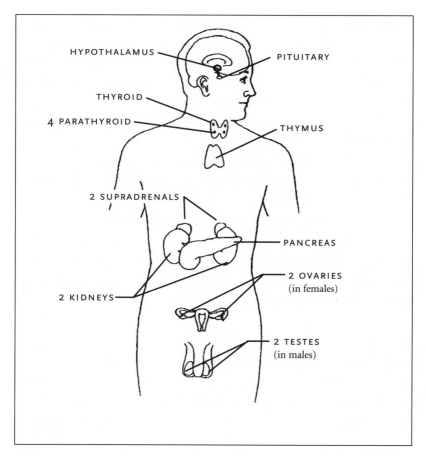

**Figure 3.4 Endocrine glands**

### Pineal

The pineal gland is a small gland about the size of a pea located near the center of the brain between its two hemispheres. It works in harmony with the pituitary and hypothalamus to control the body's hormonal systems and 24-hour rhythms. The pineal gland is sensitive to different levels of light, produces melatonin, and governs our sleep-wake cycle. As such, it is the body's internal clock, and is sometimes referred to as the "third eye". It is also responsible for directing the body's signals for thirst, hunger, sexual desire, and biological aging.

## Hypothalamus

The hypothalamus gland is situated just above the pituitary gland. It is considered to be the seat of our emotions and the control center for the involuntary or autonomic nervous system, which functions night and day, governing all vital processes in the body.

## Thyroid

The thyroid gland consists of two conjoined lobes each about 1½ inches (4 cm) long and ¾ inch (1.9 cm) wide, situated just below the Adam's apple—one lobe on either side of the trachea or windpipe. The thyroid gland secretes the hormone thyroxin to regulate the metabolism rate of the cells of the body—how fast they work, or function. Cold hands and feet, low energy, and graying hair are some of the symptoms of a stressed thyroid gland. Thyroid health is directly related to the hormone health of the body in general, and to efficient liver function in particular.

## Parathyroid

There are four parathyroid glands, two on each side of the trachea (windpipe), just behind the thyroid glands. The parathyroid glands secrete the hormone parathormone, whose function is the regulation of calcium and phosphorus levels in the blood and bones. When calcium levels are low, the body uses parathormone to extract calcium from bones and teeth, increase absorption of calcium from the intestine, and decrease elimination of calcium from the kidneys in order to meet the calcium needs of the body.

## Thymus

The thymus gland is located behind the sternum or breastbone. It manufactures thymosin, which promotes the formation of lymph glands, T-lymphocytes (a type of white blood cell scavenger), and antibodies that help to eliminate foreign substances from the body.

## Adrenal

There are two adrenal glands, similar to little caps, located one on top of each kidney. Each adrenal gland is actually two glands, secreting steroid-type hormones and adrenaline. Some of the functions of the adrenal glands include: working to maintain a healthy acid/alkaline balance by regulating mineral balances within the body; regulating fluid levels in the body; regulating protein metabolism, blood sugar levels, and the breakdown of fat; and promoting the formation of red blood cells. Adrenaline is produced to reinforce the sympathetic nervous system's effect on the body. Its effect is most noticeable as the "fight or flight" response when the body is under physical or emotional stress.

## REPRODUCTIVE SYSTEM

The reproductive glands include the ovaries in the female, and the testes in the male. The ovaries produce ova, or eggs, during the reproductive part of a female's life, and the hormones estrogen and progesterone, which promote the production of feminizing cells in the female body. The testes produce sperm for the fertilization of the female's egg, and the hormone testosterone, which promotes the production of masculinizing cells in the male body.

Even with an appreciation of how wonderfully our bodies are designed to produce health, why is disease on the increase? When we compare its capability with present day disease statistics, something is obviously wrong. So let's take a look at the subject of disease itself—what it is, and what causes it.

# 4 | WHAT IS DISEASE?

~

*There are no specific diseases:*
*there are specific disease conditions.*

FLORENCE NIGHTINGALE

~

DISEASE, OR "DIS-EASE," is defined as a lack of health. It results when any cell is not fulfilling one hundred per cent of its designed duty, whether due to trauma, toxicity, lack of communication, or a combination thereof. If we are not operating at full efficiency and vitality—physically, mentally, emotionally, or spiritually—we are experiencing some degree of dis-ease. When the body is in any state of dis-ease, it is out of balance. Disease occurs as a result of stress.[1] One or more stressors cause cells to change their form, then to change their functioning ability, and eventually to die.

## STRESS

Stress to the body can be physical, emotional, and nutritional; from deficiencies, toxicities, or imbalances.

*Physically*, our cells can be stressed by traumatic damage to the tissues of the body through injury, or by being deprived of exercise, sunshine, rest, or cleanliness.

*Emotionally*, we stress our bodies through negative attitudes and beliefs. Stressful relationships and difficult working or living situations add to this. Fear, worry, guilt, anger, resentment, impatience, and the lack of a positive outlook produce acids that take a heavy toll on the reserves of our bodies. These emotions draw a great deal of energy. It is not the events that happen to us, but our *attitudes* or *reactions* to the events that cause symptoms of stress to manifest in the body.

*Nutritionally and chemically*, we stress our cells by eating an improper diet, consuming chemicals in drugs, impure water, and food additives, and by breathing unclean air. This upsets the body's normal healthy acid-alkaline balance, and moves it into an acid condition. All these things, if continued long enough, contribute to a deterioration of bodily function and vitality. Trapped wastes and poisons from processed, cooked, and denatured foods and beverages inevitably cause reduced efficiency and disease. Without adequate nutrients, cells are unable to carry out their proper metabolic functions. In addition, their ability to communicate with the rest of the body is impaired.

*Electrically*, we stress every cell in our body by exposing ourselves to the invisible but unnatural and harmful electromagnetic force fields (EMF) generated by electrical devices such as: machinery, power lines inside and outside our homes, radios, televisions, computers, phones, electric shavers, and hair dryers. Our bodies are electrical, and anything that interferes with the free flow of electricity and communication around our bodies or within and between the cells, contributes to disease.

Disease is caused by how we live, and the environment we live in. The extent to which various stressors overload the body, combined with genetic weaknesses that were passed on to us by our parents, determines how soon, how serious, and where diseases are likely to develop in our bodies.

## GETTING MORE SPECIFIC—
## OXIDATION AND FREE RADICALS

Health is lost at the cellular level. Anything that interferes with the efficiency of cellular function causes dis-ease. When there is enough cumulative disruption of cellular function, disease symptoms appear.

Oxidation in the body is a process that is similar to the rusting of iron, or a sliced apple turning brown. Oxygen, while being necessary for life, can also become reactive and cause breakdown in the cells. In its atomic and stable form, oxygen has paired electrons in its outer ring. When something causes one of those electrons to be lost, there is an odd number of electrons in the outer ring, and the unpaired electron becomes unstable. It becomes a free radical. This free radical wants to pair with another and become stable again. It's like a single guy or gal wanting to be paired up, and while doing so, breaking up a stable marriage. In the process of becoming stable or paired again, free radicals attack other molecules. This is where the danger in living systems lies, because this process becomes a chain reaction. These reactions can take place in less than a millionth of a second. At any one time there can be millions of free-radical-attacking and neutralizing reactions going on within the body. Every time a free radical is neutralized it may have caused damage to some part of the body. Over time, the cumulative action of unrestrained free radical activity, or oxidation, manifests as aging. Although it started much earlier inside the body, it eventually becomes visibly evident as unhealthy tissue or disease symptoms.

Any food that is unnatural or changed from how nature made it can cause oxidation within the body. When food is cooked so that its enzymes are destroyed, processed with chemicals, or exposed to air for a period of time, it becomes an oxidizing agent in the body. All drugs, chemicals, and toxins are strong oxidizing agents.

## GENETIC TENDENCIES

When we are born, we inherit a genetic combination of physical characteristics and capabilities—strengths and weaknesses—from our parents and ancestors.

The Pottenger cats experiment, explained later in chapter 5, in which the impacts of processed foods on four generations of cats were studied, leads us to understand that if our parents were both healthy, with bodies relatively clear of toxins at the time we were conceived, then this tendency toward health would have been passed on to us. Likewise, if our parents had toxic bodies from consuming overcooked or junk food, alcohol, nicotine, drugs, or medications, then the cells that formed our bodies would contain toxic elements as well. We would be starting life with toxic and genetically weaker cells. We would have a tendency toward developing diseases in the weakest tissues and organs of our bodies. This combination of genetic tendencies, family nutritional habits, attitudes, and beliefs nurtured in the early years results in certain diseases being manifested more often in some families.

*We inherit **disease tendencies**, but*
*we do not have to develop the diseases.*

## WE CAN CHANGE OUR GENES

The body has awesome corrective capabilities. It only knows how to strive to be healthy; but it needs our cooperation. Dr. Bruce Lipton, cell biologist, has broken through the traditional paradigm regarding genetics. He explains that our beliefs and perceptions govern our biology at the cellular level. By changing our beliefs and perceptions, we can actually change our gene structure and what manifests in our lives.[2] When we take personal responsibility for our health, educate ourselves to understand what is helpful and what is harmful to the body, and change our lifestyle practices and beliefs, we begin to help the body heal. In time, it will reward us with increased vitality.

When we are young, our health is formed by the nutritional and attitudinal environments provided by our parents. In adolescence, we start to make our own choices. As adults, our health is created by our beliefs, and by the lifestyle choices we make. Although we may have been born with weaker tissues in some organ or area, a disease does not have to develop. If the body is supplied with a positive environment of nutrition, attitudes, and lifestyle practices, it can strengthen and repair itself; we can remain in health.

We must first be aware of what causes diseases and why they develop. We need to know which foods are good for us and which are harmful. We must become knowledgeable and aware of what strengthens the body and its immune system, and what weakens and breaks it down. We must then take consistent action to assist the body in building health.

### DON'T GERMS AND VIRUSES CAUSE DISEASE?

There is a universal belief that germs and viruses are the *cause* of disease; but this is not true. Louis Pasteur, for whom the pasteurization process is named, first put forward the idea that germs from outside the body are the cause of disease. Living in France at the same time as Pasteur was another scientist who was also conducting research on the cause and development of disease. This man was Antoine Béchamp. Pasteur actually "borrowed" part of Béchamp's research and publicized it as his own. Dr. Guylaine Lanctôt explains it thus:

> Pasteur was ambitious, an opportunist. He was also a genius in the art of promoting himself, and he plagiarized, and then vulgarized, the work of Béchamp. He stole the idea of small organisms being responsible, but he only revealed a small part of Béchamp's discoveries. Pasteur proclaimed that these small organisms only came from the outside. He forgot to mention that, once exposed to air, germs and

other morbid (abnormal) microzymes lose their virulence very rapidly. And this deceit has been perpetuated ever since.[3]

It has been said that Pasteur, on his deathbed, admitted to his colleagues that an individual's natural immunity is more important than germs in the matter of disease. He had been unable to grow his germ cultures on healthy, fresh fruit, and instead had to grow them on rotting soup.

Dr. Joel Robbins teaches that two conditions must be present in order for disease germs to enter into, or develop in, living tissue: first, something besides the germ must have previously weakened the tissue; and second, there must be acidic debris present in the tissue for the germs to live on. They cannot exist in a balanced acid-alkaline environment, neither can parasites. The conclusion is logical. If our bodies are relatively free of toxic wastes, serious disease bacteria cannot develop within us. No harmful bacteria, parasite, or virus can proliferate in a body that does not have a build-up of toxic waste. A body that has healthy levels of cellular oxygen and a strong immune system will remain a healthy body.

### How the Body Deals with Germs and Viruses

The body has a built-in natural intelligence. It knows how to fight germs and viruses. When it comes to disease, there are three principles that must be understood:

1   All forms of disease are caused by accumulations of acid and toxic waste in the body's systems, the first and foremost of which is the colon. Disease starts in the colon.

2   The body initiates all acute diseases like colds, flu, fever, skin eruptions, diarrhea, scarlet fever, and measles, in attempts to reduce the accumulation of stored waste material. Chronic diseases, such as diabetes, arthritis, bronchitis, heart disease, and cancer, are caused by the continued build-up of waste in the system, and the suppression of acute disease cleansing attempts by wrong treatment.

3   The body has the ability to return to health provided it is given the proper nutrition and conditions to do so.

We don't "catch" diseases. We cause them! We create them by the way we live. We don't "catch" a cold or flu. We actually "earn" it by fostering toxic waste conditions in our bodies, as a result of our lifestyles. When we continue to suppress illnesses with drugs and antibiotics, the body eventually develops degenerative disease conditions because it has not been allowed adequate opportunity to detoxify and heal naturally.

## THE DISEASE PROCESS

### Slipping Toward Poor Health

Disease is simply the process our body goes through when its requirements for efficient functioning are not being met. As this happens, it reluctantly moves from a state of health into illness. In the circumstance of not having its full requirements for efficient operation supplied on a regular basis, it is unable to maintain complete health. Deficiencies have the tendency of compounding into problems. It is somewhat similar to your car. You can operate its engine for brief periods when it is low on oil, but in time, the engine will overheat and be ruined. It cannot continue to operate efficiently without all its service requirements being supplied on a regular basis.

If illnesses are stopped by the stimulative use of drugs, and wrong living habits continue, the toxins that the body was attempting to eliminate via the illness process will be driven deeper into the body, setting the stage for more chronic disease. As toxic accumulations collect in the body because of harmful lifestyle choices, wrong food intake, and insufficient elimination, the standard of health drops to a lower level. This can be likened to a person who is having increasing weights added to a pack on their back. As the weight increases, his or her ability to move quickly, efficiently, and easily becomes more difficult. When stimulation and wrong living habits are discontinued, the body begins to heal and reverse the disease process.

A lower level of health is telling us that our body needs help; its organs and glands are losing their ability to function efficiently.

## Toxic Buildup Causes Disease

A toxin is defined as any substance that is harmful to the body, which the body cannot use in any way for life-maintaining purposes, and which costs the body energy and nutrition to eliminate.[4]

Always striving to survive and to build health, the body works to eliminate poisons from its system. It does this through *stimulation*. It is what happens when the body's metabolism is increased. Caffeine is an example of a toxic stimulant. The burst of energy, or "lift" we feel after drinking coffee, is the result of the body being stimulated to rid itself of the caffeine. Likewise, sugar is a stimulant and a toxin because it contains no nutrition and must be combined with other nutrients, such as calcium from the body's stores, to eliminate it from the body.

Toxins and most stimulants are negatives to the body. The energy required to eliminate them comes from the body's energy and mineral stores, and not from the stimulating substances. Continued stimulation costs the body its health. Stimulating, or "revving-up" the body, causes it to burn out faster. This is similar to running the engine of our car at a high RPM all the time. If toxic intake is greater than the body's ability to eliminate it, a gradual lowering of our vitality and state of health results. In addition, toxins reduce our cells' ability to make energy. As this is happening, the body tries to make up for our transgressions. It takes compensating action in its efforts to maintain its biochemical and electrical balance. Remember the example of a U-tube; as liquid is removed, levels remain balanced, but at lower levels. The same process happens with energy in our bodies.

## The Seduction of Gradualism

In humans, a lowered standard of health occurs slowly; we become accustomed to it and tolerate it. Health weakens so gradually that we do not notice until something serious develops. As the body's vitality weakens, the person increases the use of stimulants such as caffeine, nicotine, red meat, sugar, salt, or drugs to feel energy and a sense of well being again. It is difficult to realize that this is harming the body, so the person continues to increase stimulation thereby weakening the overall vitality of the body.

We have been conditioned to believe it is normal to slow down, and to develop aches, pains, and diseases as we grow older. It has become usual and commonplace, but it is not natural, and it is not necessary. This is similar to a frog, which when placed in a pot of cold water, will stay there while the water is heated, accepting the change in temperature until it eventually cooks and dies. Another example is of an overweight person who suddenly dies from a heart attack. The person tolerated the extra weight and ignored the toxic burden it represented. Excess fat creates a heavier blood circulation load. This requires the heart to work harder and increase blood pressure to service the body. The person may even have had pains in the chest and arms, or difficulty breathing. These are all signs the body gives to warn that serious problems lie ahead if corrective action is not taken.

When the body's warning signals are ignored, at some point one of two things happens. Either health degenerates to a point where the body is unable to reverse it and return to health, or the person decides to change lifestyles, and work with the body using nature's way to regain health and vitality. Figure 4.1 illustrates this process.

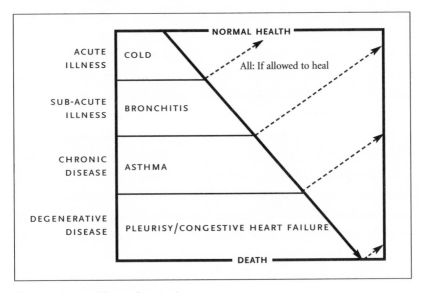

**Figure 4.1 Stages of disease degeneration**

As stated earlier, the body's first priority is survival. If it has adequate reserves of nutrition and energy, it will then direct its efforts to healing. Think about it. Without proper food to supply adequate nutrients on a regular basis, the body is forced to rob from its own stores to carry out metabolism and bodily processes needed for survival. An example of this is osteoporosis. As the body's reserves of acid buffer minerals are depleted, it turns to the use of calcium from the bones as a neutralizer. If fed a diet that is deficient in adequate nutrition and loaded with toxic substances, the body simply is unable to eliminate the toxins and clean out metabolic wastes properly. As health problems arise, if drugs are taken to eliminate symptoms, their toxicity actually adds to the problem. The natural cleansing process of the body is suppressed and it is forced to degenerate toward more chronic disease. As toxicity increases in the storage areas, vitality decreases, parasites increase, and degeneration and eventual mutation of cells occur. Cells become altered and are no longer able to reproduce themselves in their original healthy form; they reproduce as diseased cells. If this toxic process continues, the body dies. Cancer cells, for example, are a result of this process. Cells that were healthy have now changed structure and function. They have mutated. Whereas healthy cells utilize oxygen, cancer cells use carbon dioxide. They function similar to plant cells, and increase in size by storing the body's own toxic wastes. The cancer spreads as oversized cells automatically divide and multiply.

When faced with too many toxins to eliminate, what choice does the body have? If it is not given adequate times of rest without the need to digest and assimilate food, and given adequate opportunities to cleanse itself, the body has no choice but to store the toxins in the cells where they will do the least harm *for the time being*. It hopes that it will get the opportunity to eliminate them at a later date. Examples of conditions resulting from toxic storage include atherosclerosis (fatty deposits inside arteries), arthritis (deposits of toxins and unnatural calcium in joint tissues which result in degenerative changes of those tissues), fibromyalgia (toxins and unnatural calcium in muscle tissue), and gout (storage of uric acid as far from the heart as possible).

*Disease is the price we pay for our body's effort to survive longer in the face of our wrongdoing.*

The body stores toxins in tissue cell areas where they will do the least harm because it would die much sooner if toxins were allowed to remain in the blood. Even cancer is part of the body's effort to survive longer.

## HOW DISEASES CAN DEVELOP

To illustrate how diseases can develop, two areas are presented as examples: the first is a common, but often overlooked, *cause* of disease; the second is a *result* of a disease process that is often undiscovered until it is life-threatening.

### Root Canals, Tooth Infections, and Disease

Dr. Weston Price was a dental research specialist who conducted thousands of tests with infected and root-canal-filled teeth. Over a period of 25 years, he stitched one hundred healthy teeth and thousands of diseased teeth extracted from human patients, under the skins of rabbits. In addition, he isolated the bacteria from pulverized specimens of root canal filled teeth, cultured the bacteria, and injected them into hundreds of laboratory animals, mostly rabbits. His astonishing results were published in 1923.

Dr. Price discovered that infected teeth, tonsils, tonsil tags, sinuses, and similar areas of infection contain bacteria that can travel to a gland, organ, or other tissue and set up a new infection site. A complete discussion and summary of his findings is presented in the 1993 book written by Dr. George Meinig, *Root Canal Cover-Up*. The reason why Dr. Price's findings were "covered up" was that influential colleagues among the health professionals of his day disputed his findings and overrode and silenced his voice.

Dr. Meinig summarizes Dr. Price's discoveries as follows:[5]

- Bacteria that caused tooth infection penetrated most of the remaining tooth and were not killed during the root canal therapy.
- These bacteria were found to be polymorphic; they mutated and became smaller in size, thrived in the absence of oxygen, and became more deadly, while the toxins they produced became more poisonous.
- As bacteria incubated and multiplied, they spread to other parts of the body and set up new infection sites in the weakest areas.
- In almost every case, when a root-filled tooth of a patient with a degenerative disease—even a tooth that showed no apparent problem on X-ray—was extracted and embedded in an animal, that animal would often, but not always, develop the patient's disease.
- Toxins produced by bacteria in root-filled teeth, when separated from the bacteria and injected into an animal, also reproduced the same disease the patient had.
- A wide variety of degenerative diseases such as endocarditis and other heart diseases, kidney and bladder diseases, arthritis, rheumatism, mental diseases, lung problems, pregnancy complications, and almost any degenerative problem, can be transferred to rabbits from bacteria in extracted teeth that were diseased or root-filled.
- The same problems can result from cavitations (infected areas of the jawbone near an infected tooth, or sockets not properly cleaned out when a tooth is extracted).
- After extraction and proper cleaning of the sockets of problem teeth, a large percentage of patients recovered from their illnesses.
- When sound, uninfected, natural teeth, or other sterile objects were implanted in animals, no adverse health effects were experienced.

When a tooth begins to decay and a cavity is formed, a hole is created in the outer hard layers of the tooth, and decay spreads into the dentin. When decay spreads into the pulp, the only way to save the tooth is to remove the remaining pulp down to the bottom of the roots, and pack the resulting spaces with a filling compound. What has not been widely realized, however, is that the tooth is now dead; the nerves, arteries, veins, and other tissue have been removed.

When viewed under an electron microscope, dentin is shown to be a labyrinth of honeycomb tunnels. By removing the nerve and cutting circulation to a tooth, a perfect home for bacteria to incubate and multiply is created, safely out of reach of the body's defense mechanisms. Because the body's blood supply to the inside of the tooth no longer exists, there is no way for cells of the immune system to come in and attack bacteria hiding in these spaces. Bacterial toxic wastes, which prove to be more harmful than the bacteria themselves, are able to exit the tooth via the root-filled openings and the lateral accessory canals, traveling to all parts of the body by means of the circulation system. They then tend to make their homes in the weakest organs and tissues. Over time, as the body becomes stressed, the bacteria and their toxins overload and weaken the immune system, hastening the onset of degenerative diseases. The host person becomes sick and dies before his or her time.

Dr. Price found that bacteria which had caused tooth infections penetrated most of the dentin tubules. After a root canal had been cleaned, he found that bacteria were still able to gain access to dentin tubules via the space between the filling compound and the tooth, since there is always about 5% shrinkage of the compound after it has been placed in the root canal.

Dr. Price also found that about 25% of the patients he treated, who had root-filled teeth, remained in good health provided they were not

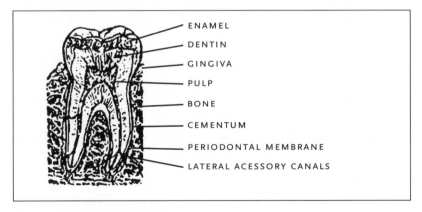

Figure 4.2  Cross section of a tooth

subjected to stressful problems such as an accident, influenza, or the death of a close family member. These individuals had excellent immune systems, excellent diets, and had parents and grandparents who were also healthy. If a patient was under stress, however, or when their immune system was battling one or more degenerative illnesses, or if there was a history of chronic disease in the family, Dr. Price favored avoiding treatment of infected teeth and recommended the removal of any which had root canal fillings.

## WHAT IS CANCER?

Cancer! The BIG C! The very word strikes fear into the patient who has been told that he or she has it. People say, "I *got* cancer," as if some cancer bacteria or virus had decided to settle into their body at random. They were picked. Bad luck! Cancer is looked at as a death sentence. And because cancer is not understood, that is often the end result. What is cancer? If disease is not something we "catch," how does cancer fit into this understanding? Can cancer actually be cured, or avoided altogether? Cancer is not the beginning of a disease. Cancer is the result of a disease process that has been going on in the body for a long time.

> Cancer does not just happen. Normal healthy cells don't just spontaneously, metamorphose into abnormal cells unless deprived, debilitated, poisoned and damaged.[6]
>
> Nobody develops cancer, except that over many years their health slowly and progressively succumbed to 20–40–60–80 such causes interacting and working together.[7]

Cancer is the result of the body storing toxins in its effort to survive longer. If the body did not store the toxins, encased in a tumor for example, they would be free to range throughout the body in the bloodstream, thereby causing the death of vital tissues and organs much sooner.

Cancer has a multitude of contributing factors, such as: heredity, beliefs, attitudes, habits, excesses, nutrition, environmental pollutants, and stresses, as well as various carcinogens like radiation, pesticides, toxic chemicals, dioxins, and asbestos—to name a few. It is an enzyme deficiency and an autointoxication disease. It is a failure of the body's cells to obtain all the building materials essential for their construction and functioning. It is also the result of excess toxicity, which affects and eventually destroys cells, or transforms them into abnormal, wild, growing cells.

### Cancer's Common Denominators

After he lost his brother to cancer, Ron Gdanski began to research the subject, and eventually wrote a book entitled *CANCER Cause, Cure, and Cover-up*. His research concluded that fermentation of sugars at the cellular level is present in all cancers:

> Cancer is caused by the cellular environment. Genetic defects do not create the capacity for human cells to metabolize nutrients without oxygen. Limiting the oxygen supply or disrupting the citric acid cycle leads to fermentation ...
>
> As soon as oxygen reaches the cells, the citric acid cycle can be re-established, fermentation stops, and microbial life destroyed.[8]
>
> Cancer, above all else, is a cellular oxygen deficiency disease. The research of Dr. Otto Warburg, a Nobel Prize-winning biochemist in the 1930s, concluded that the prime cause of cancer is impaired cell respiration.
>
> Cancer, above all other diseases, has countless secondary causes. Almost anything can cause cancer. But, even for cancer, there is only one prime cause. The prime cause of cancer is the replacement of the respiration of oxygen (oxidation of sugar) in normal body cells by fermentation of sugar.
>
> All normal body cells meet their energy needs by respiration of oxygen, whereas cancer cells meet their energy needs in great part by fermentation....
>
> In every case, during the cancer development, the oxygen respiration always falls, fermentation appears, and the highly differentiated

cells are transformed into fermenting anaerobes, which have lost all their body functions and retain only the now useless property of growth and replication. Thus, when respiration disappears, life does not disappear, but the meaning of life disappears, and what remains are growing machines that destroy the body in which they grow.[9]

Lack of cellular oxygen is directly related to acidity of body systems, and this subject will be covered in detail in chapter 10. Terminal cancer patients are approximately 500 to 1000 times more acidic than normal healthy people. Cancer will not occur in a pH-balanced body.

### Recovering from Cancer

It is not enough to just *kill* the cancer. If the environment within the body is not corrected, cancer can return. This explains the medical terminology "in remission," meaning that cancer cells have been reduced to a very low or non-identifiable level *at that time*. However, if cellular oxygen remains at low levels, body terrain conditions still exist for cellular fermentation and therefore development and proliferation of cancer cells.

Any program to eliminate cancer must address the basics of diet in order to reduce body acidity and turn off the cellular fermentation process that allows cancer to develop in the first place. Alkaline minerals must be restored in the body, and all medium to high glycemic foods strictly avoided.

Recovering from cancer involves eliminating all possible causes that may have created it. Diligent and persistent detoxification measures are a top priority. A concerted campaign to eliminate parasites needs to be mounted. All the "wrongs" for the body must be stopped in favor of the "rights." Mental and emotional factors must be addressed. Deficiencies of enzymes and essential cell nutrients must be corrected through proper diet and supplementation. The body pH must be restored to a healthy balance as a top priority to increase cellular oxygen levels. Friendly bowel bacteria must be replenished. Attention must be given to rest, relaxation, and sleep, to allow the body opportunity to heal. The body's immune system must be strengthened.

### The Power of Fresh Juices

When it comes to natural, power-packed nutrition and healing, it is hard to beat freshly made vegetable juices. A man I know who was in the final stages of cancer made a miraculous turnaround in his health when, as a last resort in attempts to address his growing anemia problem, he began to make and drink a fresh vegetable juice combination he had read about in Dr. Norman Walker's book on juicing. Many natural approaches to eliminating cancer center on the use of fresh juices. A well-known therapy is *The Breuss Cancer Cure*, which involves a 42-day fast on nothing but vegetable juices and teas. In my opinion, the main reason fresh vegetable juices have such a positive effect is because of their alkalizing properties.

### Marine Phytoplankton

Along with a healthy diet, possibly the most powerful and totally natural breakthrough in aiding the body to heal may be marine phytoplankton. This most basic of earth's foods was only developed as a food supplement in 2004. It is showing very encouraging results in replenishing the body's nutritional resources at the cellular level. (More on phytoplankton in chapter 16.)[10]

### Cut, Burn, or Poison

It was recently reported that less than 1% of the US National Cancer Institute's budget is allocated to nutritional studies.[11] This is disappointing because it is well known that poor nutrition creates chemical imbalances in the body. Time after time, it seems that funding for research and development programs that address the causes of cancer is totally ignored by those in authority positions.

Politicians like to use terms such as "declaring war" on diseases. But to return a body to health, the solution is not to find an aggressor against a disease. The solution is to build a solid defense system within the body so that disease has no appropriate medium in which to exist. From an economic viewpoint, politicians are able to justify large expenditures during wartime, hence their bellicose rhetoric. This leads people in a totally wrong direction as far as true health is concerned.

The presently accepted medical approaches for dealing with cancer are to use surgery, chemotherapy, or radiation. These measures destroy tumors but do not eliminate the causes. They do nothing to rebuild resistance, promote healing, and restore health. In fact, they add considerably to the stresses the body must then attempt to cope with in its already weakened state. Almost the entire focus of our western cancer research programs is on eliminating the cancer, not the cause.

The main cancer treatments of surgery, radiation, and chemotherapy are, in effect, options of cut, burn, or poison. Surgery cuts part of the body away. Radiation burns tissues. Chemotherapy, using chemicals such as mustard gas or warfarin (also used as rat poison), poisons the cells to kill them. Although in some cases, depending on how advanced the cancer is, initial improvement is gained, the long-term prospects are not good because the cause or reason that the cancer developed in the first place, has not been dealt with. Further, the body must also deal with the trauma and/or toxins from the medical intervention.

The body's cellular communication system is like an electronic network. The body uses this network to maintain balance in all areas. How do medical interventions affect this communication system? Consider two scenarios: first, a city with electrical wiring that connects and supplies power to all streets, businesses, and houses; and second, a computer with its complex circuitry. In either case, if you were to cut, burn, or apply corrosive chemicals to a part of the circuit, you know what the result would be. Now visualize the body as if it were filled with circuits of tiny wires, so that all parts can communicate for maximum operating efficiency. Ask what the result would be if you cut, burned, or corroded a section of its electrical circuits. Wouldn't this just add to long-term problems?

Also consider a city sewer system with collection and filtration centers to remove, regulate, and contain sewage. The body has its own channels of waste removal that utilize the blood and lymphatic systems. What would happen if you cut out a section of a city's sewage system?

### The Purpose of a Tumor

A cancer tumor forms as a filtration and storage center for the removal and containment of poisons so they will not circulate throughout the body, causing an early death. To simply remove the tumor does nothing to address the causes of why the body formed the tumor in the first place. Tumors are not body mistakes. They are examples of body wisdom at work, making a desperate stand to protect us from the effects of poisons we have allowed into our bodies. Nevertheless, if we do not take corrective action to help the body, sooner or later the tumor will be unable to contain the growing number of cancer cells; they will metastasize, or spread, to other parts of the body and eventually take over.

Overcoming cancer and rebuilding total health requires the restoration of all forces, agents, and processes that resist, fight off, protect from, and cure disease. It also requires addressing and removing emotional blockages. The body needs to have its workers, enzymes and bowel flora, and health-building nutrition re-introduced, and the toxins removed. There is no other cure. An encouraging story to illustrate this can be found at: www.shesacancersurvivor.com.

Now that we have looked at the general causes of disease, let's examine the specifics. What could we be doing wrong that is causing us to develop diseases, or at least become less healthy than we could and should be? In the next chapter we'll read about two studies that gave us answers many years ago. We'll also examine what has changed in disease statistics, food production, food consumption, and the environment since 1900.

# 5 | HEALTH AND DISEASE

∾

*One-quarter of what you eat keeps you alive.*
*The other three-quarters keeps your doctor alive.*

Hieroglyph found in an ancient Egyptian tomb

∾

## COOKING DESTROYS THE LIFE IN FOOD

Two unrelated studies were conducted in the 1930s to determine whether there were health consequences to consuming either cooked or raw foods. Although largely forgotten for sixty years, the findings of these studies present conclusive evidence regarding the harmful effects of cooked food.

### The Influence of Cooked Food on the Blood of Man

In 1930, Dr. Paul Kouchakoff directed a study at the Institute of Clinical Chemistry in Lausanne, Switzerland, to determine the effects of cooked and processed foods versus raw and natural foods on the immune system of man, as evidenced in blood analysis after eating these foods. The research findings were remarkable. They found that eating food in its raw and natural state, or eating foods that were not overheated or refined, caused no changes in the blood composition of subjects tested. However, when cooked or refined foods were consumed, the subjects' blood showed a marked increase in the number of white blood cells. Researchers termed this reaction, "pathological leukocytosis." Their findings were presented to the First International Congress of Microbiology in Paris in 1930, under the title *The Influence of Cooking Food on the Blood Formula of Man*.[1]

White blood cells, also called leukocytes or immune cells, are a component of blood and part of the body's immune system that help defend the body against infections or foreign materials. The conclusion of Dr. Kouchakoff's study was that eating cooked foods or foods that have been processed, preserved with chemicals, pasteurized, or homogenized, causes the body to divert its immune fighters to the digestive tract to deal with what it views as toxic substances. In the process, the rest of the body is left less protected. Also, it must attempt to eliminate the harmful substances as well as cope with the lack of nutrients contained in processed foods.[2]

### The Pottenger Cats Experiments

In 1932, Francis Pottenger Jr., a medical doctor in California, wanted to determine the effects of eating raw or cooked food. Experiments were conducted with 900 cats over a ten-year period. The results were profound, because they clearly demonstrated why diseases and structural abnormalities develop.

Cats were divided into groups and fed diets according to the following:

| | | |
|---|---|---|
| MEAT STUDY | Diet A (ALL RAW) | ⅓ raw milk, cod liver oil, ⅔ RAW meat |
| | Diet B (⅔ COOKED) | ⅓ raw milk, cod liver oil, ⅔ COOKED meat |
| | | |
| MILK STUDY | Diet A (ALL RAW) | ⅓ raw meat, cod liver oil, ⅔ RAW milk |
| | Diet B (⅔ COOKED) | ⅓ raw meat, cod liver oil, ⅔ PASTEURIZED milk |
| | Diet C (⅔ COOKED) | ⅓ raw meat, cod liver oil, ⅔ EVAPORATED milk |
| | Diet D (⅔ COOKED) | ⅓ raw meat, cod liver oil, ⅔ SWEETENED CONDENSED milk |
| | Diet E | RAW, METABOLIZED MILK, VITAMIN D milk from cows fed on (1) dry feed, and (2) green feed |

Table 5.1  Pottenger cats experiment diets

Mother cats and their offspring were observed for health changes. Only raw food diet males were used for breeding purposes so as to maintain consistency of fertilization.

### Study Findings

Dr. Pottenger found that only diets containing raw milk and raw meat were adequate for maintaining the optimal health of the cats from generation to generation. Cats on an all-raw diet had good bone structure with wide palates and plenty of space for their teeth, excellent bone density, shiny fur, and freedom from parasites and disease. They reproduced with ease, and were gentle and easy to handle.

Cooking meat, or substituting heat-processed milk for raw milk, resulted in physical degeneration that increased with each generation. Degeneration proceeded more quickly on Diets C and D of the Milk Study. Diet E-1 produced unexpected results—rickets and early death of male kittens. Study cats on the deficient diets suffered from most of the degenerative diseases encountered in humans, and died out completely by the fourth generation.

Dr. Pottenger noted that changes in facial structure and the onset of degenerative disease in cats on deficient diets paralleled the human degeneration that Dr. Price had observed in primitive tribes that had abandoned traditional foods for trade foods containing sugar and white flour.[4]

Study cats and their descendants fed entirely on raw meat and raw milk remained in excellent health during their lives. Death resulted only from old age or injuries sustained in fighting. None of the raw food cats died from disease. In contrast, 100% of the cats fed overcooked or treated food and milk suffered an increasing degeneration of their bones, teeth, and reproductive ability. Their disease conditions continued to increase. Figure 5.2 briefly summarizes the results of the study.

Observations from the deficient diet cats include:

- Spontaneous abortion ranged from an average of 25% in the first generation to about 70% in the second generation.

| | RAW FOODS | | DENATURED FOODS |
|---|---|---|---|
| | Raw Meat | Raw Milk | Pasteurized Milk / Evaporated Milk / Condensed Milk / Cooked Meat |
| **1ST GENERATION** | | | |
| | remained healthy | remained healthy | Developed diseases and illnesses near end of life |
| **2ND GENERATION** | | | |
| | remained healthy | remained healthy | Developed diseases and illnesses in middle life |
| **3RD GENERATION** | | | |
| | remained healthy | remained healthy | Developed diseases and illnesses in beginning of life; many died before 6 months of age |
| **4TH GENERATION** | | | |
| | remained healthy | remained healthy | No 4th generation was produced: either 3rd generation parents were sterile, or 4th generation cats were aborted before birth |

Table 5.2   Pottenger cats experiment results

- Pregnant females often had difficulty giving birth and lactating; many died in labor.
- As time went on, females had more difficulty becoming pregnant.
- Normal sexual personality traits reversed; females became more aggressive, males tended to become more passive.
- In both sexes, physical characteristics became more neutral.
- Sexual interest between cats of the same sex increased.
- Kittens born of deficient diet mothers weighed, on average, 16% less than kittens born of raw diet mothers.
- Intestinal parasites and vermin were common.
- Allergies became worse from one generation to the next.
- Skin diseases increased from about 5% in normal cats to over 90% in third generation cats.

- Infections of glands and organs were common.
- Arthritis and nervous problems developed and became progressive.
- Bones became soft and pliable.

In summary, first generation cats fed processed food began to develop diseases and illnesses near the end of their lives. Second generation cats developed diseases and illnesses in the middle of their lives. Third generation cats developed diseases and illnesses at the beginning of their lives, and many died before six months of age. No fourth generation was produced! Either third generation female parents were sterile, or they aborted their offspring before birth. This was clear and indisputable evidence of genetic deterioration from one generation to the next. A startling observation from this study was that, even though *one-third* of the food on the deficient diets" was raw, the generational health of the cats continued to deteriorate!

The good news is that part of the experiment also proved that if the diet was corrected soon enough, disease conditions could be reversed. When cats that had been fed cooked meat were returned to a raw meat diet, their physical conditions continued to improve until, by the fourth generation, the animals regenerated to a state of near-normal health.[5]

Now, that's food for thought! It gives us a great deal of insight into the increase of degenerative diseases, and the decreases in fertility, in our human population.

### Conclusions from these studies

Almost all we need to know about why disease conditions can develop is contained in the results of the Pottenger Cats Experiments:

- Cooking destroys the life-giving, and life-sustaining, properties of food. Enzymes are destroyed, and the viability of certain acids is seriously reduced.
- Disease conditions result, over time, from eating a diet of mostly cooked and processed food.

- Disease conditions and genetic weaknesses occur earlier in each succeeding generation.
- Physical, emotional, skeletal, sexual, and behavioral changes become more pronounced and prevalent with each generation.
- The only solution for vibrant, disease-free health is to revert to a diet of raw, or mostly raw, food.

### Difference between Cats and Humans

Later studies have found that heating destroys taurine, an essential amino acid for cats which they must have to remain healthy. Similarly, humans require the essential amino acid lysine which becomes bound when exposed to heat in cooking. (See page 287 for more on amino acids.)

Just like the Pottenger cats, the human body is designed for whole, natural, unprocessed food as nourishment. However, as clearly illustrated in Figure 2.1, there is a distinct difference between cats and humans. Whereas carnivores are physically designed to consume mostly meat, humans are not. The over-consumption of animal proteins produces excess acids in the human body, and as we will learn in chapter 10, this condition sets the stage for diseases to manifest. As an example of how deadly an exclusive diet of cooked meat is to humans, Arlin, Dini, and Wolfe, in their book *Nature's First Law: The Raw-Food Diet*, relate how some American prisoners during the Vietnam war were condemned to death by being fed a diet that consisted of only cooked meat. Many did not live past one month. This is very significant considering that an average person may live up to one hundred days on a complete fast.[6]

## HEALTH AND DISEASE SINCE 1900

Why are we sicker now than people were a century ago? Until the early 1900s, the incidences of cancer, diabetes, heart attacks, and obesity were rare among the general population. And, in the 1800s, doctors who observed native populations in Africa, Kashmir, and northern Canada reported that cancer seemed nonexistent."[7] It is now evident to everyone in the western world that diseases of all kinds are rampant, and treatment of diseases has become a problem as well as a huge industry. "In 1904, only 1 out of 24 Americans had cancer in his lifetime." Now "the cancer rate is 1 out of 2 in men and 1 out of 3 in women."[8]

The World Health Organization report of June 4, 2000, listed "healthy" life expectancies of people in nations around the world. Japan and Australia ranked number 1 and 2 respectively, Canada was 12th, and the United States of America was 24th, right after Israel in 23rd spot. Dr. Christopher Murray states:

> The position of the United States is one of the major surprises of the new rating system. Basically, you die earlier and spend more time disabled if you're an American rather than a member of most other advanced countries.[9]

It is becoming increasingly evident that the disease symptoms that are developing are no longer just about old age. As with the Pottenger cats, young adults and children are becoming part of the statistics. This degenerative picture is by no means restricted to North America; it is being seen in other nations as well. For example, according to the Russian Academy of Science, the Russian population is getting sicker and dying faster than ever before; only 30% of births are considered "normal," and 53% of the remaining 70% of babies born suffer from a chronic affliction or disease. Life expectancy for Russian men is now down to 56.1 years.[10]

By the 1990s, one out of five Americans under the age of 17 already had a chronic disease; 22% of Americans suffered from allergies; 60% had defective vision; 50% had chronic digestive disorders; and 9 out of 10 suffered from clogged colons.[11]

A 1992 Danish research study of 15,000 men in the United States, Europe, Asia, Africa, and other parts of the world concluded that average sperm counts had dropped significantly from 1938 to 1990. Further analysis of this study concluded that the declines were seen overall in the United States and Europe but not in non-Western countries.[12] It is probable that similar statistics apply to viability of female ova as well. In the United States, fertility rates continue to decline and age-related spontaneous abortion is on the increase.[13]

There is an increasing incidence of illness and disease in children being born today. Have you noticed the recent awareness and concern in schools about children with life-threatening food allergies? This was not a serious problem fifty years ago. Since 1900, more research has been conducted and more knowledge has been gained on the subject of disease than at any time in history. In western nations, there are now more doctors and hospitals per capita than previously. But, why are we less healthy than our ancestors?

## OUR EATING HABITS AND FOOD HAVE CHANGED

### Food Consumption[14]

Although compiled for the United States, the following statistics probably apply quite generally to most of North America.

Between 1900 and 1980, the consumption of:
- fresh fruit and vegetables decreased from 40% to 20%
- fresh citrus fruit decreased 50%
- processed citrus fruit increased 2500%
- butter decreased 75%
- lard decreased 66%
- unprocessed potato and sweet potato decreased 40%.
- whole grains decreased 50%
- beef consumption increased 75%
- poultry increased 350%
- dairy, not including butter, increased 25%
- cheese increased 400%
- fat and oil increased 150%
- margarine increased 800%
- corn syrup increased 400%

- sugar increased 50%. The average person consumes 150 pounds of sugar per year.
- processed fruits (other than citrus) and vegetables (canned, packaged, et cetera), increased 400%

> **Note:** *Fresh fruit consumption data is probably more applicable to southern regions as raw fruit is now available to us year-round, although much of it is picked unripe to facilitate shipping.*

Between 1940 and 1980, the consumption of:
- eggs decreased 25%
- food coloring increased 90%

Between 1960 and 1980, the consumption of:
- Soft drinks increased 300%. The average person now consumes 38 gallons (144 liters) of soft drinks annually, and one-fifth of our sugar intake is in soft drinks.

Other statistics tell us that since the early part of the 1900s, the consumption of whole grain products and potatoes is half of former levels, whereas the consumption of animal and dairy products is now significantly higher. It is estimated that the average American will eat 15 cows, 24 hogs, 12 sheep, 900 chickens, 1,000 pounds of fish, and 25,250 pounds of dairy products in their lifetime.[15] As we will learn in chapter 6, this extremely high intake of cooked protein is a very unhealthy trend because it causes stress to the body's organs, glands, and tissues, and how it depletes nutrient reserves.

There is a clear relationship between changes in the consumption of processed food and the increase in degenerative diseases. The contradictory statistics of more disease in the presence of apparently "better" healthcare are baffling. What are we doing wrong? What are we missing? Are there any answers to this dilemma? Or, are we just meant to get sick and suffer more as we grow older, as well as watch our children suffer with diseases? Why is there this contradiction?

It is important to note how people are also quickly moving away from drinking healthy water:

> In 1970 the average consumption of tap water was about 68 gallons per year per capita; and the consumption of soft drinks was 24.3 gallons. By 1989, water consumption decreased to 37 gallons per capita while the consumption of soft drinks rose to 42.2 gallons. Alcoholic beverage consumption was at 39.1 gallons per capita. The American public is currently consuming more soft drinks and alcohol than water!... Fast foods, alcoholic beverages, white sugar, white flour and soft drinks all have one thing in common: they do not supply the essential nutrition we need for health.[16]

### Food Production

The commercial food we now consume is grown in soil that has been seriously depleted of its minerals because of continuous farming without crop rotation or rest. In addition, there is a total dependence on chemical fertilizers and pesticides to grow produce. Depending on the soils they are grown on, there can be a significant difference between commercially grown and organically grown vegetables. One study concluded that organically grown foods were richer in minerals than commercially grown products. By comparison, there was 87% less content of magnesium, potassium, manganese, iron, and copper in conventionally grown foods.[17]

It is now a proven fact that when soil is made healthy with organic humus and natural minerals, plants become healthier and more pest-resistant. They do not contain "weakness attractors" for pests.

Even though we may be eating adequate quantities of fruits and vegetables, if they are not grown organically, or if they have been irradiated, our bodies are not receiving the nutrition required to build and maintain health. We are consuming incomplete nutrition because the food lacks the natural vitamins, minerals, amino acids, and enzymes necessary to maintain life and build vitality.

**Food Processing**

The following food preparation processes are listed in order of nutritive value, from best to worst:[18]

- Raw
- Juiced, and consumed immediately after preparation
- Dehydrated, or dried, without chemicals or additives (2–5% loss of nutritive value)
- Frozen (5–15% loss)
- Lightly steamed, so that the vegetable is still a little crunchy (15–40% loss)
- Cooked (40–100% loss, depending of length of time cooked)
- Leftovers
- Microwaved (90–99% loss)
- Commercially canned
- Fried, and deep fried
- Processed foods with additives (contain toxins and have zero nutrient value)

Food industries process food so that it can be sold to consumers. In our fast-paced world, we have been conditioned to expect food that is conveniently packaged, easy and quick to prepare, has a long shelf life, and tastes good. Tantalizing taste is now the main criterion for choosing food.

Food loses its nutrient value when it is processed. For example, refined white flour contains only two or three nutrients, compared to more than fifty in whole-wheat flour. Whenever food is heated to temperatures in excess of 112°F (44°C), most of the natural enzymes in it are destroyed. Original, living, natural food becomes more or less unnatural dead food, lacking life force energy. Enzymes contained in raw food function as catalysts to assist with the digestive process and with other functions in our bodies. Without live enzymes in food, our bodies must manufacture them from vitamins and minerals in our own tissues to be able to digest the nutrient-deficient processed foods we eat. Whenever we prepare foods by canning or overcooking, we are killing the live enzymes. When we consume these foods, we are depleting our body's nutrient reserves.

### Taste Enhancers

Many ingredients, referred to as additives, are combined with foods to increase eye and taste appeal. There is much research data on the harm that chemical food additives do to human health. Taste-enhancers are aptly called "excitotoxins." These particular chemicals are in many of our processed and prepared foods. They include monosodium glutamate (MSG), aspartame (Nutrasweet®), cysteine, hydrolyzed protein, and aspartic acid. Briefly stated, excitotoxins stimulate brain cells to death on a selective basis. They cause brain damage by exciting neurons to such a degree that various neurological malfunctions develop. Disorders can include headaches, seizures, hypoglycemia, strokes, tumors, Parkinson's disease, Alzheimer's dementia, Huntington's disease, and Lou Gehrig's disease (ALS). An in-depth analysis and explanation of the dangers of food additives and their effects can be found in Dr. Russell Blaylock's book *Excitotoxins: The Taste that Kills.*

### Microwave Ovens

Foods that have been subjected to microwave radiation are dangerous to our health. Microwave ovens heat food with high-frequency microwaves that force water molecules to heat up by violently vibrating them. This causes a fracturing of the molecules, and a rearrangement of the chemical composition of the food. Besides irradiating food, electromagnetic fields and invisible microwave emissions can bypass the built-in shielding in microwave ovens, and can leak through aging door seals, allowing them to travel to other rooms of the house.

The history of microwave ovens dates back to World War II, when the Nazis began research and development of these devices. They were searching for ways to overcome the logistical problems of producing edible food in a short time, and to be able to reduce the amount and bulk of cooking fuels that would be required to support their planned operations for the military invasion of Russia.[19] At the end of the war, the United States' War Department and the Soviet Union obtained the German microwave research and some of the devices. They took them home for further study. Adding to the German research from the early forties, the Russians continued to research the biological effects of microwave ovens and microwave-cooked food. Their findings led them, in 1976, to issue an international warning concerning the biological and environmental dangers of using such ovens and similar electronic frequency devices.[20]

German and Russian researchers found[21] that cooking food with microwaves:

- Produces cancer causing agents.
- Destroys nutritive values.
- Reduces the food's vital energy field content by 60–90%.

Humans who had direct exposure to microwaves but had not eaten irradiated food experienced:

- Long term cumulative loss of vital energies.
- Destabilized metabolism.
- Cell damage.
- Degeneration of electrical nerve impulses.
- Nervous and lymphatic systems damage.
- Hormone destabilization.
- Brainwave disturbances.
- Psychological disorders.

Conclusions on the effects of eating irradiated food included:

- Long term permanent brain damage.
- Alteration or loss of hormone production.
- Permanent damage within the human body.
- Stomach and intestinal tumors.

- Increase of cancer cells in human blood.
- Immune system deficiencies.
- Loss of memory, concentration, emotional instability, and a decrease of intelligence.

The use of microwave ovens is almost universal in restaurants and homes in North America. Considering the foregoing information, it is likely that serious damage at the human cellular level is being wrought throughout the western world. Yet, as with many other aspects of our food, medicines, and environment, the cumulative effects of microwaves are gradual; when the onset of illness occurs, it is very hard to make the connection with the original cause. For these reasons, in my opinion, the use of microwave ovens, and eating food and drinks that have been heated in them, is not advised.

### Genetically Altered Food

Genetically altered food is food derived from plants or animals that has had its genetic structure altered by splicing in genes of another species. Such produce is also referred to as "bioengineered" or "transgenic." Scientists are experimenting with these processes in attempts to increase yields, increase plant resistance to toxins and pests, increase nutrient levels, and improve taste. In 2000, 25% of the U.S. corn crop and 55% of the soybean crop were of genetically modified varieties.[22] A livestock example is pigs that are being injected with genetically engineered growth hormones to make them grow faster and 40% larger.

Genetically altered produce has now found its way into many foods in our stores. Do you know what you are eating? Do you know whether the tomato has fish genes, or your corn has genes from bacteria? Is this a problem?

Often, problems with this kind of experimenting can be observed in nature first. As an example, it is now being discovered that pollen from genetically modified corn can kill monarch butterflies.[23] There is long-term concern that pollen from bio-engineered crops will spread and kill beneficial insects as well as create strains of superweeds that are totally resistant to pesticides.

Genetic engineering is changing the composition of foods, and most North American consumers are uninformed on the issue of bio-engineered crops. In Britain and Europe, there is widespread awareness and opposition to the introduction of genetically altered foods. European and Asian nations are beginning to require labels on all foods containing genetically modified ingredients. Commercial interests in North America are fighting this trend because they realize that once labels identifying foods as genetically altered appear, consumers will start avoiding them.

On the surface, one might think that altering foods genetically is better for the farmers and better for consumers. But, look a little closer. Food that has been natural since its time on earth began has now had its genetic structure changed by humans. A problem develops: if the food's genetic structure has changed, so has its electrical structure. The human body thrives only on natural food. It can only be nourished, or recharged, by electrically compatible matrices. The cells of our bodies cannot utilize unnatural, processed, altered, or distorted electrical matrices without succumbing to disease.

Bottom line? Avoid genetically altered foods.

### Our Environment Is Changing

The world's environment has changed radically over the last 50 years, particularly in regard to the air we breathe and the products we consume. It is much more toxic than it used to be. Scientists estimate that, from earlier times on earth, the average oxygen content of air has decreased from 38% to between 19% and 21%.[24] In some larger cities where pollution is highest, the oxygen content of air is lower than this. This is quite troubling because adequate intake of oxygen is critical to life and health. The Compressed Gas Association of Arlington, Virginia issued a safety bulletin stating that when breathing air content is 15–19% it results in decreased ability to perform tasks, and "may impair coordination and may induce early symptoms in persons with heart, lung, or circulatory problems."[25]

Not only is the oxygen content of the air many of us are breathing deficient, but industrial emissions and engine exhausts are continually polluting the air as well. Industrial chemicals such as pesticides, fungicides and insecticides, plastics, radiation, and synthetic products are changing the natural health-giving properties of our food. They introduce toxins to our bodies that our ancestors did not have to cope with.

Some industrial chemicals, detergents, and food dyes are classified as hormone disrupters because they are estrogen mimics. Our bodies mistake synthetic estrogens for the real thing, accept it, and process it, which causes an imbalance of our natural hormones. Red Dye #3, for example, which is used in hot dogs and other processed foods, contains synthetic estrogen. The plastic coating in many food cans contains a powerful estrogen mimic. In the wild, we are now finding that animals, birds, and fish exposed to pesticides and industrial chemicals are having difficulty producing healthy offspring. They are developing shrunken male sex organs, and many are developing both testes and ovaries. These sexual organ changes are leading to behavioral changes, reproductive loss, and early mortality in offspring.

Oxygen deficiency, air and chemical pollution, and denatured foods place great stresses on our organs and cells. Our bodies are being forced to cope with pollution and inferior nutrition as never before. And although the human lungs, liver, and kidneys are able to filter out toxins within reason, they were never meant to do so to the extent they are being required by our present-day changing environment.

## NUTRITION AND PHYSICAL DEGENERATION

After completing his research on root canal and dental infections, Dr. Weston Price decided to study individuals and animals that did not have tooth or gum disease, and then determine what caused such diseases to evolve. During a nine-year period he and his wife traveled around the world seeking out primitive cultures that were living on native foods. They studied several tribes from different races. Their findings were very revealing. In his book *Root Canal Cover-up,* Dr. George Meinig summarizes Dr. Price's work as follows:

> Invariably, no matter what their native diets or where they lived, these people had excellent teeth, extremely low decay rates, very little—if any—crookedness of teeth, and no impacted teeth. Most were magnificent specimens of health, having few illnesses, physical or mental. The equivalent of jail was non-existent, because these natives proved to have great mental and emotional stability.
>
> On the other hand, when these same people came in contact with our civilization through the establishment of trading posts, rampant tooth decay took place. First generation children developed severe crookedness of teeth, and many of the same diseases and malformations exhibited in modern civilization, including cleft palates, harelips and clubfeet.
>
> The items primitives received in trade were much the same everywhere: a few pieces of clothing, some trinkets, certain vegetable oils, jams and jellies, white flour and sugar. No matter where in the world these primitives lived, ninety percent of the total items they received in trade consisted of white flour and sugar.
>
> These two foods accounted for their severe degeneration and downfall. It was clearly demonstrated that most of the diseases, which developed after adopting these foods, were not caused by genetics, but were caused by environment.[26]

The two totally unrelated studies by Dr. Price and Dr. Pottenger, done many years ago, clearly illustrate that humans and animals thrive and live in health when they eat diets of natural, unprocessed foods. But, when they eat foods that have been processed, denatured, and preserved with additives, they develop degenerative diseases.

## IT TAKES LIFE TO GET LIFE

Around the year 325 AD, the Roman Emperor Constantine and his Council of Nicea decided to simplify the collection of scriptures into what is now known as the King James Version of the Christian Bible. Many original books did not "make the cut," as the Council recommended that at least 45 documents be removed.[27] This screening process, or even censoring, later became known as the Constantine Conspiracy.

In 1946, a discovery of lost manuscripts was made in forgotten caves in an area known as Qumran, between Israel and Jordan, near the Dead Sea. Nearly one thousand documents had been hidden there for safekeeping. Among the Dead Sea Scrolls was the Book of the Essenes, from which the following quote is taken:

> Kill not the food which goes into your mouth.
> For if you eat living food, the same will quicken you,
> But if you kill your food, the dead food will kill you also.
> For life comes only from life, and death comes always from death.
> For everything which kills your foods, kills your bodies also.[28]

How can it be said any more plainly?

Why haven't we known this before? Or, if someone did know, why haven't we been told about it? Isn't that what doctors and the healthcare system are supposed to be about?

Let us have a closer look at our western conventional medical care system and its history to understand how it developed into what it is today.

# 6 | CONVENTIONAL MEDICAL CARE

∾

*If the doctors of today do not become the
nutritionists of tomorrow; .... the nutritionists
of today will become the doctors of tomorrow.*
ROCKEFELLER INSTITUTE OF MEDICAL RESEARCH

∾

## HEALTHCARE OR DISEASE CARE?

CONVENTIONAL MEDICAL CARE treats *symptoms* of disease. True
healthcare works to correct the *causes* of disease. And, although the present allopathic system is often referred to as "traditional medicine," it is
not. True traditional medicine is healthcare that uses natural methods,
foods, and herbs, and has been practiced since the beginning of civiliza-
tion. Today's medical system, which is barely a century old, attempts to
treat disease with chemicals, surgery, and radiation technologies. It is not
*health* care. It is *disease* care.

What are the beliefs underlying the conventional doctor-patient relationship? We usually seek medical help only when we are sick, hurt, or
suspect that something is wrong. We go to our doctor believing that he or
she will "fix" it. If, after a period of time, we don't experience relief, we lose
faith in that doctor and want to look for another one who might eliminate
our symptoms and make us feel better. If we have pain or discomfort, we
want something or someone to take it away. The doctor asks questions

and examines us to determine what "disease" or body malfunction is present. Often, a prescription for a pharmaceutical drug is written. For more serious problems, continuous and multiple drugs may be prescribed. If there is cancer present, treatments usually focus on surgery, chemotherapy, or radiation.

## THE TRAINING OF DOCTORS

Medical doctors are educated and trained to look for disease, and to use pharmaceutical drugs as the treatment of choice. They receive almost no instruction in the nutritional aspects of disease prevention. A 1999–2000 survey of 122 medical and osteopathic schools in the United States found that, in the 98 schools responding, only an average of between 6 and 30 hours of nutrition courses was required, including material integrated into other courses. The report noted that "exposure" to nutrition is required as part of the curriculum.[1] A 2000–01 survey of 116 medical schools reported that only 39 of the schools responding require a separate nutrition course.[2] Dr. Andrew Weil, author of *Spontaneous Healing*, says that conventional doctors are "nutritionally illiterate."[3]

After leaving medical school, doctors receive their ongoing education about the efficacy of new drugs from pharmaceutical company representatives, whose main objective is to convince doctors to sell their products. Dr. Bruce Lipton notes that "medical doctors are caught between an intellectual rock and a corporate hard place," and calls them "pharmaceutical patsies."[4]

## MEDICAL THINKING IS CHEMISTRY-BASED

Conventional medicine, with its drug-treatment mindset, typically views the body only as a chemical entity. This thinking is 80 years out of date, and based on the Newtonian physics view that the universe is composed of matter. This completely ignores the energy factors of health proved by quantum physics since 1925.[5] All living things have *living* chemistry. Drugs contain no life, and are therefore incapable of *creating* life; in fact, they are often harmful.

The pharmaceutical industry bombards the public via the media, urging people to "ask your doctor if this drug is right for you." Yet the same advertisements list multiple possible harmful side effects that may be experienced. Meanwhile, there are increasing reports of illness and deaths caused by certain prescription drugs. A recent example is the drug Vioxx; usually prescribed as a pain reliever, it is reported to have caused 40,000 deaths in the United States and between 4,000 to 7000 in Canada.[6]

The medical system is inseparably linked to the pharmaceutical industry and the use of drugs. The contradiction is that, even though drugs will make a healthy person sick, we expect a sick person to become healthy by taking drugs. It doesn't make sense.

It is interesting to note that while society as a whole perceives illicit drugs to be dangerous, we have been conditioned to accept the constant and extended use of pharmaceutical drugs as acceptable and supportive to the health of our bodies. The truth is—all drugs are toxic.

## OUR OWN TREATMENT OF ILLNESS

When we use over-the-counter drugs or natural remedies to treat our illness symptoms, do we really know what we are doing? Do we understand what a drug, herb, or vitamin pill does in our body? Do these measures help or hinder the body? Are they helping it function according to its priorities, or are they forcing the body to expend energy, changing its natural healing priorities in order to relieve our uncomfortable symptoms? Are we trading immediate symptom relief for longer-term loss of vitality? We need to know the difference between treating symptoms and working to restore health by addressing the causes of disease.

When we closely examine our behavior and reactions to being sick, we realize that we give very little thought to how we can stay healthy. For the most part, we take our health for granted until it is almost gone. Unfortunately, we have also come to expect disease as a natural part of growing older. But we do not understand why young people become seriously ill. Somehow that doesn't seem right.

In short, most of us do not understand how the body operates, and we do not take personal responsibility for staying healthy. We want a quick fix without having to suffer, to take time off the job, or to change our habits of eating, drinking, exercising, and thinking.

## RISKING OUR HEALTH

When we become ill and seek medical treatment, we place our lives in the hands of someone else. Except for unexpected trauma situations, do we really want to give total control to someone else?

The medical term used to describe a condition induced in a patient by a treatment given by a health practitioner is "iatrogenic." A July 2000 article in the *Journal of the American Medical Association* (JAMA) presented statistics to show that doctors are the third leading cause of death, after heart disease and cancer, in the United States.[7] From a separate study commissioned by the Nutrition Institute of America, a more recent article entitled "Death by Medicine" by Drs. Null, Dean, Feldman, and Rasio concludes that the American medical system is the "leading cause of death and injury in the United States." It lists the total number of iatrogenic deaths in the United States as 783,936 compared to the 2001 heart disease annual death rate of 699,697, and annual cancer death rate of 553,251.[8]

Rather sobering, don't you think? One would expect that, with its ranking in medical technology near the top of all nations, the U.S. would place among the best in the health of its citizens. Unfortunately, this is not the case. According to the JAMA article, the U.S. ranked on average, from seventh to thirteenth among nations of the world for 16 health indicators, ranging from birth problems through to life expectancy. The year 2000 World Health Organization report ranked the U.S. twenty-fourth in health-expectancy among nations of the world despite it being the most prosperous.[9]

## HOSPITAL INFECTIONS

The Chicago Tribune conducted a study of the files of 5,810 hospitals in the U.S. in the year 2000. The report found that, "nearly three-quarters of the deadly infections—about 75,000—were preventable, the result of unsanitary facilities, germ-laden instruments, unwashed hands and other lapses." It estimated that approximately, "50% of doctors and nurses in hospitals do not clean their hands between patients." The conclusive finding was that preventable deaths from hospital germs are now the fourth leading cause of death among Americans. Many germs are becoming "super bugs" that are resistant to antibiotics.[10] Similar problems exist in Canada, Britain, Australia, and New Zealand.[11]

## TREATING SYMPTOMS

We are confused about what causes disease. Our medical system doesn't know either! Typically, we think diseases just "happen" to us, similar to the bad luck of being dealt a losing hand in a game of cards. For a large percentage of the diseases described in medical books and literature, we find the cause listed as "unknown." If we don't know what the cause of a disease is, how can we know what to do to treat it? We invariably end up only treating the symptom. Treating a symptom is like taking the battery out of a smoke alarm when it has sounded instead of looking for the source and cause of the smoke.

Is it possible the headache we feel is signaling that something is out of balance with the body's metabolism? Or could it have something to do with our emotional state? What is something as simple and basic as indigestion telling us? The body is talking to us; but are we listening? Are we trying to correct the underlying causes? We should be.

## SYMPTOMS VERSUS CAUSES

Illness symptoms have been given names such as: headache, indigestion, stomach ache, diarrhea, constipation, hayfever, asthma, eczema, sinusitis, arthritis, high blood pressure, and cancer. They are called diseases, but are more correctly "dis-ease indicators." These indicators are signals, or symptoms, of more serious problems within the body. They are the body's effort to get our attention, telling us that it needs supportive help to correct underlying conditions of imbalance which, if left to continue, will develop into serious disease conditions.

When we take medication to make a discomfort go away, we trade short-term gain for long-term pain, lower levels of energy, and ill health in the future. We should, instead be focusing our attention, not on the annoyance of the symptom, but on what the symptom is trying to tell us. What have we been doing wrong that is causing the body to complain? The symptom is not the problem; it is our friend. If we pay attention to this communication and cooperate with it, our bodies will work to correct the deeper conditions and save us from greater suffering and poor health in the future.

Our thinking should be:

- What does my body need to be able to correct the *cause* of this distress?
- What is it lacking?
- How can I avoid contributing to the distress?
- If I take this or that remedy, will it help or hinder my body?
- Will it make my body healthier, or will it lower my body's nutrient and energy reserves and further weaken my immune system?
- Am I working *with* my body or *against* it?
- Am I helping my body or abusing it?

Symptoms arise because of deficiencies, toxicity, and imbalances within body fluids and cells. Only the removal of causes will bring about true and lasting health.

## HOW DO DRUGS WORK?

In life-threatening situations, the use of certain drugs may be necessary to save or prolong life. Notwithstanding this caveat, pharmaceutical drugs are manufactured chemicals; they are not natural to the body. They lack living energy and have electrical configurations that are incompatible with those of the body. Drugs are toxic, and cannot be incorporated into the body's cellular structure to build tissue and promote health.

Drugs cause the body to react. It reacts in a protective manner to eliminate the toxic substances. Drugs work because the poisons they contain create a stress in the body that is more serious than the symptom for which they were taken. In this process, the symptom is relieved. For example, acetylsalicylic acid, used as a painkiller, causes bleeding in the stomach or small intestine. Another top-selling painkiller causes similar stress in the liver. They relieve a symptom because they create a greater stress in another area of the body that forces it to divert its attention to the new threat. The body always tries to deal with the most serious problem first.[12]

Strong poisons taken into our bodies are viewed as life-threatening. The body draws on all its energy resources, including the energy that is keeping us conscious, if necessary, to eliminate the threat. It goes into triage mode, and shuts down all our awareness centers. This is what happens when systemic anesthetics are administered before a surgical operation. If too much anesthetic is given, the energy required to eliminate it is greater than the body has and the person dies. That is why the work and monitoring of the anesthetist is so critical. He or she must walk the fine line between the unconsciousness or death of the patient.

Antibiotics kill both harmful bacteria and friendly bacteria; they do not discriminate. The body requires friendly bacteria to maintain a healthy balance in the colon, and to manufacture certain vitamins and antibiotics of its own. Our intake of antibiotics is not only from prescription sources. Approximately 2.4 million pounds of antibiotics are given each year to farm animals—mainly cattle, pigs, and chickens—as a preventative to infection. This is more than eight times the amount administered to humans.[13]

Jane Goodall, in her book *Harvest for Hope*, warns of the dangers and short-term folly of eating farm-raised seafood. According to her research, commercial seafood farms use massive amounts of pesticides, antibiotics, and disinfectants to combat disease in the crowded environments where the fish and tiger prawns are raised. To make them grow faster and larger, their diet includes growth hormones. Farmed salmon are fed pink dye to colour their flesh. In addition, these chemically-laden farms are devastating surrounding sea life, causing deadly water pollution and ruining the land on which the seafood farms are set up, with the consequent ruination of fishermen and farmers who depended on these areas for their livelihood.[14]

When we eat these animal and seafood products, antibiotics, and growth hormones and chemicals, end up in our body systems. Over time, bacteria are becoming increasingly resistant to antibiotics. Scientists are warning that this could pose increasingly serious problems for humans, as available antibiotics are rendered ineffective against certain new bacterial strains.

Drugs only deal with symptoms. They do not correct the cause of symptoms. Natural and complete healing does not take place with drug use. In order to deal with a toxic drug, the body is forced to put the cause of the pain or infection "on hold." If the body has enough energy after the episode, the symptomatic condition returns at a later date as the body attempts to heal and correct the basic problem again. If the drug is too devitalizing, the symptom may not return because the body no longer has sufficient energy to mount another healing attempt. That is, the symptom cause has been suppressed, but may return later as a more chronic disease. There is no free ticket. We cannot get something in health without consciously working for it. We can take the quick fix, but there is a consequence to pay later. That consequence is usually reduced quality of life as we grow older.

Ask yourself this: Does it make sense that a person can be poisoned back to health? The problem with drug treatment is that it diverts the body's attention from working on its own priorities for healing. Drugs send the body down a spiral, increasing in speed—like a whirlpool— toward degenerative disease. Eventually, as the body becomes less able to defend itself and correct the cause of malfunctions, it succumbs to critical disease.

## WHAT ABOUT VACCINATIONS?

A vaccine is a preparation of dead or weakened disease-causing organisms. It is injected into the body to produce immunity against the disease that the organisms cause. But do vaccines really do that? Are they effective?

A British physician, Edward Jenner, performed the first recorded vaccination in 1796 when he inserted a small amount of cowpox from an infected dairy maid into the cut arm of a healthy eight-year-old boy. Forty-eight days later, smallpox matter was injected into the boy with no effect.

Today, vaccines exist for many diseases, and are mandatory in many countries. We have been led to believe that they are safe. But according to Neil Miller, "… findings on seven of the more commonly administered vaccines—for poliomyelitis (polio), diphtheria, measles, German measles (rubella), mumps, tetanus, and pertussis (whooping cough)—do not support this conclusion."[15]

Two books on vaccinations, by Neil Miller and Viera Scheibner respectively, were written after extensive studies of vaccine research. They present convincing evidence, not only of the ineffectiveness of vaccines, but of the dangers inherent in their use. These books are a "must read" for any parent or prospective parent. They also shed light on some of the afflictions contemporary adults may be suffering from. Here is how Viera Scheibner summarizes her research:

> I did not find it difficult to conclude that there is no evidence whatsoever that vaccine of any kind - but especially those against childhood diseases - are effective in preventing the infectious diseases they are supposed to prevent. Further, adverse effects are amply documented and are far more significant to public health than any adverse effects of infectious diseases. Immunizations, including those practiced on babies, not only did not prevent any infectious diseases, they caused more suffering and more deaths than have any other human activity in the entire history of medical intervention.[16]

While modern medicine leads us to believe the reduction of epidemic diseases like smallpox and polio is due to the introduction of mass vaccination programs, the research of Miller and Scheibner found this to be totally unsubstantiated. They found that infectious diseases, which were rampant in Europe even a century ago, had declined up to 90% before any vaccine had been used in large sections of the population. Diseases such as bubonic plague and scarlet fever disappeared entirely on their own without any vaccination programs at all. These reductions were largely attributed to improvements in nutritional and sanitary measures.

In brief, some of Miller's findings are:[17]

- The polio death rate was decreasing on its own before the vaccine was introduced (1923 to 1953).
- In five New England states, cases of polio increased after mass inoculations (1954 and 1955).
- 87% of all polio cases were caused by the polio vaccine (US Federal Center for Disease Control figures, 1973 to 1983).
- The measles death rate decreased by more than 95% in the U.S. and Britain before the vaccine was introduced (1915 to 1958).
- Among all U.S. school-age children in 1984, 58% of all measles cases were contracted by people who had been vaccinated against the disease.
- Two separate scientific studies found the rubella (German measles) vaccine, introduced in 1979, to be the cause of Chronic Fatigue Syndrome (also called Epstein-Barr Virus). In children, the virus can stay in their systems for years and can be passed on to adults through casual contact.
- The pertussis (whooping cough) death rate decreased by more than 75% before the vaccine was introduced.
- In the U.S. in 1984, among all children between the ages of 7 months and 6 years who contracted pertussis, 46% had been vaccinated against the disease.
- In a study of 103 children who died of SIDS (Sudden Infant Death Syndrome, or crib death), conducted by Dr. William Torch of the

University of Nevada School of Medicine, it was found that 70% had received the DPT (combined diphtheria-pertussis-tetanus) vaccine within three weeks of their deaths.

• Scientific evidence links vaccinations to chronic fatigue, autoimmune disorders, AIDS, learning disabilities, and other health problems.

Viera Scheibner notes that the annual death rate in Europe prior to 1940 from diphtheria was "negligible (less than 300 deaths per million)." After this date, when mass vaccinations against the disease were begun, "unprecedented" diphtheria epidemics followed in "fully vaccinated subjects." Mass vaccinations against tetanus and whooping cough also began in many countries in the 1940s, and were followed by outbreaks of the "so-called provocation poliomyelitis."[18]

The evidence appears very clear that vaccinations are an unnatural assault on the body, which compromises and weakens the immune system. The long-term effects of all vaccines are unknown.

Dr. Guylaine Lanctôt, author of *The Medical Mafia*, is very blunt regarding health authorities' claims that vaccines protect us against contagious illnesses and epidemics. She calls this "the big lie." Her research concludes that:[19]

• Vaccines are ineffective in protecting against illnesses and can make the person more susceptible to the illness being vaccinated against;

• People who are vaccinated can transmit the illness, even if they are not ill themselves;

• Certain vaccines such as tuberculosis, tetanus, German measles, diphtheria, influenza, and hepatitis B are useless for various reasons, yet repeated use of these is widespread;

• Innumerable complications result from vaccines, ranging from allergies and neurological disorders to sudden death of infants;

• Frightening and unforeseen effects result, such as the permanent and hereditary changing of the genetic code, and the creation of new uncontrollable illnesses, such as AIDS.

Research findings now available from many sources are indicating that vaccinations interfere with the body's immune system development and make people more susceptible to diseases, not less.

There is a growing body of evidence suggesting that childhood diseases, most of which are harmless, are critical stages in the development of a strong, fully functioning immune system. An immature immune system needs to develop naturally, by fighting off the illnesses that occur in childhood. Vaccines shield the body from exposure to minor illnesses, but may also be stunting its immune system and introducing other viruses and bacteria that the immune system cannot overcome.

Some ingredients that may be found in vaccines are:[20]

- Phenol (carbolic acid), distilled from coal or coal tar.
- Formaldehyde, a known cancer causing agent, which is commonly used to embalm corpses.
- Mercury (thimerosal), a toxic heavy metal and a neurological poison, which accumulates in the brain.
- Alum, a preservative.
- Aluminum phosphate, a toxin used in deodorants. Aluminum is a neurological poison that accumulates in the brain.
- Acetone, a solvent used in fingernail polish remover; very volatile, passes easily through the placenta.
- Glycerin
- Sodium chloride
- Pig or horse blood
- Cow pox pus
- Rabbit brain tissue
- Dog kidney tissue
- Monkey kidney tissue
- Chicken or duck egg protein
- Other decomposing protein
- Various chemicals

The decision to vaccinate a child rests with the parents. Parents are encouraged to read the research on this subject to understand the risks of vaccinations. They can learn about their right to refuse vaccinations for their family. For example, in Canada, there are no laws that can force a person to be vaccinated against their will. Health officials, however, fail to inform the public of these rights.

The question of taking vaccines is also an issue for adults. There is such a media blitz, especially toward the elderly, to have annual flu shots; yet there is very little evidence that they are effective. In an article entitled *The Flu Vaccine Myth,* Croft Woodruff presents the case that flu vaccines may actually increase the risk of developing neurological pathologies:

> ... according to Hugh Fudenberg, MD, ... If an individual has had five flu shots between 1970 and 1980 (the years studied) her chances of getting Alzheimer's Disease is 10 times higher than if she had one, two or no shots. When asked why this was so, Fudenberg said it was due to the mercury and aluminum that is in every flu shot (and most childhood shots). The gradual mercury and aluminum buildup in the brain causes cognitive dysfunction. Is this why the number of those suffering from Alzheimer's is expected to quadruple?[21]

The evidence against vaccinations is clear, yet there is a continuing effort to make vaccine administration compulsory worldwide. Woodruff claims that this "will be a license to print money for the vaccine producers and an iatrogenic health disaster of the first magnitude." [22]

If you still have doubts after reading the foregoing information, I urge you to conduct your own independent research. Think again of the electrical nature of the body, and consider how any molecule of a vaccine can have a natural electrical matrix that is compatible with the body's cells. As with drugs, vaccines are not natural to the body.

The best defense against disease is a body that is balanced electrically and chemically and supported by healthy attitudes. When the immune system is strong, harmful bacteria and viruses are not a worry, because, as parasites, they need a toxic environment on which to feed.

## HISTORY OF DRUGS IN MEDICAL PRACTICE

If drugs are so bad for the body, why are they in almost universal use? To answer this question, we need to look at the history and evolution of how drugs developed, and how they came to be accepted for use by the medical professions throughout the world for treating ailments and diseases.

In the 1800s, pharmaceutical companies in Germany began developing and producing drugs for medical purposes on a large scale. These companies grouped together and formed a cartel. In the late 1800s this cartel established operations in the United States. It was backed by Rockefeller and the German chemical and pharmaceutical company I. G. Farben in alliance with Dupont, Standard Oil, and Ford.

The Food and Drug Administration, or FDA, was formed in 1906 to establish credibility and keep public opinion positive toward the use of pharmaceuticals. It was set up to be an independent government organization whose purpose was to test all foods and drugs, and remove from the market any products it considered to be unsafe. It was given the power to approve drugs and natural supplements as either safe or unsafe.

At that time, all medical schools in America taught the use of only natural remedies for healing. Students did not learn to use drugs for treatments and therefore doctors did not prescribe the pharmaceutical companies' products. This was not good business for the cartel. Its solution to this problem was to form the Council of Medical Education in 1910, through the American Medical Association. This became the body that accredited medical schools. Schools that were accredited received funds from the government, but were also required to comply with the Council's requirements. Those that did not apply for accreditation were forced to close. The Council's call for the discontinuance of all courses teaching natural healing methods and the institution of courses teaching drug therapy were the finishing strokes. Within the AMA an anti-natural-healing arts, pro-medical arts propaganda committee was formed. Its function was to distribute literature against the professions of practitioners that were not approved AMA members, for example, chiropractors.

In 1972, the AMA formed the Professional Standard Review Organization to ensure that doctors would use the accepted modes of drug therapy. This committee has the right to enter any medical office and revoke the doctor's license if AMA protocols are not being followed. This has been done many times in the U.S. and Canada, all the while labeling those medical doctors "quacks." It happened to Dr. Leo Roy whom I quote in this book.

The final stroke of genius was to ensure that the general public could afford the expensive drugs and treatment procedures. Government health insurance was set up, but only for orthodox medical treatment. Health insurance companies were convinced that the medical association treatment methods were the best and that natural healing methods were ineffective.

With these organizations in place, the pharmaceutical cartel's control was complete, and tremendous profits were assured.

## CODEX ALIMENTARIUS

In recent years, there has been an upsurge of interest in "alternative" medicine, with its preference for non-invasive and natural therapies, including herbal supplements. The pharmaceutical cartel saw this coming many years ago. In 1962, a commission called Codex Alimentarius (Latin for "food code") was established by the World Health Organization and the United Nations Food and Agriculture Organization. Its directive was to develop international food standards to protect consumer health and to facilitate fair trading practices in foods. About half its members, however, are directly or indirectly related to the pharmaceutical industry.

The Codex commission now meets every year behind closed doors. Its primary goal is to eliminate natural health supplements from the market. Their decisions, on behalf of the pharmaceutical cartel, are passed on to the United Nations General Assembly, and recommended to become binding law for all member countries of the United Nations.

Codex Alimentarius has been leading a vigorous effort to protect the pharmaceutical business from the increasingly popular and effective, safe, non-patentable, natural health supplements. The process has been quite insidious. Dr. Matthias Rath, an outspoken leader in the natural health freedom movement, states:

> No one of healthy mind would support a ban on natural health just like that. The drug Cartel therefore needed to provide a pretence for the yet undecided politicians why they should outlaw natural health therapies. That pretence was the invention of non-existing vitamin side effects. Of course, these side effects only exist in the imagination of the pharmaceutical interest groups and on the drawing boards of their global PR-machinery. Vitamins, minerals and amino acids are the building blocks of life and the body can eliminate any surplus of them without any problems.[24]

Much of the Codex agenda with regards to natural health supplements is now law in parts of Europe, Australia, and New Zealand. Codex dietary supplement rules are in effect in Norway and Germany. For example, in Norway, the sale of vitamin E is restricted to no more than 45 International Units, the maximum for vitamin C is 200 mg per tablet, and coenzyme Q10 is now classified as a drug and is dramatically higher in price. In Canada, when the 'sleep booster' tryptophan was reclassified as a drug, the price escalated by 500%. Eventually, the cartel wants to make even home-grown herbs illegal and require all natural supplements to have a Drug Identification Number (DIN). As drugs, if they are allowed to be sold, they will be much more expensive.

Once approved, the Codex Alimentarius recommendations will form an international code of standards that will force nations adopting them to "harmonize" with its heavily restrictive rules. Further information on Codex may be found at www.friendsoffreedom.org.

Today, it appears that our health is under attack from new viruses, more diseases, and more pervasive economic interests that want to restrict our access to natural therapies. What can we do to protect ourselves? The first step is to understand what we are doing wrong so we can strengthen the environment within our own bodies. Knowledge leads to personal empowerment.

# 7 | WHAT ARE WE DOING WRONG?

~

*In the presence of trouble, some people grow wings;*
*others buy crutches.*

HAROLD W. RUOPP

~

## WHY DO WE BECOME UNHEALTHY?

WE BECOME unhealthy because we fail to give the body what it requires to function properly, and don't know how to interpret the signals it is sending to us. We don't consider them to be important. We don't give our bodies the loving respect and honor they deserve. Our attitudes and lifestyles are not health conscious. It is not until we lose our health, or nearly lose it, that we decide to search for answers.

When one part of the body is stressed, whether physically, nutritionally, or emotionally, the efficiency of the whole body is compromised. All parts are important to the body. If one part suffers, the whole body suffers.

When a plant such as a flower or a tomato is not growing properly, we check to see if it is getting the proper amounts of water, nutrients, light, and temperature. When these are in proper balance, we expect the plant to thrive. We wouldn't think of feeding the plant alcohol, nicotine, sugar, salt, coffee, or frying grease. This principle applies to our household pets as well. Dogs and cats fed a diet of processed foods, cooked table scraps, and sugary treats succumb to afflictions such as obesity, heart disease, and arthritis the same way we do. Cats that are able to forage outside on a regular basis for mice—raw food containing natural enzymes and amino acids—are much healthier. Why should the human body be any different? If the body is deficient in pure water, nutrients, enzymes, or sunlight, or has to deal with an abundance of toxic matter, it starts to show signs of dis-ease. It becomes physically stressed. If the stressful condition continues for too long, the body's recuperative ability is compromised and degenerative disease is the logical and inevitable result. But if we respect the body by giving it what it requires for efficient operation, it will work to reward us with good health.

## WHAT WRONG THINGS ARE WE DOING?

### Not Accepting Responsibility for Our Own Health

We seem to take our health for granted. When we have health problems, we have been taught to look to someone else, or to take medication, to make us feel better. We typically ignore self-responsibility. In order to take responsibility for our own health, we must become knowledgeable about the basics of what the body requires to be healthy.

### Weakening the Digestive System

A healthy digestive system is fundamental to a healthy body. We can never have optimum health without efficient digestion, and we cannot have efficient digestion without an adequate supply of enzymes and sufficient stomach acid.

*One of the first indications of enzyme depletion in the body is the incidence of a digestive problem.*

Our digestive systems become weakened when the body has been deprived of its nutritional needs for years on end. The digestive organs become less efficient in their job of digesting, absorbing, assimilating, and delivering energy to cells. It is not just what we eat that is important, it is what we are able to digest. Consuming dead foods that have no enzymes, wrong combinations of foods, toxic foods, stimulants, drugs, alcohol, overeating, and drinking with meals adds to the load the digestive system has to cope with. This produces stress, and depletes the body's energy and stored reserves.

Following are some practices that cause stress to our systems.

### Ignoring the Acid-Alkaline Balance

This subject is explored in detail in chapter 10, but a few comments are made here as an introduction.

Fundamental to digestion and health is acid-alkaline balance. In health, the cells of the body are slightly alkaline. In a disease state, cells are acidic. The more acidic cells become, the sicker we are and feel. The greatest causes of body acidity are stress and tension from negative emotions, such as anger and fear. Also detrimental are the acid-producing foods and beverages we consume as well as the air we breathe each day. Ninety percent or more of the typical diet of most people is acidic. The normal waste products of cellular metabolism are also acidic.

An acid based diet consisting of overcooked foods, junk foods, sugar, dairy products, excessive meats, soft drinks, alcohol, nicotine, and drugs places an ever-increasing stress on the body. In order to maintain healthy blood alkalinity, the body is forced to rob nutrients from its own tissues. As an example of how acidifying some foods are, Dr. Robbins cites the example of one meal of well-done steak with all the trimmings as requiring nine meals of fresh raw fruits and vegetables to balance out the acid introduced into the body from the meat.[1]

Most liquids we drink are very acidic. A single 12-ounce (355 ml) glass of a cola-type soft drink upsets the acid-alkaline balance of the digestive system so much it requires 32 glasses of pure water to bring it back into balance.[2] Figure 7.1 lists some commonly consumed beverages and the amount of water required to neutralize their acid content:

| Beverage (Glass or cup) | pH Value | Glasses of $H_2O$ to Neutralize |
|---|---|---|
| Coffee | 5.2 | 12 |
| Decaf coffee | 5.0 | 12 |
| Beer | 4.2 | 18 |
| Wine | 3.6 | 20 |
| Concentrated juice | 3.2 | 24 |
| Cola | 2.5 | 32 |

Table 7.1  Acidity of common beverages

As we learned earlier, toxin storage is also acidifying to the body. The body must expend energy for digestion as well as elimination of ingested toxins. If it is unable to eliminate the toxins because of insufficient nutrition and congestion in the organs, the body has no alternative but to store them in the cells where they will do the least harm for the time being. The body hopes it will get the opportunity to eliminate stored toxins at a later date.

An example of toxin storage can be seen in how the body deals with common table salt, sodium chloride. Refined salt, unlike natural sea salt, is unnatural and cannot be used by the body as a nutrient. In excess, it is toxic and harmful to the body. The body makes every attempt to eliminate it. But, until it can be removed via the normal channels of elimination, and through the skin via perspiration, it must be stored. In order to keep this toxic chemical from killing the cells, the body retains water to dilute its concentration. That is why we feel thirsty after a salty meal and experience some swelling of the tissues; the body is using extra water to dilute the salt.

Our body needs alkaline minerals to balance acid, and the only source of alkaline minerals is from the food we consume, or the correct supplements we take. Most raw fruits and vegetables are alkaline. These must be regularly supplied to the body in an adequate quantity to maintain a healthy acid-alkaline balance. A healthy diet should consist of approximately 80% alkaline-forming foods and 20% acid-forming foods. The average person in western cultures eats the reverse of this combination. Is it any wonder that we are getting progressively sicker, and that degenerative diseases are increasing and appearing at younger ages?

As long as our diet remains predominantly acidic, the alkaline deficit problem will be progressive and will lead to more chronic disease. The more acidic our cells are, the poorer our health is; eventually, when the cells become too acidic, death results.

### Combining Foods Improperly

Very few people understand or practice the proper combining of the foods they eat. Yet this is so basic to digestion, the health of the body, and how energetic they feel. Animals in nature, feeding on natural raw foods, eat only one food at a time and never experience digestive discomfort. This is the ideal way to eat and the healthiest for the body. We have been conditioned to eat several different foods at the same meal.

The proper food combination principle is quite simple. In order to be digested properly, proteins require an acid medium in the stomach, while carbohydrates or starches require a more alkaline medium. When concentrated proteins and starches are consumed at the same meal, for example, meat and potatoes, or cheese sandwiches, the acid and alkaline secretions tend to neutralize each other. In a weakened digestive system, this causes food to ferment and putrefy, producing toxic by-products. In the process, one can experience indigestion, heartburn, bloated feelings, gas, and nausea. As an example of this, mix baking soda and fresh lemon juice together and notice the bubbling and frothing; the gas produced is caused by an acid mixing with an alkali.

Aside from the acid-alkaline stomach digestion consideration, we must become aware of the time that different foods take to digest. This is important because combining a fast-digesting food, like sugar, or fruit that has sugar in it, with a slow-digesting food, like bread or meat, sets up fermentation in the stomachs of those who manufacture inadequate amounts of enzymes and hydrochloric acid. This causes indigestion, which creates toxins that are hard on the body. Some people say they can't eat melons. The probability is great that they would have no difficulty digesting melons if they ate them alone, and not with or after other foods. Melons complete the digestive process in the stomach very quickly, but when combined with other foods, they cause fermentation.

The common practice of eating fruit or desserts containing sugar with or after meals is a classic "no no" in proper food combination. It is just asking for trouble.

The following are examples of approximate times for some foods, when eaten alone, to complete digestion in the stomach and pass into the small intestine. Although digestion times vary with the individual, and according to the health of the stomach, these times can be used as general guidelines as to how much time to leave between meals to allow for complete digestion.

- *Melons* (Watermelon, cantaloupe, etc.)                10–20 minutes
- *Most fruit* (Apples, oranges, pears, cherries, etc.)   20–40 minutes
- *Sweet fruit* (Bananas, fig, dates, dried fruit, etc.)  30–60 minutes
- *Green and low starch vegetables*                       1–1½ hours
- *Starchy vegetables* (Potatoes, corn, carrots, etc.)    1½–2 hours
- *Light starch* (Grains, flours, etc.)                   2–3 hours
- *Proteins* (Vegetable: nuts, seeds)                     3–4 hours
- *Proteins* (Animal: meat, fish)                         4–6 hours

Improperly combined foods can take as much as eight hours to leave the stomach and pass, in various degrees of fermentation, into the small intestine. The small intestine then has difficulty absorbing the required nutrients, because each step in the digestive process depends on the completeness and efficiency of the step before. Fermentation in the digestive tract results in flatulence and lower bowel gas. If this toxic air is not eliminated by "off-gassing," it is absorbed into the body.

The process of normal digestion requires a considerable amount of energy. When foods are incompatibly combined at the same meal, the body must direct more energy than normal to the task of digesting and clearing it through the system. Excessive amounts of enzymes are used, which results in lower energy production. This is why we often feel sleepy after a large or improperly combined meal. Food excesses switch blood flow from the brain to the stomach in order to address the difficult digestive task. It is no wonder that many people feel they have so little energy.

Their bodies are likely being forced to focus on processing the toxic overload created in their stomachs on a regular basis.

The simplest and most efficient digestive principle for the body is to digest no more than one concentrated food at a time. A concentrated food is any food that is not a fruit or a vegetable, or one that has been processed or refined.

The following list gives a simplified general understanding of the guidelines to follow for proper food combinations.

Foods that combine well:
- Proteins + Salads (no starch)
- Carbohydrates + All vegetables
- Most dairy products + Salads (no starch)

Foods that combine poorly:
- Concentrated Proteins + Carbohydrates
- Fruit + Other foods

Foods best eaten alone:
- Melons
- Most fruit (except apples, which will mix with non-starchy salad vegetables)
- Milk (if eaten at all)

If people ate foods in correct combinations and had efficient digestive systems, there would be no need for antacids. Food would be fully digested, broken-down, absorbed, and assimilated by the body in an efficient manner, without undue stress. Waste products from digestion would be eliminated from the body in well-formed stools, and would not contain undigested fragments. People would be healthier, feel healthier, and have more energy.

### Overeating
We sometimes eat too much food at one time for our digestive systems to handle. Many people overload their plates, go for seconds and thirds, and

eat until all the food is gone. They eat until they feel "stuffed," or even until their stomachs hurt. It should not be surprising that many men and women have large "bellies." Their stomachs have been stretched and stuffed repeatedly, and their colons have become clogged with impacted wastes.

Overeating is stressful to the body. It is like flooding an engine with too much fuel. When too much food is consumed, the stomach and pancreas are unable to supply the quantity of enzymes and digestive juices required to properly digest it. The result is that food sits in the stomach longer than it should, and does not digest completely. Toxins are produced. The stomach, small intestine, and liver are burdened. Metabolic and toxic waste products are produced in quantities that the intestines may not be able to eliminate completely. When this happens, the body has no alternative but to store the wastes as fat and pockets of toxins. These toxin pockets are what can develop into tumors and disease. The body is simply acting in a defensive manner in order to survive. If toxins from wrong foods and overeating were allowed to remain in the blood stream or vital organs, we would die quite quickly.

Richard Weindruch suggests that a balanced, calorie-restricted diet should do wonders for the health and longevity of humans.[3] His comments are based on studies which showed that by restricting their diets, the lifespans of fish, insects, and rodents increased by 40% and more. In a study with monkeys, several measures of health such as percentage of body fat, blood pressure, and glucose, insulin, and triglyceride levels were improved by caloric restriction.

A good objective for us to work toward is to leave the stomach 20% empty at each meal. This lightens the digestive load, greatly improves the absorption and assimilation of nutrients, and leaves adequate time and energy for the body to properly eliminate waste products. By eating less food, even more often if we feel we need to, all systems of the body will work more efficiently. In turn, we will have increased energy. We will feel lighter and livelier. All of this can contribute to better health and longer life.

## Using Stimulants

A stimulant is defined as, anything put into or done to the body that the body cannot use for life maintaining purposes at that very moment; anything which will cause an expenditure of energy by the body, giving the body little or nothing in return.[4]

Stimulants cause the body to increase its metabolism. It does this primarily by producing adrenaline, which causes the liver to release stored glucose into the bloodstream. Cells then convert the glucose into energy. With this burst of energy and increased blood circulation, the body works to eliminate the poisons that were ingested. Stimulants cause the body to go into an abnormal reaction. Essentially, they "rev-up" the body. They get us going and make us feel like we have more energy, but it is false energy. It is because of the increased metabolism that we feel an energy lift. The stimulant itself contributes no energy to the body. Stimulants are detrimental because they actually cost the body nutrients and energy in order to cope with the stress induced by them. The overuse of stimulants stresses the body by drawing on energy that could be used to improve health. They deplete mineral reserves from our tissues and bones. This leads to lower vitality and disease as we grow older.

Many people get through the day by consuming stimulants in order to have energy and feel better. The most common are: caffeine, nicotine, sugar, salt, and meat.

*Coffee* drinkers force their bodies to run in high gear. Coffee's caffeine belongs to the family of alkaloid poisons; it has no food value. In order to rid itself of this poison, the body draws energy and minerals from its emergency reserve system. In this process, stomach temperature is raised, stomach acid increases, enzyme production is decreased, digestion becomes more difficult, heart rate is increased, blood vessels in the brain become narrower, lungs work harder, the nervous system is irritated, the adrenal glands, liver, and pancreas are stressed, and overall metabolism is increased 15 to 25%. Caffeine stresses the body and causes it to overwork and wear out sooner.

*Nicotine* contains highly toxic irritants and poisons, which are extremely acidifying and harmful to the body. It overworks the adrenal glands and heart, constricts arteries, and reduces circulation in all parts of the body and acts as a whip to the nervous system. It can be related to numbness of the hands and arms, gum disease, high blood pressure, indigestion, colitis, stomach ulcers, diarrhea, nausea, colds, sore throats, shortness of breath, bronchitis, and many other illnesses. One or two cigarettes per day can block the healing processes in a sick body. Nicotine is such a detriment to healing that at least one doctor I know, Dr. Leo Roy, refused to work with patients who continued to smoke.

*Refined sugar* contains no nutrition for the body. During its manufacture, sugar becomes devitalized, demineralized, and robbed of any life-giving qualities it once possessed. Sugar robs mineral and energy reserves from the body while giving nothing in return. It upsets the calcium–phosphorus ratio in the body.

Society's increase in sugar consumption is matched by an increase in many diseases such as diabetes, hypoglycemia, and obesity. Even though these diseases are clearly due to excess sugar intake, sugar continues to be added to almost every processed food on market shelves. Many soft drinks contain eight tablespoons of sugar plus phosphoric acid! Researcher Nancy Appleton reported that 69 illnesses and diseases are caused by the consumption of refined sugar. She concluded that sugar excesses ruin our health.[5]

As if sugar isn't bad enough, artificial sweeteners, which have been introduced into over 5000 food and drink products, are absolute poisons. During his 30 years of research on Alzheimer's disease, Dr. H. J. Roberts[6] showed that artificial sweeteners containing aspartame, sold under various brand names, cause Alzheimer's, multiple sclerosis, lupus, chronic fatigue syndrome, fibromyalgia, plus a host of other disease and dysfunction symptoms. This is because the aspartic acid and phenylalanine in artificial sweeteners are neurotoxic without the other amino acids found in protein. They cross the blood brain barrier and deteriorate the neurons of the brain. Methanol (wood alcohol) in aspartame is released when temperature exceeds 86°F (30°C), and converts to formaldehyde and formic acid, both of which are potent poisons. When aspartame is ingested, this always happens because normal body temperature is 98.6°F (37°C).

Common *table salt*, sodium chloride, is salt that has been refined, processed, and depleted of its minerals. It is toxic and addictive to the body. Refined salt is a chemical compound that contains no food value. It cannot be digested or assimilated. It accumulates in the body, is very acidifying, and causes disorders and diseases similar to those mentioned earlier. It is harmful to the heart and has been linked to high blood pressure and hardening of the arteries. It places great stress on the kidneys and replaces calcium and potassium in the body, which may lead to osteoporosis and heart disease. On the other hand, natural whole sea salt (not refined sea salt; there is a big difference), has many health benefits. Food should only be seasoned with whole sea salt after cooking, as heat harms the salt.

*Red meat* produces strong acids in the body even though it contains nutrition. Animal proteins contain sulfur, nitrogen, and phosphorus that produce strong acids.

One can stimulate the body for only so long before it begins to tire and break down. For example, if you are riding a horse and want it to go faster, it will respond to the stimulation of a whip. However, stimulating it in this manner to keep going at a rapid pace will only work for so long. Eventually, its energy reserves deplete and it becomes exhausted. Repeatedly whipping a horse to make it run faster can kill it. It is the same with our bodies. They work as long and as efficiently as they can, attempting to respond to our needs and wants. Under the repeated whip of stimulation, they too eventually become exhausted, break down, and die.

The good news is that if we stop introducing stimulants into our bodies and start eating alkaline, mineral-rich foods, get adequate rest and exercise, and remove negative attitudes, our bodies will replenish their reserves and move toward improved health and vitality.

### Eating Junk Food

Junk food is called "junk" because it does not provide quality nutrition. It actually robs nutrition from the body and contributes to degenerative disease conditions. It is missing part of the complete package of nutrents required for health. Eating a regular diet of junk food leads to vitamin, mineral, amino acid, and enzyme deficiencies. Junk foods are dead because they lack their live enzyme components. Further, most of them have been refined, processed, and overheated. In addition, chemicals have been added as taste enhancers and preservatives. Junk food is toxic and stressful to the body.

### Too Much Cooked and Processed Food

Cooked and processed food places hardships on the body. Enzymes, which are in raw food to assist in its breakdown, are destroyed when food is heated above 112–120°F (44–49°C). Some researchers say this process begins at as low as 102°F (39°C). This deficiency causes the body to use enzymes and nutrients from its own stores to produce the digestive and metabolic enzymes needed. Cooking food for three minutes or longer above 118°F (48°C) also denatures proteins, breaks down natural fibers needed to maintain the health of the intestinal tract, and significantly reduces the availability of vitamins and minerals.[7] When we consume the majority of our food in cooked and processed form, we deplete our body's energy reserves, thereby reducing its ability to produce health. In short, we shorten our lives.

The refining of food destroys enzymes and many natural nutrients. For example, refined white flour products like bread, cookies, and pasta are almost totally depleted of nutrients. They take more from the body than they give. When eaten, they quickly convert to sugar, causing the body to take nutrients from itself to complete the digestion process. Over time, the depletion and deficiency of minerals such as calcium, magnesium, potassium, and phosphorus result. This leads to disease conditions.

Most processed foods have had chemicals added to make them last longer without spoiling. An additive is, by definition, a food embalmer or preservative. It does to food what formaldehyde does to embalmed corpses.

Products that are "enriched" are no better. Actually, they are worse because most additives are toxic, requiring the body to expend energy and nutrients to eliminate them. In the refining process, hundreds of nutrients are removed, and then a few synthetic chemicals added back. The food industry calls this enrichment. The products are not enriched; they are actually depleted and made more toxic by the synthetic additives. A 1970 study in which rats were divided into groups and fed products made with whole wheat flour, white refined flour, or enriched white refined flour, found that the rats continued to thrive on whole wheat, while the ones fed white bread became malnourished.[8] Animals that were fed enriched white flour products died first because the enrichment of this flour is from synthetic vitamins and minerals. Raw whole wheat contains approximately fifty main nutrients whereas refined white flour contains no more than two or three.

### Too Much Protein

Our bodies use protein to make, repair, and replace tissue. The structural materials of cells are proteins reinforced by minerals. Contrary to popular opinion, the body does not use protein from its tissues for energy. In times of starvation, the body is able to utilize protein tissue for energy, but this is done as a last resort because it is very expensive in terms of the nutrients and energy required. Excess protein consumption causes increased metabolism, produces excess acids, and if continued over time, it causes the pancreas to become overworked, enlarged, and fatigued.

Once we have finished growing and have reached adulthood, the body's requirement for protein drops. The period of greatest need is during the first six months of life. Babies thrive best on breast milk from their mothers, which contains only about 1.6% protein. As a comparison, dairy products are 9–18% protein, and meats are 18–24% protein—much too concentrated.

When protein is cooked, it cannot be converted into complete amino acids, which the liver needs. Eating too much cooked protein, especially animal protein, requires great amounts of pancreatic and stomach enzymes. It causes strong acid formation, liver congestion, kidney stress, adrenal gland fatigue, vitamin and mineral deficiencies, and an overall depletion of health. Scientific evidence from the medical community has determined that the highest meat and dairy consuming nations in the world have the highest levels of illness and disease. Results of *The China Study*, described as "the most comprehensive study of nutrition ever conducted," concludes that chronic degenerative diseases occur at significantly higher rates where diets are richer in animal products.[9]

The typical North American diet supplies 90–150 grams of protein per day. Authorities are now recommending as little as 20 grams per day, with vegetable protein being seen as more beneficial than animal protein. Consuming 47 grams or more per day will result in a net loss of calcium from body stores with long-term adverse effects on all body systems.[10] When we reduce our intake of animal proteins, our requirement for vitamins and minerals decreases.

Good quality proteins are found in hemp, spirulina, chlorella, nuts, seeds, whole grains, carob powder, vegetables, kelp, and dulse. Eggs and meats, which could include fish, chicken, turkey, and lamb, should be eaten in moderation. Meat should be farm-raised, without the use of antibiotics, hormones, or drugs. The fat of meat should not be eaten, nor the skins of chicken and turkey. Cooking should be by steaming, broiling, or baking. Whatever can be cooked in an oven should be; stovetop temperatures are too high. Keep in mind that all cooked protein has a change in composition, becomes incomplete, and places undue stress on the body, which can eventually lead to disease.

### Too Many Dairy Products

The consumption of dairy products is harmful to the health of the body. Besides having a protein content that is too high, dairy products are pasteurized and trigger mucus secretions in the body. Pasteurized milk contains no enzymes and is acid-forming. The high temperature of pasteurization kills enzymes in milk and denatures its minerals. The body cannot utilize unnatural minerals. The denatured calcium that the body is unable to eliminate is deposited on the outside of bones and between joints, where it causes bone spurs and arthritis, or in the tissues, where it causes fibromyalgia. It is a myth that milk is a good source of calcium for the body. Pasteurized dairy products, in the process of being metabolized and eliminated, actually draw calcium out of the body.

Pasteurized dairy milk contributes to many disease conditions such as: intestinal cramps, diarrhea, constipation, intestinal bleeding, skin conditions, bronchitis, ear infections, tooth decay, arthritis, and asthma. I know of a young mother who was unable to digest milk products. One week, when her new son was five weeks old, she ate a piece of cheese pizza and an ice-cream cone. By the end of that week, her son, who was breastfeeding, began bleeding with each bowel movement. When she went to the hospital she was told to stop breastfeeding and to put her baby on formula, and if the problem did not correct itself, they would have to operate on the child to determine where the blood was coming from. She was reluctant to do this because she was very aware of the value mother's milk has in building a strong immune system for a baby. She did some research on this problem and discovered that milk can cause intestinal bleeding in individuals who are allergic to milk. So this mother studiously avoided eating any dairy products and continued to breast-feed the child. In a few weeks the problem cleared completely and did not return. When a doctor told her that it would be "one chance in a million" that her consumption of dairy products could be the cause of the bleeding, she replied, "Well, I guess I'm that one in a million," as she walked away.

As an illustration of how poor pasteurized dairy products are as food, consider what happens to newborn calves when they are fed pasteurized milk instead of raw, untreated milk. They die at between one and six months of age. And we feed these products to our babies and children and expect them to thrive. Further, we continue to consume these products as adults. We are the only species that continues to drink milk after we have been weaned.

### Milk and Milk Products[11]
Due to man's intervention, milk can contain disease-producing contaminants. Some of these include:

* Antibiotics (administered to increase milk production)
* Detergents

- Viruses
- Toxins
- Impurities in the containers
- Pesticides
- Radioactive isotopes

Ideally, milk, no matter what its form—raw, skimmed, partly skimmed, pasteurized or otherwise—is not for human consumption. It was created for calves. Even adult cows don't drink it. While most people cannot digest milk, they can digest other dairy products. This is because the milk has been partially digested by certain bacteria during their conversion to other products such as buttermilk, yogurt, and cottage cheese. However, know that these generally have been exposed to heat and contain many, if not all, of the following:

- Pesticides
- Antibiotics
- Hormones
- Dyes (made from coal tar)
- Salt
- Preservatives
- Emulsifiers
- Calcium chloride
- Hydrogen peroxide
- Bleaching agents (all chemicals)
- Synthetic vitamins

Ice cream manufacturers are not required by the FDA to label what is in their product. The following is a partial list of legal ingredients in ice cream:

- Milk in any form (whole, skim)
- Cheese whey

- Calcium hydroxide
- Disodium phosphate
- Gelatin or gum
- Antioxidants
- Neutralizers
- Buffers
- Bactericides
- Stabilizers
- Emulsifiers
- Sodium carboxymethylcellulose (a known carcinogen)
- Polyoxyethylenes
- Propylene glycol alginate (paint thinner)
- Corn syrup
- Artificial flavors (chemicals)
- Chocolate replaced with amylphenyl acetate, vanillin, aldehyde c18, veratraldehyde, n-butyphenyl ethylacetal, propylene glycol.
- Strawberry replaced with alcohol, propylene glycol, glacial acetic acid, aldehyde c16, benzyl acetate, vanillin, methyl cinnamate, methyl anthranilate, methyl heptine carbonate, methyl salicylate, ionine beta, aldehyde c14, diacetyl, ethanol.

Should you still be sold on having the occasional ice cream treat, eat either homemade (use honey instead of sugar), or a brand of ice cream that doesn't use any chemicals, petroleum products, or additives. These brands have nothing to hide, and proudly list the ingredients on the label.

If you must eat dairy products, the choices that can be consumed on a limited basis are:

- Cheese (unprocessed and/or made from unpasteurized milk only; the whiter and less sharp the cheese the better)
- Cottage cheese
- Yogurt (homemade is best without sweeteners or additives)
- Butter (unsalted)

### Soy and Soy Products

Commercial manufacturers have done it again. If something doesn't have a natural niche in the food market—create one! It doesn't seem to matter whether the product is good for health, just as long as it sells and people are convinced they need it. Certain health benefits, compared to other products, are claimed. If it doesn't taste good, the product is "enhanced" with artificial flavorings such as MSG. Unfortunately for the health of many people, this has been the case with soy products. What has been made to appear as a healthy alternative to meat and dairy actually has many more sinister attributes than good ones. The longer-term effects from eating it are not pleasant. Read on.[12]

Soy products, except fermented ones like tempeh, miso, and soy sauce, were not used as foods until their recent commercialization. In fact, a few centuries ago, soy was not considered fit to eat in Asia. Even now,

> … except in times of famine, Asians consume soy products only in small amounts as condiments, and not as a replacement for animal foods—with one exception. Celibate monks, living in monasteries and leading a vegetarian lifestyle, find soy foods quite helpful because they dampen libido.[13]

Originally, soybeans were only used in crop rotation to fix nitrogen into the soil. Soy was not used as a food because of the high content of antinutrients it contains. Only through a long fermentation process are the toxins in the soybean broken down to make it digestible. Products being marketed to us such as tofu, soy milk, infant formula, soy ice cream, soy cheese, and soy sausage have not undergone the fermentation process. In their report on the Third International Soy Symposium, regarding the US Food, Drug, and Cosmetic Act, held April-May 2000, Sally Fallon and Mary Enig state:

> All food additives not in common use prior to 1958, including casein protein from milk, must have GRAS (Generally Recognized As Safe)

status. ... To this day, use of soy protein is codified as GRAS only for limited industrial use as a cardboard binder. However, the soy industry public relations campaign has been a huge success. "The competition—meat, milk, cheese, butter and eggs—has been duly demonized by the appropriate government agencies. Soy serves as meat and milk for a new generation of politically correct vegetarians. ... Soymilk has posted the biggest gains, soaring from $2 million in 1980 to $300 million in the US last year. ... Soy is now found in most supermarket bread.[14]

Let's dig a little deeper to understand what some of these "antinutrients" are, and what effects they have on our bodies. The following outlines some of the main areas of concern with soy products.

Soybeans contain:

- Hemagglutinin, a clot-promoting substance that causes red blood cells to clump together.
- Goitrogens, substances that depress thyroid function.
- High levels of phytic acid, which can block the uptake of essential minerals in the intestinal tract, and which can cause growth problems in children.
- Trypsin inhibitors that interfere with protein digestion, and may cause pancreatic disorders.
- High levels of aluminum, which is toxic to the nervous system and the kidneys.
- Phytoestrogens, that disrupt endocrine function, have the potential to cause infertility and to promote breast cancer in adult women, as well as being potent anti-thyroid agents.
- Potent enzyme inhibitors that block the action of other enzymes needed for protein digestion, and which can produce gastric distress, reduced protein digestion, and chronic deficiencies in amino acid assimilation.

In addition, soy products:

- Increase the body's requirement for vitamins D and B-12.
- Contain denatured proteins formed during high temperature processing—soy protein isolate and textured vegetable protein.
- Contain MSG, a potent neurotoxin formed during processing, and which is also added to the products to enhance flavor.
- Contain carcinogenic nitrites formed during processing.

In their report on The Third International Soy Symposium, Fallon and Enig presented an interesting overview of the soy question.

> Soy processors have worked hard to get these antinutrients out of the finished product, particularly soy protein isolate (SPI), which is the key ingredient in most soy foods that imitate meat and dairy products, including baby formulas and some brands of soy milk. SPI is not something you can make in your own kitchen. Production takes place in industrial factories where a slurry of soy beans is first mixed with an alkaline solution to remove fiber, then precipitated and separated using an acid wash and finally neutralized in an alkaline solution. Acid washing in aluminum tanks leaches high levels of aluminum into the final product. The resultant curds are spray dried at high temperatures to produce a high protein powder. A final indignity to the original soybean is high-temperature, high-pressure extrusion processing of soy protein isolate to produce textured vegetable protein (TVP). ... Nitrites, which are potent carcinogens, are formed during spray drying, and a toxin called lysinoalanine is formed during alkaline processing. Numerous artificial flavorings, particularly MSG, are added to soy protein isolate and textured vegetable protein products to mask their strong "beany" taste, and impart the flavor of meat.[15]

In the same report, Fallon and Enig relate an interesting story to explain how problems with soy first came to public attention in 1991, in Whangerai, New Zealand. When tropical bird breeders Richard and Valerie James purchased a new kind of bird feed based largely on soy protein, they noticed that their birds "colored up" after just a few months, compared to the normal 18–24 months. As the birds aged, problems such as decreased fertility, deformed offspring, and premature deaths developed, which resulted in a steady decline of the aviary population. Autopsies on dead birds revealed that the birds' digestive organs were in a state of disintegration. Subsequent research of studies dating back to the 1950s done by Mike Fitzpatrick, the toxicologist the Jameses hired, revealed that similar disorders, including increased cancer and infantile leukemia, were linked to the consumption of soy protein. These studies had found that genistein, which is in soy, causes the disruption of endocrine functions in animals. Analysis of the bird feed revealed high levels of phytoestrogens, mainly genistein. With the discontinuation of the soy-based feed, the birds gradually returned to normal reproduction and behaviors.

Fallon and Enig go on to point out how further research revealed serious problems in humans who consumed soy.

In 1992, the Swiss health service estimated that 100 grams of soy protein provided the estrogenic equivalent of the pill. … But it was the isoflavones in infant formula that gave the Jameses the most cause for concern. In 1998, investigators reported that the daily exposure of infants to isoflavones in soy infant formula is 6 to 11 times higher on a body weight basis than the dose that has hormonal effects in adults consuming soy foods. Circulating concentrations of isoflavones in infants fed soy-based formula were 13,000 to 22,000 times higher than plasma estradiol concentrations in infants on cows milk formula. … Fitzpatrick estimated that an infant exclusively fed soy formula receives the estrogenic equivalent (based on body weight) of at least five birth control pills per day. By contrast, almost no phytoestrogens have been detected in dairy-based infant formula or in human milk, even when the mother consumes soy products.[16]

Fitzpatrick's research confirmed problems Richard and Valerie James were encountering with their own two children, and which other parents were recounting to them about children fed soy-based formula. These included extreme emotional behavior, asthma, problems with immune systems, pituitary insufficiencies, thyroid disorders, and bowel irritations.

Another report, presented to the Third International Soy Symposium by Dr. Lon White, revealed findings from a study of Japanese Americans residing in Hawaii. The study showed:

> a significant statistical relationship between two or more servings of tofu a week and "accelerated brain aging." Those participants who consumed tofu in midlife had lower cognitive function in late life and a greater incidence of Alzheimer's disease and dementia. "What's more," said Dr White, "those who ate a lot of tofu, by the time they were 75 or 80 looked five years older."[17]

After reading these research findings, what do you think of this so-called healthy alternative to meat and dairy? When you compare this information with the discussion of hormones and xenoestrogens in chapter 9, you will recognize and understand the reasons for many of the health problems that are manifesting in children and adults today.

### Too Many Wheat Products

Modern strains of commercial wheat have been "re-engineered" and contain up to five times the gluten and one-third the normal protein compared to original strains. Gluten is difficult for the body to completely digest. It clogs and congests the capillaries of the circulatory system. It is, as the name implies, like glue. It thickens the blood, similar to what happens when you mix water and flour to make paste. As alternatives, choose products made from other grains such as brown rice, rye, and barley, or ancient wheat strains such as spelt and kamut. Among the best are millet and quinoa.

### Five White Poisons

Five white foods—sugar, salt, white flour, white rice, and pasteurized milk—are often referred to as the "five white poisons." This is because they contain little, if any, nutrition, and all produce acid in the body. They draw on the body's nutrient resources while being digested. None of these foods should be included in one's diet because they are health depleting. They are incomplete foods.

### Drinking Liquids with Meals

When liquids of any kind are consumed with meals, they dilute the digestive secretions and interfere with digestive efficiency. This causes the body to secrete greater quantities of acid or alkali to achieve adequate concentrations to break down food in the digestive tract, which lengthens digestion time and uses more energy. Water should be consumed approximately thirty minutes before meals, and not until two hours after consuming a carbohydrate meal, and three to four hours after consuming a heavy protein meal.

### Using Too Many Condiments

Condiments such as refined salt, distilled vinegar, and most relishes, sauces, and seasonings are not real food because they contain toxins and very little, if any, food value. They cost the body energy and nutrients to digest and eliminate. As alternatives, some healthfood store condiments and raw or fermented vinegar may be used sparingly.

### Not Chewing Food Thoroughly

As previously outlined, the digestion of starch begins when it is mixed with saliva in the mouth. Quickly swallowing food reduces the efficiency of the digestion process and places a stress on the body. Ideally, food should be chewed 20 to 40 times before swallowing.

### Drinking Unhealthy Water

Tap water often contains chlorine and fluoride, which are very toxic to the body. Chlorine also kills friendly bacteria in the bowel, and when it combines with organic substances, it forms cancer-causing compounds. Tap water can also contain pesticides and other chemicals. Water from city systems should be passed through a good filter unit before drinking. Raw fruit and vegetables naturally contain 75%–90% water. These should be our main source of healthy water for the body.

## Bathing in Chlorinated Water

When chlorine is absorbed through the skin, it upsets the body's natural chemistry. The comments about drinking chlorinated water also apply to bathing in it. Aquasmart Technologies Inc., a Canadian company that makes filtration devices, states: "More chlorine is absorbed through the skin during the average shower than by drinking two quarts (approximately two liters) of water." To counteract this problem, a carbon filter unit can be purchased to install on the bathroom showerhead.

## Ignoring Good Bowel Management

The colon is thought by many to be just a temporary holding area for wastes, but it is so much more. Many books on bowel management make the statement that disease and death begin in the colon. Incompletely digested and inefficiently eliminated wastes putrefy in the large intestine, producing poisons which are then reabsorbed into the blood stream and transported throughout the body. When the "sewer system" of the body is sluggish and inefficient, it also blocks the removal of toxins from other parts of the body, such as the liver, glands, and lymphatic system, causing them to become congested. Toxic wastes are then stored in the tissues. Over time this results in autointoxication, self-poisoning by toxic substances generated within the body. Dr. Bernard Jensen makes this very clear:

> The colon is a sewage system, but by neglect and abuse it becomes a cesspool. When it is clean and normal we are well and happy; let it stagnate, and it will distill the poisons of decay, fermentation and putrefaction into the blood, poisoning the brain and nervous system so that we become mentally depressed and irritable; it will poison the heart so that we are weak and listless; poisons the lungs so that the breath is foul; poisons the digestive organs so that we are distressed and bloated; and poisons the blood so that the skin is sallow and unhealthy. In short, every organ of the body is poisoned, and we age prematurely, look and feel old, the joints are stiff and painful, neuritis, dull eyes and a sluggish brain overtake us; the pleasure of living is gone.[18]

In the previous quote, Dr. Jensen indicates that every organ and gland is poisoned from the colon. Figure 7.2, adapted from various sources,[19] illustrates the connection of the colon to various organs and glands of the body via nerve reflexes.

Compare Figure 7.2 (a healthy colon) with Figure 7.3 (an unhealthy colon). Notice the distorted and malformed sections in Figure 7.3. By overlapping the sections, you will be able to identify which areas of the body are suffering due to the weak, diseased bowel conditions.

By studying these two diagrams, one can gain a newfound respect and appreciation for the "lowly" colon.

Bowel health and regularity are of vital importance. The efficiency of digestive and pancreatic functions can simply be deduced by the absence of any symptoms of faulty digestion, and from the normality of our stools. Normal stools are brown in color, firm but not hard, and do not contain undigested food particles. There should be as many bowel movements as substantial meals eaten each day. There should be no digestive complaints such as abdominal cramps, burping or gas, burning feelings in the stomach, and heaviness or fatigue after meals.

Moving from an unhealthy bowel situation to a healthy one requires detoxification, changes toward a healthy diet, and supplementation with herbs and enzymes if necessary. Enemas may be used as necessary to clear stagnant and impacted feces from the colon. Colonic irrigations are much more effective than enemas. The use of digestive enzymes and acid supplements to aid the digestive process, as well as bowel flora supplements to introduce healthy bacteria back into the intestines, are also recommended. Raw fruit and vegetable intake, which provides more fluid and fiber for the colon, should be increased. Regular exercise, rest, and the reduction of emotional stress are also important.

A primary key to improving our health is improving our digestion; health begins in the stomach. Good bowel management leads to improved health.

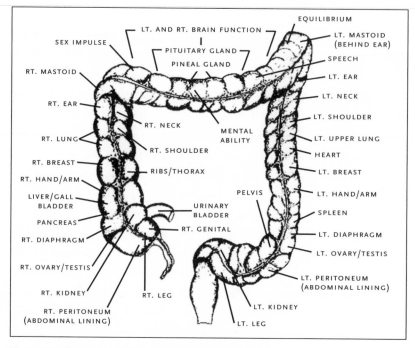

**Figure 7.1  Colon nerve reflex connections to glands and organs**

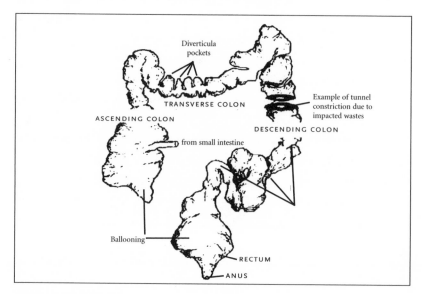

**Figure 7.2  Unhealthy colon**

134

## Using High Dosage Vitamin and Mineral Supplements

All fruits and vegetables, if grown in mineral-rich soil and ripe when picked, contain a wide and balanced range of vitamins and minerals. This is the natural way we are intended to obtain them. The body cannot normally utilize large doses of separate vitamins and minerals. Synthetic or refined vitamins are toxic to the body, and it reacts to eliminate them. Along with enzymes, vitamins and minerals are meant to work together as a synergistic team. If high doses of a supplement are taken, a nutritional imbalance can be created in the body.

## Eating Irradiated Food

The routine exposure of fresh food products to radiation has been implemented in many countries for the purpose of extending its marketable life and killing harmful bacteria and parasites. This process kills everything alive within the food, including its natural enzymes. It also reduces the effectiveness of many vitamins. That is why food can remain in storage or in the refrigerator for long periods of time without spoiling. Nutritionally, irradiated foods are similar to cooked foods.[20] When eating fruits and vegetables that have been imported from another state or country, one should supplement with digestive enzymes to assist digestion. Whenever possible, one should buy locally-grown products.

## Using Drugs

Drugs are unnatural chemicals which can alter normal functioning of the body in some way. Drugs are toxic, very acidic, oxidizing, and cost the body energy and nutrients to neutralize and eliminate them. Antibiotics also kill friendly bacteria in the bowel that are needed for health. While drugs alleviate symptoms such as pain, they do so by causing a greater stress in another internal area of the body. Since the body only concentrates on the area of greatest threat and stress, the symptom for which the drug was taken is relieved; the body refocuses its attention. However, the cause of the original pain or discomfort has not been removed or corrected. The symptom has only been suppressed temporarily.

### Not Exercising Regularly

Without adequate exercise, there is poor circulation of blood and inadequate movement of lymph fluids. Blood must be able to efficiently carry oxygen and other nutrients in order to nourish cells and tissues. Exercise improves the removal of metabolic waste products and toxins from cells via the lymph system, and promotes muscle tone and the overall health of all body systems.

### Not Getting Enough Rest and Sleep

Healing takes place *only* when the body is resting or sleeping. Sleep is our time of "battery recharging," when all conscious physical, mental, and emotional activity is suspended. This is when the body concentrates on cleansing, replenishing energy stores, and healing. Most of the energy we enjoy during the day is manufactured during the previous night's sleep. Adequate sleep is also required for mental and emotional health. The amount of sleep required by a person depends on how toxic the body is and how much energy is being expended during waking hours. A detoxified body with a low stress lifestyle requires less sleep time to rest and rejuvenate.

Much of the discussion in this chapter has centered on foods and behaviors that are harmful to the body. Next, we are going to see how other factors in our lives and environment also harm us.

# 8 | ARE WE BEING POISONED?

∿

*A truth's initial commotion is directly
proportional to how deeply the lie was believed ...
When a well-packaged web of lies has been
sold to the masses over generations,
the truth will seem utterly preposterous
and its speaker a raving lunatic.*

DRESDEN JAMES

∿

## IS SOMETHING POISONING US?

Is SOMETHING poisoning us? In one word—YES! Something is poisoning us like never before, and what we don't know can surely hurt us.

If a criminal wanted to blow up or burn down a building, but avoid suspicion by being well away from the area when it happened, he would plant a delayed action device. That's the way heavy metals, noxious chemicals, and pesticides work—very insidiously! They are very harmful to the human body, but they do their work in such a way that it is hard to connect the weakened immune system and developing diseases with the original or continuing exposure to the real culprit.

Evidence and research findings regarding these poisons are now beginning to be made public in spite of industrial and medical attempts to ignore, cover-up, or refuse to look at the facts. Our job is to become informed so that we can protect our own health and the health of our loved ones, our friends, and others. We can be part of the small but growing number of people who question, make informed decisions, and demand change.

## HEAVY METALS

Metals are presenting an increasing hazard to our health. Heavy metals are defined as chemical elements that have a specific gravity or density at least five times greater than water. The ones most often implicated in human poisoning are mercury, nickel, lead, arsenic, and cadmium. Aluminum, although lighter, is another metal that causes many problems in the human body. Other heavy metals like copper, iron, zinc, chromium, and manganese are required by the body in small amounts, but can be toxic in large quantities. Our concern in this discussion is with the main toxic heavy metals. They can enter our bodies through food, water, air, and the skin, from industrial, pharmaceutical, agricultural, and dental sources. In our systems, heavy metals compete with and displace other essential minerals such as, calcium, magnesium, and zinc, thereby reducing cellular and organ functions throughout the body and causing imbalance and disease.

### Mercury

Mercury has been labeled the most toxic non-radioactive metal known to humans.[1] What is surprising about mercury is that its toxicity was well known in the 1700s, when they realized that people who worked in the beaver felt hat industry were becoming very ill, and would go mad as a result of breathing toxic mercury fumes. These people became known as "mad hatters."

In the mid-1900s, residents of Minamata, Japan became very ill, with many of them dying after eating fish and shellfish contaminated by mercury that had been dumped from a chemical plant into Minamata Bay. This problem became known as the dancing cat disease because of the tremors and uncontrollable muscle spasms observed in the fish-eating, poisoned cats of Minamata. Now, throughout most of the world, afflictions from mercury poisoning are referred to as Minamata disease. There have been other mercury poisoning incidents to alert us to its dangers, but industry, and dentistry in particular, continues its use.

Dental "silver" amalgams and seafood, especially fish, are now recognized as the number one and two sources of mercury poisoning. Coal-burning power plants release a large amount of mercury into the environment.[2] Mercury poisoning is a global problem, because winds carry it around the world, even to the Arctic. Once in the air, it is inhaled, and starts accumulating in the food chain. A World Health Organization report from 1997 stated that mercury accumulates at the top of the aquatic and marine food chains, and that fish are the major source of dietary exposure. Many species of fish, especially tuna, swordfish, shark, and bottom-feeders, as well as shellfish, are now considered unsafe to eat. Even in the supposedly clean environment of Greenland, one in six Greenlanders now have potentially harmful blood levels of mercury from eating contaminated fish and whales.[3]

What makes mercury so devastating to our health is its ability to travel to all parts of the body, causing dysfunction, degeneration, and destruction of cells. Our immune systems weaken until we gradually slow down and then begin to age rapidly.

### Mercury Poisoning From Dental Amalgams
Silver amalgams, used to fill cavities in teeth, are mixtures of mercury, silver, copper, tin, and in some cases, zinc. All of these elements are toxic. Up to 50% of an amalgam's content is mercury. It is toxic in even small doses.

Dental amalgams are unstable compounds. They corrode, and the corrosion releases mercury into the body continuously. It is constantly being "off gassed," or released as vapor in the mouth, and absorbed via the lungs and intestinal tract, where it enters the blood stream. Dr. Murray Vimy, Clinical Associate Professor at the University of Calgary and Practitioner of Dental Medicine, published articles in more than forty medical journals around the world on the dangers of mercury. Tests and experiments with mercury and amalgams, which he conducted, established that mercury travels throughout the body via the blood to cells, where it is converted to inorganic mercury, which is an "extremely dangerous poison." It settles mostly in the kidneys, liver, and brain. He stated that mercury is more toxic than lead or arsenic. It is a time-released poison that is so slow and gradual there is little awareness of it happening. We rarely connect illness symptoms we experience with amalgams that were put into our teeth many years before.

In his publication, *Toxic Teeth: A Guide to Mercury Exposure from "Silver" Fillings*, Dr. Vimy says:

> It is now established that dental mercury fillings constitute the largest single source of inorganic mercury exposure to the general population, larger than all other environmental sources combined.
>
> Experimental evidence clearly shows that kidney function is reduced by 50% one month after dental filling placement and continues to decline at 60 days. ... The loss of 50% kidney function is comparable to losing one kidney. ... mercury exposure has been called the 'great masquerader'. The similarity of mercury related symptoms to other medical conditions makes it very difficult for physicians to arrive at the correct diagnosis. ... Mercury's primary mode of action is as an enzyme poison and the net effect is metabolic sickness.[4]

Mercury contributes to a lowering of the body's ability to fight disease. It weakens the immune system and lowers resistance to the process of degeneration. Drs. Hal Huggins, DDS, and Thomas Levy, MD wrote the book *Uninformed Consent: The Hidden Dangers in Dental Care*. This is an excellent book that I encourage everyone to read. It is full of facts and revelations from Dr. Huggins' own research and experience as a dentist. He has spoken extensively around the world since 1973 on the dangers of mercury amalgams, root canals, and cavitations. Because he has made these warnings public, he is less than popular with many of his colleagues in general, and with the American Dental Association in particular. The quote at the beginning of this chapter seems quite apropos with respect to Dr. Huggins.

Some of the facts that have been learned from the research and experience of Drs. Vimy and Huggins, plus reports from the World Health Organization, are that mercury:

- Has a particular affinity for the brain and central nervous system. It interferes with nerve impulses, resulting in such symptoms as uncontrollable shaking, muscle wasting, partial blindness, deformities in children exposed in the womb, learning difficulties, poor memory, and shortened attention spans.
- Creates autoimmune responses by attaching to normal cell membranes, which causes enough physical change that the body no longer recognizes these cells as its own, and so begins to attack them; hence the development of diseases such as Lupus, Multiple Sclerosis, Parkinson's, and Myasthenia Gravis.
- Damages chromosomes, thereby altering DNA structure and genetic code, which can cause birth defects in offspring.
- Attaches to red blood cell hemoglobin binding sites, thereby reducing oxygen-carrying ability of red blood cells, which then leads to chronic fatigue.
- Can kill or change the function of friendly bowel bacteria, which allows candida to proliferate and dominate.
- Seriously reduces immune function; white blood cell counts increase significantly, as is the case with leukemia.
- Interferes with the body's endocrine system. Such interference is linked to low body temperature, cold feet, disturbed emotions and behavior, and suicidal tendencies.
- Interferes with enzyme function, digestion, and assimilation.
- Can increase blood pressure.
- Is linked to fertility problems in both males and females.

Each of the metals that compose mercury amalgams is poisonous, but they also react in combination to form more toxic products. Dr. Huggins states that the new high-copper amalgams (about 30% copper) release mercury 50 times faster than the older conventional amalgams.

If you have mercury amalgams in your teeth and at present feel that you are healthy, do you need to have your amalgams removed? The best, and shortest way of answering this question, is to give you the same reply that Dr. Huggins gave to Dr. Levy when he asked the same question: "Only if you want to stay healthy."

### Other Sources of Mercury

Although they are the most serious, amalgams and seafood are not the only sources of mercury that we may come in contact with. Mercury is fairly widely used in commercial products such as: cosmetics, contraceptive creams and gels, lubricated condoms, spermicidal preparations, eye drops, contact lens solutions, red tattoo pigment, and vaccination shots. To identify mercury in products, look for "mer" in the ingredient names, for example, *Mer*curochrome, and thi*mer*osal.

### Until Amalgams Can Be Removed

It is wise to minimize excessive chewing, and consuming hot liquids, until one is able to have mercury amalgams safely removed and replaced. Mercury in amalgams is unstable and not tightly bound to other metals. Actions like pressure and heat cause it to be released much more quickly. Tests have shown that mercury is released about 15 times faster when chewing, and over 150 times faster after drinking a hot liquid.

### Removing Mercury from Our Mouths

Because of the potential for the release of mercury into the mouth and air, the removal of silver amalgams must be done carefully, by a dentist who has been trained in techniques for safe removal. The action of the high-speed drill on the material being removed generates heat that dramatically increases the off-gassing of mercury, which can then be inhaled by both patient and dentist. Unless good air suction and a rubber dam are used, the little flying fragments will be inhaled and swallowed. Failure to take these precautions causes an immediate and serious poison overload in the body which can then lead to one or more of the disease symptoms listed above.

Research has shown that the best replacements for mercury-containing amalgams and crowns containing metal are non-conductive composites.

Here is some good news. Dr. Huggins reports that a number of so-called incurable diseases respond positively after all the offending dental materials have been removed from the mouth. Disease symptoms that have shown definite links to toxic metal poisoning are: fibromyalgia, epilepsy, leukemia, arthritis, diabetes, eye problems such as nearsightedness and astigmatism, high blood pressure, Bell's palsy (especially after the removal of nickel crowns), breast cancer, Parkinson's disease, allergies, blood cell abnormalities, Lupus, Alzheimer's disease, AIDS, Multiple Sclerosis, ringing in the ears, headaches, serum cholesterol levels, digestive problems, and memory difficulties.

### Root Canals and Cavitations

Some persistent disease conditions will not clear up until bacterial growth and hidden infections are completely removed from root canal and cavitation sources as well. Just because root canal teeth, and gums over the places where teeth were removed, appear to be healthy, based on visual inspection and X-ray, that does not mean they are not a source of significant poisoning of the immune system. If you suspect the possibility of problems in this area, get more detailed information, such as the book by Dr. George Meinig, listed in the "Resources and Recommended Reading" section at the end of this book. Also, consult a dentist who specializes in mercury-free dentistry. Dr. Huggins' website, www.hugnet.com, has a wealth of information on all dental-related areas of concern.

### Nickel

Nickel is worthy of special mention because, although it is one of the most durable metals, it is also one of the most carcinogenic metals in the world. Yet it is often used as a main component, over 70%, in making crowns, bridges, braces, and partial dentures. Information has been available in scientific literature for many years regarding studies that have demonstrated how cancer and birth defects can develop in animals when they are exposed to nickel. Dr. Huggins points out that dentists often call the nickel alloy used in dentistry stainless steel, as it sounds better.[5]

### Chelation—Removing Heavy Metals from the Body

Metals in tooth fillings and crowns can be removed and replaced with non-conductive composite materials. However, removing toxic heavy metal residues that have built up in the body from dental, food, and environmental sources are more difficult. It is generally agreed that to remove heavy metals from the body, it must be done through some form of chelation. A chelator is an agent, or a combination of agents, that binds to heavy metals and carries them out of the body in the urine or feces. One chelator in wide use is ethylenediaminetetraacetic acid (EDTA), a man-made amino acid, which is dripped into the blood via an infusion through a vein. Oral chelators such as zeolite, cilantro, chlorella, the sulfur amino acids—methionine, cysteine and cystine—plus all sulfur containing foods, are preferred from a strictly natural health point of view. Exercise that produces perspiration, saunas, and steam baths in combination with the foods indicated above, are also helpful in eliminating heavy metals.

## HARMFUL CHEMICALS

Synthetic chemicals and their combinations pose a serious threat to health. It is reported that 80,000 chemicals are in use today, and that this number increases yearly. Many are known to be carcinogenic and immune-suppressing. Many others don't even have testing data on basic toxicity. Harmful chemicals can be found in daily-use items such as packaged and processed food, household cleaners, cosmetics, and fragrances. Volumes could be written on this subject alone, but a few of the more widely-used chemicals and their common sources are covered here so that readers can take precautions to minimize exposure to them.

## Chlorine

Chlorine is used as a bactericide in drinking water, and as a bleaching and cleaning agent. In small concentrations it is supposed to be non-toxic, or perhaps is apparently so. In strong solutions or as a pure gas, it is a deadly poison. Chlorine kills bacteria efficiently, but it doesn't discriminate; once inside the body, even in small concentrations found in municipally-treated water, it also kills the good bacteria in our colons. When absorbed through the skin from baths, showers, and hot tubs, it upsets the body's natural chemistry.

By-products of manufacturing processes that use chlorine, and com-pounds formed when chlorine interacts with organic matter, called organochlorines, are a serious threat to our health and the environment, both as potent carcinogens (dioxins and PCBs) and as xenobiotics. They are considered so serious that President William Clinton, the World Health Organization (WHO), and the United States-Canadian Joint Commission (IJC) have called for a phase-out of the use of chlorine and chlorinated compounds.[6]

However, "calling for it," and actually seeing it done, are two different things. One needs to take steps to minimize exposure to chlorine. We do this by drinking water that has been filtered, showering and bathing in filtered water, avoiding the use of hot tubs with chlorine-treated water, and not using, or being very careful when using, cleaning products that contain chlorine.

## Fluorine

Fluorine is considered the most chemically active non-metallic element of all the elements. It is never found in nature uncombined, yet humans have created it as a separate element. Our bodies can handle it in the naturally combined forms, but not when it is isolated. Fluorides, which are com-pounds of fluorine and another element, are listed by the U.S. Agency for Toxic Substances and Disease Registry to be among the top 20 substances that pose the most significant threat to human health. They have the same toxicity level as lead.[7] Like chlorine, fluorine kills good bacteria in the colon, and research studies are linking fluoride to low-thyroid conditions, neurological impairment, genetic damage, and cancer. While fluorine is in wide use in North America, most other countries in the world prohibit its use. The main exposure to fluoride is in municipal drinking water and toothpaste, as a supposed deterrent to tooth decay. Many studies, however, have found that the contrary is true; when water fluoridation is discontinued, the incidence of dental caries actually decreases.[8] Fluorides can also be found in Teflon pans, pesticides sprayed on fruit, and some beverages and food items. To minimize exposure, use only filtered drinking water, thoroughly wash fruit before eating, read labels, and avoid any products that contain fluoride.

### Pesticides

According to the World Health Organization, more than 3 million people become ill and 220,000 die worldwide annually because of pesticides. Pesticides harm humans and animals alike. In the U.S., it is reported that more than one-third of the calls to animal poison centers result from pets exposed to pesticides.[9]

There are more than 865 active ingredients registered as pesticides, which are, in addition, formulated into thousands of pesticide products available in the marketplace. About 350 pesticides are used on the foods we eat, and as protection for our homes and pets.[10] And while the U.S. Environmental Protection Agency attempts to monitor pesticide exposure levels for human health risk, it subscribes to the guideline that "the dose makes the poison"; as long as the exposure is low enough, it does not cause serious harm. But is that the case?

According to a National Academy of Science report, 70 pesticides known to cause cancer in animals are allowed in commercial foods.[11] Pesticide chemicals can accumulate to toxic levels in body fat. Many of them are linked to the disruption of nervous, endocrine, and reproductive systems. Animals exposed to some pesticides are showing problems such as male animals not reaching sexual maturity, development of both testes and ovaries at the same time, thyroid problems, birth defects like crossed bills in birds, club feet, and missing eyes.

Pesticides are toxic, but the risk depends on what chemicals are in their formulation, and the amount, length, and kind of exposure; whether they are ingested in food, absorbed through the skin, or inhaled; and the body weight, age, and health of the person exposed.

Great care should be taken when handling pesticides or insecticides. Breathing and skin protection should be used. Any such household chemicals must be stored away from children. Washing and peeling can help to remove some residues from fruit and vegetables, but others are systemic, found within the fruit or vegetable themselves. As far as food is concerned, the only way to be sure it is pesticide-free is to buy certified organic, or to grow your own. Drinking water should be filtered because chemicals of all descriptions make their way into our wells, rivers, and lakes.

## Tobacco Smoke

It is well known that smoking and second hand smoke cause cancer and heart disease. It can also lead to other conditions such as: stroke, lung disease, chronic bronchitis, miscarriages, underweight babies, sudden infant death syndrome (sids), meningitis, and osteoporosis. Over 4,000 different chemical compounds, including heavy metals and pesticides, have so far been found in tobacco smoke. More than 50 of these are known carcinogens and others are suspected mutagens which can cause harmful changes in the genetic material of living cells.[12] Visible tobacco smoke represents only about 5 to 8 percent of the chemicals released from a burning cigarette. The rest are invisible. Some of these chemicals include: lead, carbon monoxide, vinyl chloride, hydrogen cyanide, benzene, ammonia, acetone, and nicotine. Nicotine is a powerful nerve stimulant, is extremely toxic, and is the most addictive drug known. It is so powerful that if two or three drops were taken internally at once, it would kill the average person. Anyone who smokes tobacco is putting themselves and those around them, as well as their future offspring, at risk.

The most important thing a smoker can do to improve their own health, and the health of those who live and work with them, is to stop smoking.

## NOXIOUS ENERGY FIELDS

Most of us are somewhat aware that electronic equipment like television sets, computers, microwave ovens, heating pads, electric blankets, cell phones, electric razors, and high tension power lines give off radiation or electrical waves that may be harmful. But do we really understand the health implications of electromagnetic radiation? Knowledge of noxious energy fields emanating from certain earth locations is just beginning to be understood. We have man-made electromagnetic force fields (EMF), as well as natural ones from the earth, known as geopathic forces. Both can be harmful to our health.

While researching the subject of heavy metals, I came upon the work of Dr. Gloria Dodd, who has been practicing holistic veterinary medicine since 1960. She is one of those rare people who is both a seeker and an "outside of the box" thinker. She has studied with medical naturopaths in Germany, South America, and the United States, is an international speaker and teacher, and has done extensive pioneering work of her own. The following information is from Dr. Dodd's experience regarding the health of animals and people, especially with respect to electromagnetic force fields:

> Why do animals get sick? There are as many causes as there are for why people get sick. In my experience of observing the many animals who have come to me since I opened my practice in 1960, and my education in both orthodox and holistic philosophies, I have come to the following conclusion: We get sick from any and all things that weaken the body's protective electromagnetic force field or life force.
>
> We have to stop thinking of our animals (and ourselves) as physical beings alone. All things exist in *physical* and *energy* forms. I have proven this to myself by photographing the electromagnetic field (EMF) of dogs, cats and people with a Kirlian camera. This is a special technique that exposes the film with electricity in a light free environment. I have also measured the magnitude of the EMF by using a

sophisticated, electronic machine made in Germany. By both methods I have compared the EMF of "healthy" individuals to those having known organ illnesses. In the Kirlian photograph, the sick animal and person show "holes" in the EMF and the amplitude of their EMF is very weak compared to the continuous, strong EMF of a healthy body.

What weakens the EMF and causes illness and pain?

1   Inheritance of a genetic code that is flawed and produces a weakened constitution. This may produce impaired organ function, immune response or coping with stress. Yes, animals do suffer illnesses due to stress as we do.

2   Environmental toxins—chemicals in the food, water and air that are foreign to the metabolism of the body. To this I add the toxic affects of drugs and vaccines.

3   Trauma to any part of the body but especially to the head, which deranges the natural flow of Chi or Life force. This touches every cell in the body depriving it of the needed energy for health.

4   Noxious energy fields where we work and live. These are EMF of the earth known as Geopathic forces and man-made noxious EMF.[13]

It has been discovered that radiation from the center of the earth comes to the surface through geological faults. And, although they are now thought to be weakening, Hartman lines and Curry grid lines, discovered by Drs. Hartman and Curry, which form parallel magnetic lines vertically and horizontally around the earth, can also be harmful, especially when they intersect an underground stream.

Not all earth energies are harmful. Other energy emanations, such as Schumann waves, are naturally occurring, beneficial electromagnetic waves that oscillate between the Earth and certain layers of the atmosphere. NASA had to install equipment to generate these waves in their manned satellites[14] to offset their absence in space after astronauts returned to earth feeling distressed and disoriented. Jet lag is also linked to the weakness of Schumann wave energy at high altitudes.

Earth areas where energies are harmful are called geopathic zones. Areas that are health enhancing are called geomantic zones. There are also neutral zones.

Geo-energies can cause health problems where two different frequencies cross and combine, disrupting the body's bioelectric system. When you think about it, this makes sense because we know that our bodies are electric, they operate on electricity, and produce an electrical force field, referred to by some as an aura. Our physical and mental health is actually electrical health. The whole field of "energy medicine," including acupuncture, physical energy healing with hands, or the religious practice of "laying on of hands," as well as the use of electronic machines such as the Quantum Xrroid, Harmonic Translation System, Advanced Biophoton Integrator, SE-5, SCENAR, and the Tennant Biomodulator that you will read about in chapter 11, is concerned with returning the body's electrical energy back to homeostasis.

## Geopathic and Geomantic Zones

I met with a person in Vancouver, Canada, who had first-hand knowledge about stressful geopathic zones. Because the gentleman prefers to remain anonymous, I will refer to him as TS. Over several years, TS, who was in his 30s at the time, had become increasingly ill to the point he could no longer stand it. He had a very severe form of arthritis called Reiter's Syndrome that produces pain, swelling, redness, and heat in the joints. His immune system was getting weaker and weaker. His skin and hair quality was poor, his digestive system bad, and he was continuously on powerful drugs. He was sleeping about 22 hours each day, just to escape from the pain. TS was extremely depressed, to the point that he tried to commit suicide several times because he could no longer stand the torment of living. Nothing he or his doctors did brought any relief or improvement in his condition.

After one of TS's unsuccessful suicide attempts, a friend who had some knowledge of geopathic stress began to wonder if that might be a contributing cause of his extreme illness. He got an expert to check out his property. This man discovered that the lot TS was living on was the worst he had ever encountered. There was a wide watercourse underneath the property, combined with crossing earth radiation lines. The expert built a device he called a "white energy emitter," and placed it on the property. This not only neutralized the geopathic zone but also turned it into a geomantic or health-producing zone. In the words of TS, "In five days I felt 3000% better!" Subsequently, the expert worked with TS to restore his health with food and supplements.

The recovery itself was incredible. When I met him, it had only been sixteen months since he had started on his new program of nutrition, and been free of geopathic stress. He was now on an all-raw food diet. He used no heat in his house. Nor, he told me, did he suffer from the high heat other people had suffered the previous summer. We sat and talked in his kitchen with the door wide open to the outside, watching the pouring rain. The temperature was 47°F (8°C). I was dressed in a T-shirt, shirt, sweater, and jacket. TS wore just a light T-shirt with his arms bare. He was absolutely warm and comfortable, but after two hours, I had to cut our visit short because I was getting cold. Being bathed in the positive geomantic energies and being nourished with high-vitality raw food, his body had returned to homeostasis.

While I think the story about the geopathic zone and its subsequent neutralization interesting, TS's own personal example of recovery, astounding health, and the efficient way his body was now functioning spoke volumes to me.

It is estimated that we are subjected to 100–200 million times more electromagnetic radiation than our ancestors were![15] That is quite a statement, and quite a problem. Further, as our modern technological society "progresses," this will only increase.

## PROTECTING OURSELVES

After reading these accounts, you may be wondering, what can we do to protect ourselves? Good question. The answer is there is some good news.

For those who care enough to be informed and take action, there is technology being developed that can go a long way in protecting us. Here are some specific steps to take:

1   Be aware of the hazards and keep them in mind as you make health your choice. Keep reading and studying to find out the truths for yourself; don't just believe without question the statements and reports put out by industry, the medical establishment, and government agencies.

2   As much as possible, avoid those things that are harmful to your health as indicated in chapter 6.

3   Work to strengthen and improve the health of your body's digestive and elimination systems.

4   As much as you are able to, correct the wrongs that are present in your life, such as mercury amalgams and smoking.

5   Choose not to use, any more than is absolutely necessary, any harmful chemicals, pesticides, tobacco, or food additives.

6   Reduce your exposure to EMF and EMR-emitting electrical devices. Regarding geopathic energies, look at animals to identify them. For example, large animals like horses, cows, and dogs will not lie down in geopathic energy areas. So if your dog won't lie on your bed where you sleep, move the position of your bed. You can buy small devices for your home, car, phone, place of work, and person that neutralize harmful EMRs. Search the Internet on subjects such as EMF and geopathic stress to learn more about modes of healing and protection.

Our bodies were designed to be healthy and to self-correct when things start going wrong. But how can we know disease is developing within us before it gets a firm foothold? The answer is that your body talks to you all the time in its own language. All you need to know is how to interpret the signals or symptoms it sends you.

# 9 | YOUR BODY
# TALKS TO YOU

∼

*The real doctor is the doctor within.*
*Most doctors know nothing of this science*
*and yet it works so well.*
ALBERT SCHWEITZER

∼

## BODY SIGNALS

A BABY doesn't learn to talk for a long time, but it begins communicating as soon as it is born. Mothers soon learn to interpret the baby's needs and wants from the noises, smiles, grimaces, and body language it uses. Our bodies have a similar relationship with us. They cannot speak in words, but they communicate satisfaction or need to us all the time. Our job is to be observant, to become consciously aware of the signals they are sending, and to understand what they mean. When our bodies are at peace, there is a feeling of ease. When they are under stress, there is a feeling of dis-ease.

## HUNGER—THE CALL FOR NUTRIENT SUPPLIES

True hunger is the body's call for nutrition, not simply a signal to have its stomach filled.

Can you recall a time, such as Thanksgiving, or a feast of celebration, when you ate a meal of cooked food until you felt "stuffed"? You couldn't eat another bite, yet after an hour or so, you were back poking around the kitchen looking for something more to eat. Why was your body turning on the hunger signal again? You had eaten more than enough food. Or had you?

What your body was telling you was, "In all that cooked and processed food you ate, you didn't give me the supplies I need to do my job. I need usable nutrition."

Dr. Francis Pottenger's experiment, discussed in chapter 5, showed that the only food that produces health and avoids disease is whole, raw, and unprocessed food. Eating a diet that consists mostly of heat-processed food depletes the body's nutrient resources and eventually results in degenerating health. The subject of what real food for our bodies consists of will be covered in detail in chapter 16.

After years of having deprived our bodies of health-building nutrition, they begin to show signs of stress, or dis-ease, to which we have given various names.

## COMMON SYMPTOMS OF A STRESSED BODY

Following are examples of common dis-ease signals the body manifests when stressed by acid wastes in its tissues. These are symptoms which tell us the body needs assistance to remove acid residues, and to build up nutrient reserves that will enable it to become healthy again.

### Allergies

An allergy is the body's reaction to an invader, an "allergen," which it identifies as foreign to the body. An allergen is any substance that a body cannot completely metabolize and use as a nutrient. For the sake of health and survival, the body does not allow these substances to stay in the blood and tissues. Allergies manifest as skin reactions, hay fever, asthma, or as reactions to certain foods.

Allergies are *not caused* by pollen, animal hair, dust, insect stings, or this and that food. In certain individuals, these substances may cause the body to trigger reactions. But, they are not the reason that the body is reacting. If this were so, why wouldn't everyone react to the substances?

A very extensive section could be devoted to a dissertation on allergies. There are many sources of information on the subject. However, my treatment here will be a simple and summary explanation.

Most people with allergies have compromised, inefficient digestive systems. Their bodies have been subjected to an overload of toxins to the point where their colons have become impacted with wastes, and other body organs and glands weakened. Normally, the adrenal glands increase body metabolism in response to any harmful substance that enters the blood, in order to remove it via the liver, kidneys, lungs, and skin. When these organs are overloaded and the adrenal glands fatigued, the body must resort to the backup system of an allergic response. Allergens are removed via mucus membranes, the skin, or the colon with diarrhea. The reason the allergen gets into the body is due to weakened membranes of the skin, sinus, throat, lungs, or intestine, in which microscopic holes have developed because of irritation and inflammation. Although very small, they are large enough to allow protein molecules from pollen and food to gain entrance into the bloodstream. Acting in the interest of survival, the body works to eliminate these foreign substances. What results is an inflammation and mucus discharge, along with itching and irritability.

A healthy body does not have allergies. It is only because of weak genetic tendencies and intestinal toxemia that some bodies must resort to the allergic response mechanism. If the organs of filtration and elimination—liver, lungs, skin, and colon—were not overloaded and congested, there would be no allergic reactions necessary. Any potentially harmful substances would be processed out of the body in the normal way.

An adult who develops allergies at various stages in life does so as a result of degenerating health from cumulative toxic input and stresses to the body. Likewise, a child develops allergies because of genetic weaknesses passed on from its biological parents. The Pottenger cats experiment demonstrated that the effects of a toxic diet are generationally cumulative and progressive, unless the nutritional input is corrected.

In order to correct allergic conditions, the body must be detoxified and strengthened by a diet of whole live foods and a healthy lifestyle. Enzyme intake must be increased. All allergens must be avoided while the body is healing. Pasteurized dairy products, in particular, should be avoided due to their mucus-forming, acidic, and denatured nutritional properties. One should seek the guidance of a health practitioner who understands allergies and who counsels the detoxification and strengthening of bodily systems.

Allergies that persist over many years indicate that the body is not producing sufficient pancreatic enzymes, and that there is an insufficient intake of digestive enzymes from raw food and/or supplements. Most allergens, be they foods, pollens, molds, or other substances, are protein-like substances. Therefore, as with proteins, they are digestible to protease enzymes. The temporary solution for controlling allergies is to use good quality enzymes, along with a natural antihistamine, as needed. I have a personal story as an illustration.

One morning a few years ago, while visiting Dr. Leo Roy, I joined him in eating a bowl of assorted breakfast grains he had cooked. It tasted good, but after a while I could feel the telltale tingling in my mouth and throat, the beginning reaction to eating egg, to which I am allergic. He had added a whole egg to the dish we were eating. Furthermore, the egg was only very lightly cooked. Raw egg acts as the strongest poison to my system. By the time I had stopped eating and had asked him about the possibility of there being any egg in the cooked grains, I had probably consumed about one-third of an egg. I was going to be in serious trouble since I didn't have the adrenaline injection kit, which had recently been prescribed for me by my medical doctor. Dr. Roy said, "No problem." He gave me several pancreatic enzymes along with a natural antihistamine liver extract, which I took several times over the next hour and a half. Although I felt discomfort, I did not develop the serious problems I had typically experienced, and which I had been warned would become progressively more life threatening as time went on. Within three hours, aside from feeling tired, my system had returned to normal. This incident was very encouraging to me because it eliminated most of my fear associated with the egg allergy. I have never had to use the adrenaline injection kit.

## Arthritis

Arthritis, the inflammation of a joint, is a degenerative disease that usually appears in mid- to older-aged adults. It is the result of chronic deposits of toxins in joint tissues, resulting in degenerative changes for those tissues.

There are two main types of arthritis: osteoarthritis, which is a chronic inflammation of joints due to the infiltration of toxins and crystals resulting in bony spurs and restricted range of motion; and rheumatoid arthritis, which is a chronic inflammatory condition of the joint tissues, with swelling, but without bone changes. Pain, swelling, and stiffness accompany arthritis. In the case of osteoarthritis, as the disease progresses, joints, especially of the fingers, become deformed.

The cause of arthritis is the over-consumption of acid-producing foods over a long period of time, resulting in an excess buildup of toxins and poisons. Because the body is unable to eliminate the toxins, it deposits them in tissues that have been traumatized or weakened. As with other degenerative disease conditions, if the body did not do this, it would succumb to the effects of the toxins and die much sooner. Here again, the disease condition is your helpmate, keeping you alive longer as the body continues to deal with the toxins and lack of proper nutrition. The body does the best it can under the circumstances.

Since the cause of arthritis is an unhealthy lifestyle, the solution or cure of the condition is a healthy lifestyle. The body will need a continuous opportunity to detoxify and build its nutritional reserves. A naturally healthy lifestyle that will eliminate arthritis includes the elimination of most meats, dairy, refined carbohydrates, sugar, salt, irritating spices, coffee, and the other harmful foods. As a regular regimen, one to three glasses of fresh raw fruit and vegetable juices should be consumed daily. When consuming citrus fruits and juices, because of their high content of citric acid which turns body and blood calcium into insoluble calcium citrate crystals, arthritic symptoms will be exaggerated during the cleansing process. However, the body is helped with wholesome nutrition and healthy lifestyle practices; over time, toxic deposits in the joints and tissues are dissolved and eliminated from the body. This takes time and persistence, however, since the conditions that cause arthritis take many years to develop.

### Bad Breath

A healthy body has sweet smelling breath that is not offensive. Bad breath, or halitosis, can have many causes. Rotting food particles in the mouth due to poor oral hygiene, decaying teeth, infection in the mouth or throat, or indigestion are the more obvious and more superficial causes. These are fairly easily observed and corrected.

Persistent bad breath that is not due to one of the causes just mentioned is an indication that the body is very toxic. It is attempting to neutralize and throw off toxins via the lungs. Body systems such as the liver and colon have become congested due to the intake of unhealthy foods, faulty digestion, and bowel stagnation, and are signaling their clear need for detoxification. When we ignore what the body is telling us and just mask the odor with toothpaste or breath fresheners, we are not working with the body to relieve the stress it is being subjected to. If we do not change our nutritional lifestyles to include detoxifying and healthier foods, we allow the overload of organs and congestion and stagnation to persist. We are inviting serious discomfort and disease in the future. To correct bad breath, one must address the causes of the problem, which are bowel toxemia and faulty digestion.

### Common Cold

A cold is the body's normal reaction to stagnant, excess toxins in the body. When the storage of toxins has reached a certain level, *and* the body still has enough stored energy, it will produce a cold to move the toxins out via mucus discharges from the upper respiratory membranes of the nose, throat, sinuses, lungs, and even ears.

The major offending foods that contribute to toxic mucus buildup are sugar and dairy products. All drugs and non-natural foods, which have been processed, denatured, preserved or flavored with additives, also contribute to the load of toxins that the body will attempt to eliminate via the mechanism of a cold.

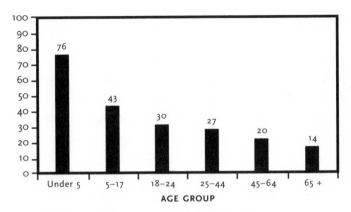

**Figure 9.1   Percentage of people having at least one cold in a year**
*Source: National Centre for Health Statistics.*

Bodies go through detoxification cycles or seasons as required, just like the rest of nature. A cold does not just happen to us. Nor do we catch it from someone else. If we do develop a cold near the time that we come into contact with others who have colds, it is because our bodies have similar toxic accumulations and available energies for the cold to happen. If this were not the case, why doesn't everyone exposed to a cold develop one? Healthy bodies have no need for the mechanism of a cold because they have very low levels of toxic accumulations.

It is interesting to note that only the very healthy, and the very ill, do not get colds. Figure 9.1 illustrates how colds typically become fewer as we age.

Healthy people do not get colds because their bodies are clear of toxic buildup. Very ill people, such as those with cancer, rarely get colds because their bodies have an inadequate supply of enzymes to react against the toxins and cannot afford the expenditure of energy that colds require. Children typically have more colds than adults because of the quantity of enzymes and natural energy their bodies have. With this capability, their bodies attempt to "clean house" in order to make them healthier. But, as time goes on, and as the input of cooked, junk, sugar, and dairy food products continues, bodies become more congested and weakened as a result of the storage of toxic wastes. This reduces the body's efficiency for producing energy from food, meaning that it is not able to stage detoxi-fication efforts in the form of colds as often as it used to.

During a cold, one should work with the body to conserve energy for healing by sleeping and resting as much as possible. Consuming water, diluted fresh fruit and vegetable juices, or broth soups made from vegeta-bles are also recommended. Continuing to eat solid food detracts from the efficiency of healing that the body is attempting since digestion requires a lot of energy. Remember that the body will not initiate a cold or flu unless it already has enough energy and nutrients stored for this purpose, so we do not need solid food at this time to "keep our energy up."

### Constipation

An inability to move the bowels at least once a day is a fairly common problem. It can have several contributing factors. Constipation is a condi-tion where stools are dense, packed together, and insufficiently elimi-nated. It is a classic symptom of intestinal toxemia. The bowels should move as often as required by the body to prevent stagnation and toxin absorption. Mucus buildup from wrong eating habits, emotional stress, and poor bowel habits can cause constipation.

A person who takes five or ten minutes to complete a bowel movement is constipated. A healthy body on a healthy diet should take only a minute or two to complete the process.

As digested food moves through the digestive tract, the walls of the colon are constantly at work absorbing moisture and nutrients out of the contents for use in the body. The colon wall acts as a two-way filter that allows the passage of body wastes, toxins, and fluids en route to elimination. The longer that digested material remains in the colon, the more moisture is absorbed from it, and the drier and more compacted it becomes.

Chemical laxatives are harsh and irritating to the bowel and should not be used. They only provide temporary relief and add to the problem. Most laxatives work because they irritate the colon. This triggers a movement of the bowel to expel the irritant. The bowel moves the irritating laxative, not the other way around. Due to irritations from laxatives, the bowel lays down more protective layers of mucus on the intestinal walls, which increases other problems. If an occasional laxative is required, one could use a herbal laxative tea purchased at a health food store. The easiest and safest aids to moving the bowels are clear water enemas and colonics.

To correct constipation, the body requires a correction of the irritating causes. It needs to be detoxified. A herbal detoxification blend can be taken regularly to achieve excellent results. Raw fruits and vegetables that contain enzymes, fiber, and water are healthy fare for the colon. The diet and digestion must be improved. Supplementation with digestive enzymes is helpful.

Additional fiber, from psyllium husks or flax seeds, for example, along with pure water, are helpful in retaining moisture and filling out the stool. Bran products should not be used as they are irritating to the bowel and add to the problem of mucus buildup in the colon if they cannot be completely digested.

When constipation is present, water intake should be increased. Just like flushing a toilet, the bowel cannot be cleaned without adequate water. A good regimen is to start the day by drinking two or three glasses of warm water. It is very helpful for the whole body if the juice of half a lemon is added to the first glass. It acts as an excellent alkalizer and cleanser.

### Diarrhea

Diarrhea results from irritation in the colon and intestinal toxemia. When we have diarrhea, we need to recognize that the body is reacting this way for a purpose and needs our cooperation. Diarrhea is the body's natural action of quickly removing harmful toxins from the intestinal tract.

Occasional or unexpected diarrhea is usually due to the consumption of toxic foods, poisons, or too much food (which becomes toxic in quantities greater than the digestive system can handle). It may also accompany intestinal flu, or periods of emotional or physical stress.

More persistent forms of diarrhea are usually a symptom that the body is unable to digest the food being consumed. This can be due to a lack of digestive enzymes, overeating and the consequent overloading of the digestive system, or a lack of friendly flora in the bowel. Chronic diarrhea can actually be a form of constipation, with the accumulation of old feces adhering to the walls of the colon in such quantities as to be actively irritating. Thick mucus then sticks to the intestinal wall and cannot be expelled. Because of the mucus buildup, the colon passageway becomes narrowed, making it necessary for the body to add more water to the waste contents and increase contractions to empty whatever can be forced out.

A healthy, properly functioning bowel contains an average of three pounds of friendly bacteria composed of over 400 kinds of microorganisms. These bacteria are essential ingredients for improving nutrition and protecting against disease. When antibiotics are taken to kill harmful bacteria in the body, they also kill many of the healthy strains. This creates severe side effects and difficulties for digestion and immunity. Antibiotics are also unconsciously consumed in meat because commercial animals and poultry are routinely given large doses of antibiotics.

For the occasional toxin, flu, or food poisoning diarrhea, we can assist the body in cleaning out the intestines by taking a clear water enema. For persistent or chronic diarrhea, we should be working to improve our diets, supplemented with digestive enzymes and bowel flora products, as well as detoxifying the colon with gentle herbs, enemas, and colonics.

### Fever

A fever is the body's natural defense against an invading virus. It is not a symptom of a disease, but is actually part of the body's anti-viral immune system. The body may also raise its temperature to speed a cleansing process.[1]

When toxins build to a certain level in the body, germs or viruses enter to scavenge on wastes and in so doing, produce toxic wastes of their own. Viruses multiply very well at normal body temperature 98.6°F (37°C). However, they are unable to live and multiply at temperatures above 101°F (38.3°C).[2] In order to keep the viruses from multiplying and poisoning the body with their wastes, the body increases its metabolism and cellular activity, which raises its temperature.[3]

When the body is left to handle a virus on its own, normal health is usually restored in a few days. However, serious problems can develop when a person tries to feel better by self-medicating with over-the-counter cold or flu remedies. The reason is because most of these contain acetylsalicylic acid or similar anti-inflammatory drugs. And while these drugs may give some temporary relief from pain or stuffiness, they also lower the body's fever below 100°F (37.8°C), thereby allowing the virus to multiply unchallenged and spread throughout the body.[4] A young or relatively healthy body may be able to handle this interference, but the elderly and those with weak immune systems may develop serious conditions such as encephalitis or pneumonia, which can lead to death.[5]

While body temperature is above 100°F (37.8°C), no food should be consumed—only pure water or dilute juices. The ill person should stay warm and rest. Temperatures up to 104°F (40°C) should be left alone. If temperature goes beyond this, ice packs and cool water sponges may be used.[6]

### Flu

Flu, or influenza, is similar to a cold but with the addition of a virus. The body generates a fever to fight the virus. During flu, there may be discharges similar to those of a cold. However, the general weakness, chills and fever, muscle and joint aches, and pain are present because the entire body is undergoing a cleansing of heavy accumulations of toxic wastes. The feelings of weakness are due to the body's utilization of available energy to focus on internal cleansing and healing activities. Toxins liberated from storage areas are being released into the blood and tissues. When the healing crisis or cycle is complete, the body returns the flow of energy to the rest of the body. Jensen and Anderson describe flu as:

> ... a turbulent detoxification reaction of the body. Every symptom of a cold or flu ... is a symptom of detoxification. What are the major symptoms of the flu? High fevers (burning of waste, and bacteria); the pores of the skin open for profuse sweating; diarrhea, the bowels dump; chills, which generate internal heat; vomiting, and coughing up and expectoration of respiratory mucus—all the cleansing actions. This is a way that the body can violently and quickly rid itself of the unprocessed metabolic waste. The waste is a smorgasbord for bacteria.[7]

The treatment for flu is much the same as that for a cold: reduce the intake of solid foods, rest, take natural fluids, and use whole food natural vitamins and mineral supplements and warm water enemas to assist with bowel cleansing. Stay warm, and let the illness run its course. Do not try to stop diarrhea, if present. Depending on the amount of toxins to be eliminated and the energy that the body has prepared in reserve, a cold or flu will usually last three or seven days, or a multiple of these. Be patient, and work with the body because it is working to improve overall health.

If we try to ease the symptoms of a cold or flu by taking medications, this blocks toxin elimination and interferes with the natural healing the body is carrying out. The body must then use extra energy to deal with the additional stress introduced by any drug taken. Cleansing is reduced and sometimes even stopped when the elimination of the toxic drug becomes a higher priority. When this happens, toxins are left in storage in various tissues, setting the stage for a more serious disease at a later time. The body does not have drug deficiencies; health cannot be forced on the body. Only the body can heal itself, and it will do so provided we don't interfere. If a disease process is already in progress, the body may lack sufficient enzymes and nutrition to correct the situation. Our part is to give the body what it needs to do its job. A healthy body has specific processes for handling every bacteria or virus.

### Gallstones

Gallstones are collections of crystals composed mostly of cholesterol and calcium salts in the gallbladder or bile ducts. They are the result of a prolonged overly-acid diet.

The liver produces bile to emulsify fat in food so it can be better digested in the intestine. The other function of bile is to raise the pH of food materials in the small intestine from acid to alkaline because the digestive enzymes in the small intestine only work in an alkaline medium. The liver produces alkaline bile for this reason.

When the diet is predominantly acid, the body will reabsorb sodium from the bile in order to conserve alkaline minerals, leaving the bile with an acid pH. As a result, the bile begins to crystallize and form stones. Acid bile can also irritate the gallbladder, causing a gallbladder attack. When acid bile is dumped into the intestine, it can burn and cause pain. Further, because the bile is now acidic, it cannot raise the pH of food from the stomach, rendering digestive enzymes in the small intestine ineffective, and resulting in nausea, bloating, belching, and flatulence.

A correction of these conditions requires the adoption of healthy eating and lifestyle practices so bile can return to alkaline again. In the meantime, highly acidic foods such as red meat, coffee, alcohol, sodas, fatty and fried foods, oils, and dairy products should be avoided. A flush using virgin olive oil and lemon juice can also be helpful and may even prevent unnecessary removal of the gallbladder.

## Heart Problems

A narrowing of the arteries as a result of deposits of minerals or fat, respectively called arteriosclerosis and atherosclerosis, causes most of the heart problems that lead to heart attacks. These problems are diet related, and along with genetic predisposition and stress, they comprise the major causes of heart disease.

### Bypassing the Bypass Operation

The present-day medical treatment for occluded arteries is a bypass operation. However, there is a natural remedy which has been reported by many to be very effective for clearing arteries. It involves placing fifteen drops of a herbal mixture under the tongue three times per day for several months.

Doug Henderson published a book about such heart drops which he entitled *Diet and Exercise is a Crock*.[8] At the time that title was selected, Mr. Henderson and his advisors were unaware of what true healing nutrition is. And while I don't agree with what the title generally implies, the book made interesting reading. After two heart attacks, a strict regimen of diet and exercise, a quadruple bypass operation, then more diet and exercise, he still ended up needing about twenty nitroglycerin tablets a day to survive. He was close to death when he was introduced to the 'heart drops' produced by Jim and Peter Strauss of Kamloops, B.C., Canada. He returned to leading a productive and active life while taking no medication other than the drops. Doug became a personal friend of mine, and I urged him many times over the five years that I knew him to take corrective measures with his diet. Unfortunately, he refused to make any of these changes in his lifestyle.

It is my opinion that, as with all other health treatments and therapies, heart drops must be used in conjunction with an improved diet and lifestyle. Otherwise, the underlying or contributing factors that caused the narrowing of arteries in the first place will still manifest as disease at a later date.

Several brands of heart drops are now available on the market, and can be found on the Internet.

### The Testosterone Connection

Eugene Shippen, MD, is a doctor who specializes in reversing the negative factors of male menopause in his patients through testing and adjusting their testosterone levels. As an adjunct to his focus of improving men's energy, health, and sexuality by returning testosterone levels to their more youthful levels, he discovered a remarkable but not widely recognized relationship between testosterone and heart health and recovery. In his book *The Testosterone Syndrome*, Shippen cites that an increasing majority of medical studies report a relationship between high testosterone and low cardiovascular disease in men, and that men are healthier and live longer when their testosterone levels are normal.[9] He states that "testosterone is the heart-protective hormone of the male body,"[10] and suggests that after reading chapter 3 of his book, most male heart patients will show the information to their doctors and demand a test of their testosterone levels.

### Hemorrhoids

Hemorrhoids, or piles, as they are more commonly known, are the engorgement and swelling of the veins of the rectum. Hemorrhoids can result from straining to have bowel movements during constipation, or from pregnancy. They can also be caused by an accumulation of backed-up blood that has not been able to circulate through a congested liver. One reason why rectal veins become inflamed and swell is because of pressure buildup between the rectum and liver to which they directly connect. The main vein, called the portal vein, does not have one-way valves such as are in the arm and leg veins. Therefore, anything that restricts blood flow, such as congestion in the liver, causes a backpressure and consequent inflammation and swelling of the rectal veins, either internally or externally.

To prevent hemorrhoid conditions, one needs to adopt a healthful lifestyle, have regular exercise, and detoxify the bowel. For relief of hemorrhoid pain, a suppository-sized piece of raw white potato can be inserted into the rectum and changed as needed. Fasting for a period of time, until symptoms subside, on fresh fruit and vegetable juices or diluted juices, will relieve the load on the digestive system, and relieve and reduce hemorrhoids.

### High Blood Pressure

The purpose of blood circulation is to supply all parts of the body with oxygen and nutrients. When unhealthy lifestyle practices make this task more difficult, the body must increase blood pressure to keep delivering life-sustaining nutrients and oxygen to its tissues.

There can be many reasons for increased blood pressure, such as the narrowing of arteries due to fat and mineral deposits; the congestion and clogging of organs from cellular waste products; a build-up of plaque, calcium, or cholesterol in the arteries; a loss of elasticity in the blood vessel walls; negative emotions; stimulants like drugs, food excesses, salt, and pollutants; lack of exercise; and blood that is too thick or too thin.

Correcting high blood pressure requires an elimination of all its causes. Stated simply, it comes down to adopting healthy lifestyle practices, feeding the body what it needs to be healthy, and improving bowel and liver function. Given the necessary workers in the way of enzymes and bowel bacteria, proper nutrition, exercise, rest, and reduced stress, the body will self-correct.

A study completed in the United States confirms that high blood pressure can be overcome very quickly using entirely natural methods. Dr. Alan Goldhamer and his research team conducted a twelve-year study with 174 patients at the TrueNorth Health Center, in Penngrove, California. Here is a summary:

It was discovered that by having patients consume nothing but pure water in a supervised environment of complete rest, blood pressures rapidly normalized. In fact, many patients who began their fasts while on high blood pressure drugs were required to quickly discontinue their medications, so that their blood pressures would not drop artificially low!

... The treatment procedure included an average water-only fasting period of 10.6 days, followed by a supervised re-feeding period of about one week with a whole, natural foods diet. In the final analysis, this safe and simple procedure demonstrated extraordinary effectiveness. By the end of their stay, all patients were able to discontinue their medications, no matter how severe their initial condition. In fact, ... the most impressive results were observed with the most serious cases. In cases of 'moderate' to 'severe' hypertension (blood pressures of 174/93 or greater), the average reduction at the conclusion of treatment was a remarkable 46/15! For these cases, which medical practitioners generally would insist need lifetime medical intervention, the average exit blood pressure was 128/78 using no medication whatsoever![11]

### Hormonal Problems

The endocrine system, also referred to as the hormonal system, comprises several glands whose purpose is to produce hormones that regulate various metabolic functions in the body. The liver and kidneys, while classed as organs, are also glands because they secrete hormones. When the endocrine glands are unable to do the jobs that they are intended, various problems develop such as growth problems, thyroid and adrenal gland disorders, diabetic symptoms due to impaired insulin production, PMS and menopausal difficulties, as well as others.

A healthy body does not have hormonal imbalances. It was designed to produce all the hormones necessary to regulate metabolic functions. To be able to produce these hormones, however, it must have its basic nutritional needs met. The liver is the master organ, gland, and processor in the body. It depends on complete amino acids from protein to manufacture hormones and enzymes required by the endocrine glands.

The two main problems with our diet are lack of sufficient digestive enzymes and unavailability of amino acids, both of which are related to cooked foods. Cooking food at temperatures above 112 to 120°F (44–49°C) kills digestive enzymes, which must be present in the stomach to break down proteins into their smaller amino acid components for digestion and assimilation. Also, when food is heated even to a sterilizing or pasteurizing point (which is much lower than baking or frying temperatures), the amino acid lysine becomes bound, making lysine and other amino acids biologically unavailable to the body.[12]

It is very important that the body be supplied with an adequate quality and quantity of raw food and/or be supplied with enzyme and amino acid supplements, so it can produce required hormones. The effects of cooked food on hormonal development were clearly demonstrated in the Pottenger cats experiments. The cats on a two-thirds cooked food diet all developed multiple growth, disease, personality, metabolic, and sexual development problems.

### PMS and Menopause

Many women in our society suffer needlessly from hormonal imbalances. To many, the "period" has become the "curse." The monthly cycle brings on PMS, and menopause, when it occurs, is accompanied by hot flashes, weight gain, fatigue, and mood swings. There is much suffering for women who go through such episodes, and sometimes, for those who live with the women experiencing them. But it wasn't meant to be that way, and it shouldn't be. Women in other cultures sail through these cycles and times of life without the problems that many women in western cultures experience. For them, it seems they have happy hormones. Why is there this difference?

Female hormonal difficulties have been turned into diseases. But they are not diseases. They are imbalances in the body's hormonal system brought on by nutritional deficiencies, stress, pharmaceutical drugs, unnecessary surgeries, and environmental toxins. An industry has been created to exploit, and unfortunately, exacerbate these problems. It is estimated that 500,000 hysterectomies are performed annually in North America, 90% of which are classified as "elective surgeries."[13] This procedure, when combined with removal of the ovaries, immediately triggers menopause.[14] Then, in attempts to mitigate and handle this onslaught and resulting changes to the body, synthetic hormones are prescribed. In 2001 alone, one hormone replacement drug, Premarin, prescribed for many hormone related conditions, generated more than two billion dollars in sales.[15] The human body cannot incorporate synthetic, unnatural substances into its tissues for optimum health.

### Prostate and Male Midlife Problems

The prostate is a walnut-sized gland of the male reproductive system, located below the bladder and encircling the urethra. It helps control urination and produces a major component of semen. It depends on an adequate supply of nutrients and balanced hormones for its health.

At some time in his life, usually around middle age, almost every man will experience discomfort and problems caused by an inflamed or enlarged prostate gland. It is estimated that over one-half of men between age 40 and 60 have enlarged prostates.[16] Some symptoms of prostate problems can be: a frequent urge to urinate, weak urine stream, difficulty beginning the urine stream, dribbling of urine, painful urination, painful ejaculation, erectile difficulties, blood in the urine or semen, and pain in the lower back.[17] These symptoms should always be taken seriously because of the possibility of the presence of prostate cancer—the second most common malignancy in American males.[18]

If prostate problems persist, advice should be sought from a healthcare practitioner who is knowledgeable in this area. In addition, I strongly suggest that men do their own research regarding prostate cancer treatment, if that has become necessary. An excellent booklet, containing condensed, very informative, and possibly life-saving information, was written by Dr. John R. Lee, and is entitled *Hormone Balance for Men*. Dr. Lee presents conclusions from documented studies showing that contrary to the prevailing conventional medical approach for treating prostate cancer, testosterone is not the culprit; estrogen is. He points out that the blame attributed to testosterone is based on false assumptions drawn from experiences with prostate cancer patients by Dr. Charles Huggins in 1941. Also, absent from many of the early prostate cancer studies was the measurement and consideration of progesterone and estrogen levels.[19] Dr. Lee successfully treated many prostate cancer patients who recovered and did not have to resort to the standard medical treatments of surgery and chemotherapy, by using diet, antioxidants, progesterone, and testosterone.[20] He also explains why the psa (Prostate Specific Antigen) count is not a reliable indicator of cancer because it is based on an erroneous understanding of the role of psa in the body. He suggests that men should endeavor to maintain healthy levels of progesterone and testosterone for both preventing and treating prostate cancer.[21]

To date, it is largely unrecognized and unacknowledged that the male body goes through a midlife hormonal change similar to that of the female body, although more gradually. This time of life is referred to as "male menopause," but should more correctly be termed "andropause." After about age 40, testosterone, the hormone of youth in the male, begins to decline at the rate of about one percent per year.[22] This is a normal part of aging, but problems begin to develop when the ratio of testosterone to estrogen becomes unbalanced, with estrogen levels rising and testosterone levels falling. As this happens, symptoms can develop such as lack of energy and stamina, inability to concentrate, depression, loss of muscle mass and strength, increased fat especially around the mid-section and breasts, increased difficulty in reading fine print, decreased libido, and erectile difficulties, to name a few.[23] Low testosterone levels are also associated with heart problems[24] and osteoporosis.[25]

Increased estrogen levels can be due to nutritional factors, stress, and chemicals in our foods and environment that act as synthetic estrogens in the human body. Estrogen in the male body is normally kept in check by weight-bearing exercise and several nutritional factors, of which three important ones are: cruciferous vegetables (cabbage, cauliflower, broccoli, kale, brussel sprouts); lycopene vegetables and fruits, especially tomatoes; and zinc. The prostate gland contains the highest concentration of zinc of any organ in the body[26] but inflamed prostates have one-tenth the zinc levels of normal prostates.[27] Since men lose zinc in every seminal emission, it needs to be constantly replaced to avoid a deficiency. One of the most concentrated vegetarian sources of zinc is raw pumpkin seeds.

Men who are experiencing some of the difficulties described above should take immediate steps to resolve them. Nutritional prostate support supplements for symptomatic relief may be found in healthfood stores. However, a hormone balance assessment may also be beneficial for longer-term health considerations, to be certain that problem causes are being addressed. Hormone levels of estrogen, progesterone, and testosterone can be easily and accurately checked with a saliva test, which Dr. Lee says is the only sure method of measuring "free testosterone."[28] One source for further information and advice on how to do this is www.help forhormones.com.

When hormone levels are returned to more normal levels, many of the declining health and physical factors of andropause can be reversed."[29]

### Synthetic Hormones

Dr. John R. Lee has done a tremendous job of breaking through the myths and dangers of synthetic hormone supplementation.[30] Over an approximate period of 25 years, Dr. Lee and other researchers have uncovered a largely western phenomenon of estrogen dominance that is affecting women especially, but also men. In simple terms, estrogen dominance is an excess of estrogen over progesterone. In a healthy body, progesterone is produced in sufficient quantities to balance out the effects of estrogen. Progesterone is also needed for many other functions in the body. The often used allopathic treatment for female hormonal problems is to prescribe synthetic estrogen hormone replacement therapy, HRT, which further increases estrogen dominance. The answer that Dr. Lee arrived at was to treat typical hormone problems with natural progesterone.

### Estrogen Mimics

Other hormone disrupter problems in our society, in addition to synthetic hormones, are xenoestrogens or xenobiotics, which produce estrogen-like activity in the body. They are found in herbicide and pesticide sprays, petroleum products, plastics, and other chemicals that pollute our food, air, and water.

Agricultural animals raised for meat consumption are injected with estrogen-like hormones to increase fat content. These synthetic hormones remain in the meat when it is consumed. Even though they may be in small amounts, it takes very little to upset the delicate hormone balance in the body. Other food products such as those made from soy contain phytoestrogens, naturally occurring estrogens that are reported to be at much higher levels than those found in meat products. Several scientific studies have linked high levels of phytoestrogens to many hormonal problems, including early puberty in girls.[31]

When we understand how such foods are grown, processed, chemicalized, and promoted to the public, these hormonal side effects should not be too surprising. Excess estrogen, or xenoestrogens, in the body can produce a myriad of undesirable symptoms. In premenopausal women, symptoms can include: fatigue, depression, weight gain, water retention, headaches, loss of sex drive, mood swings, inability to handle stress, irritability, fibrocystic breasts, uterine fibroids, endometriosis, low metabolism, symptoms of hypothyroidism, unstable blood sugar levels, sluggishness in the morning, and a craving for caffeine, sweets, and carbohydrates. Menopausal women can experience symptoms such as: hot flashes, vaginal dryness and atrophy, water retention, fat and weight gain, sleep disturbances, decreased libido, mood swings, headaches, fatigue, lack of concentration, short-term memory lapses, thinning of scalp hair, increased facial hair, osteoporosis, various body aches and pains, and dry, thin, and wrinkled skin. Estrogen dominance has also been linked to male problems, including lowered sperm counts, physical feminization symptoms such as enlarged breasts, as well as osteoporosis and prostate cancer.

### Indigestion

All digestive discomforts are a result of the abuse or overloading of the digestive organs, plus possible genetic inabilities to produce adequate quantities of digestive secretions. Factors that contribute to digestive disorders are: the lack of digestive enzymes; insufficient stomach acid; poor food combinations; overeating; drinking liquids with meals; consuming substances like soft drinks, coffee, and strong alcoholic drinks, which are irritating to the digestive linings; consuming drugs and antibiotics that are irritating to stomach and intestine linings and which destroy friendly intestinal bacteria; eating while under stress; and consuming foods and drinks that are too hot or too cold, indigestible, overcooked, fried, microwaved, refined, and chemically treated.

Countless people suffer regularly from acid indigestion, heartburn and the so-called acid reflux "disease." Billions are spent on acid-buffering agents like Tums, Rolaids, Maalox, and Alka-Seltzer, as well as high-tech drugs such as Prilosec, Prevacid, Pepcid, and Tagamet. But is all this necessary? Do we really produce too much stomach acid?

In their excellent book *Why Stomach Acid is Good for You*, Drs. Jonathan Wright and Lane Lenard carefully document research that explains the *myth* of acid indigestion, and note that except in a few rare conditions, "heartburn is hardly ever associated with *too much* stomach acid." In fact, the reverse is true. They explain that as we get older, "the most common thing that goes wrong in the stomach is a loss of acid-producing cells, which is accompanied by a fall-off in acid production."[32] On average, the stomach acid secretion of a typical 65-year-old person is one-third that of a 25-year old.[33] When stomach acid is too weak, food digestion and the absorption of minerals are seriously compromised, which can lead to deficiencies and disease conditions.

Symptoms of low stomach acid include:

- Indigestion or sourness 2 to 3 hr. after meals
- Abdominal bloating, distension
- Full, logy feeling after heavy meat meal
- Loss of former taste or craving for meat
- Excessive gas, belching or burping after meals
- Burning sensation in stomach, heartburn
- Heavy, tired feeling after eating
- Constipation
- Stools poorly formed, pale, greasy, floating

- Undigested food particles in stools
- Ridges on fingernails, slow growing nails

For temporary solutions, one should pay attention to proper food combination as a first measure. Taking digestive enzymes with meals will also help with the breakdown of food in the stomach. To increase the strength of stomach acid, tablets of hydrochloric acid (HCl) and pepsin with meals may be used. As an alternative to this, some people receive great relief from serious acid indigestion by taking one or more teaspoons of unpasteurized apple cider vinegar in a little water before meals. This encourages the stomach's natural production of HCl and, while it has an acid effect in the stomach, it leaves an alkaline mineral residue in the body. If this does the trick, it is a win-win solution.

The permanent solution to low stomach acid is to address its cause. The reason the stomach secretes insufficient acid is because the body lacks the necessary vitamins and minerals to produce it. The Roseburg study conducted by Victoria Boutenko (see *The Green Breakthrough*, chapter 15) demonstrated that increasing the natural production of stomach acid appears to be related to the intake of raw green vegetables, the requirement of which is far greater than cooked and raw food eaters typically consume. This problem can be overcome by introducing raw green smoothies into the diet.

### Intestinal Discomfort

At times, a person may experience persistent bloating, cramping and/or pain associated with the intestines but which does not seem to be associated with an upset stomach. This could be due to the ileocecal valve being locked in the closed position. When this happens, the process of waste elimination can be hindered, causing digested and partially digested food to back up in the small intestine, creating pressure. As the pressure increases, pain and tenderness in the associated area results. There is a simple procedure that someone can do to open this valve, and get things moving again, relieving the pressure.

The ileocecal valve is located in the lower right abdomen at the juncture between the small and large intestines. Place the thumb of your right hand on your navel and your little finger on the top of your right hip. Where the tip of your middle finger rests will be close to the location of this valve, just inside from the groin. Press the fingertips of both hands into this area and massage firmly in a counter-clockwise direction for about ten seconds. You may have to repeat this procedure a few times. To achieve better results, also massage the area between the ileocecal valve and the navel. As the valve is opened, you should begin to experience relief fairly quickly. Remember to drink plenty of pure water because digested food and wastes may have become dry and compacted.

Sometimes the ileocecal valve can be locked in the open position causing food and wastes to move through too quickly, resulting in diarrhea. The same procedure described above, but in a clockwise direction, can be used to close the valve if this is a problem.

### Lack of Energy

A lack of energy in general, or a decrease in the level of energy we used to have, is a sign that our bodies are not functioning as efficiently as they could. They are in an overly acidic state. There may be many reasons for this, but it is usually due to a deficiency of proper nutrients from live foods, including complete proteins, vitamins, and minerals. Other contributing factors may be the lack of oxygen and enzymes, the inefficiency of the digestive system, congestion of organs such as the liver and kidneys, congestion of the elimination systems of the lymph and colon, and adrenal fatigue. When toxic wastes are stored in the body, the cells become less efficient at producing energy. What energy is produced must be directed toward survival as a first priority. Therefore, less energy is available for muscle movement and activity. Intestinal toxemia sets in.

Fatigue is a means that the body uses to block activities that continue to deplete its life reserves. It is the body's way of letting us know we are disregarding its needs. The body may be calling for rest from the depleting negative emotions of worry, anxiety, fear, anger, hatred, and guilt, and for a healthier diet and the detoxification of acid congestion in its organs and tissues.

## Obesity

Excess fat storage in the body is the result of consuming a greater quantity of acid and toxic calories than the body can properly metabolize and eliminate. When this occurs, the body has no alternative but to store the toxins, along with the excess calories, as fat. People who have a different genetic makeup, and who eat basically the same diet but do not have a weight problem, tend to burn the excess calories and store the toxins in their organs.

Obese people have a greater risk of becoming ill or of dying from most diseases. They are more apt to become injured or have accidents. Fat storage around the mid-section, or abdominal obesity, is associated with a high risk of coronary artery disease, which can include high blood pressure, adult onset diabetes, and high levels of fats in the blood.[34]

An overweight problem can be due to eating too many calories, liver congestion, glandular malfunction, and the fluid that the body retains to dilute toxins. The most offending foods are trans fats and sugars. People who eat as little as others but seem to gain weight in spite of this are often deficient in the digestive enzyme lipase, and the food-form minerals chromium, zinc, and selenium. Lipase is required by the body to digest fat in order to utilize it as energy. Chromium is required for insulin to work efficiently in controlling hunger, regulating energy production, and utilizing fat. The secretion of healthy bile is essential for dissolving and eliminating fat.

In addition to the physical contributors of an overweight problem, there is usually an emotional component that needs to be addressed to achieve a permanent return to the body's ideal weight. "Within every big person is a big emotional issue begging for attention and resolution."[35]

Weight problems are corrected by detoxifying the body through cleansing the colon and liver, and changing to a healthy lifestyle. The body must be made less acid. The best foods that help to do this are fresh vegetable juices made from carrots, celery, spinach, beets, parsley, and a little ginger. A healthy lifestyle includes adequate regular exercise to activate the lymph system and help burn stored calories, as well as a diet that supplies all the required nutrients and live enzymes. Supplements to clean the colon, plus enzymes and complete protein products are very helpful. An overweight body is actually starving for wholesome alkaline nutrition. A person with an acidic body cannot lose weight and keep it off. It doesn't matter what diet is tried, the results will only be temporary unless acid-alkaline balance is restored.

## Pain

Pain is simply the body's way of letting us know that some of its parts or systems are under stress and in need of help and correction. Pain can be from trauma or toxic buildup. When we are injured, we understand the pain, and that the body must be allowed to heal. However, we cannot see or feel toxins as they build up. Much of the pain we experience is created by the irritation of nerve endings by poisons and toxins from metabolic wastes. Several billion cells die each day, and unless this dead matter is properly processed and eliminated from the body, it stagnates and accumulates. It decays the same way rotting carcasses do, producing poisons. A failure to eliminate stems from overload problems, which in turn cause intestinal toxemia, constipation, and the malfunction of glands and organs of elimination.

In the case of a headache not caused by trauma, there are too many toxins in the blood and the body is working very hard to keep them out of the brain and eliminate them from the blood. In the process of doing this, the blood vessels can spasm or dilate in an attempt to remove the toxins from the bloodstream faster. This causes the pain.

It is also necessary to understand that when we correct lifestyle practices and experience healing during the reversal process, there can be pain associated with this process. This is due to the release of toxins from storage, for elimination via the bloodstream and elimination channels. Toxins, whether they are going into cells for storage, or coming out of cells for elimination, cause the spasming or dilation of blood vessels.

## Skin Problems

The skin is an important organ of elimination and detoxification. It removes most of the poisons from the body through perspiration: up to

200% more abnormal minerals and metals than do the other channels of detoxification.

All skin problems such as eczema, acne, pimples, dandruff, dry skin, and psoriasis are the result of the body's elimination of toxins via the skin pores when the other channels of elimination are congested. This means the body is overly acidic. When the liver is clean, skin problems do not manifest. The excessive elimination of toxins causes the outer layers of skin to die off at a faster rate than new skin cells can be produced, resulting in dry skin. Dry skin is also an indication that essential oils are lacking in the diet. Understandably, blood circulation is less efficient in dry and congested areas. When the toxic overload is heavy, the skin becomes saturated with irritants that cause nerves in skin to react by reflex, giving us the urge to scratch. Scratching increases the flow of blood to the area. Itching is the same as a very low-level pain. We feel an urge to scratch the itchy area hard enough until there is a little pain. Pain is easier to tolerate than the itch, and in the process, circulation to the area is increased, if only for a while.

Excessive body poisons create an inflammation of the inner lining of skin pores. This makes the pores swell, narrowing their openings, even to a point where they become blocked. Oozing can develop, which may lead to eczema and psoriasis.

Soaps dry the skin, while creams and medicated ointments clog the pores, reducing their ability to carry out the elimination it is attempting. We are working with the body when we keep the skin clean and free of creams that alter the pH of the skin surface and congest the pores.

Research done by Dr. Nicholas Perricone[36] and Dr. Robert Connolly[37] has found that sugar, and foods that convert rapidly to sugar, cause an inflammation in the skin. One needs to avoid all sugars, as well as foods that contain sugar and honey, and high starch foods such as pasta, bread, potatoes, and rice.

Skin problems are a clear sign that the body requires detoxification. The first areas to work on are the colon and the liver. To correct skin problems, the conditions of intestinal toxemia and over-acidity must be addressed. The body needs the assistance of a healthful lifestyle, which would include a diet that supplies adequate enzymes, vitamins, minerals, amino acids, and essential oils. Good digestion and bowel management are necessary. Also required are adequate rest, exercise, fresh air, moderate exposure to sunshine, and skin brushing instead of using soaps and ointments.

The body produces healthy skin when its requirements are being met.

### Yeast Overgrowth (Candida)

Yeast is normally present in the colon along with hundreds of other organisms. In a healthy body, it is kept under control by enzymes and hydrochloric acid in the digestive system, and by friendly bacteria in the bowel. The main causes of yeast overgrowth are improper diet, antibiotics, steroid drugs, birth control pills, and stress; all of these can weaken the immune system and cause a depletion of healthy bowel flora.

When healthy bowel flora are depleted, yeast in the form of *Candida albicans* can multiply and invade other tissues. Antibiotics kill bacteria, but they do not discriminate between helpful and unfriendly bacteria. Acidophilus cultures in the colon, which are one of the main defenses against yeast overgrowths, are destroyed, thereby allowing yeast to proliferate. Birth control pills, because they contain steroid hormones and upset the normal hormonal balance of the body, can encourage yeast growth. Excessive and continued stress over-stimulates the adrenal glands, causing them to release steroid hormones, which can depress the immune system. Diets that are high in processed foods and sugar change the pH in our intestinal tract, making it difficult for friendly flora to survive, while providing a good environment for candida to multiply. Fluoride and chlorine in drinking water upset the balance of bowel flora as well. Anything that upsets the balance of healthy flora in the intestine sets the stage for and encourages the growth of yeast which, in turn, weakens the immune system.

Candida overgrowth can affect three general areas: gastrointestinal and genitourinary tracts, allergic responses, and mental/emotional problems. Symptoms can include sweet cravings; nasal itching, congestion and discharge; abdominal pain; belching; bloating; heartburn; constipation; diarrhea; itching; vaginal discharge; worsened PMS symptoms; prostatitis; impotence; chronic fungal outbreaks; fatigue; muscle aches; depression;

irritability; cold hands and feet; asthma; hay fever; allergies; and eczema. Some alternative health practitioners also believe fibromyalgia is often just candida in the muscles.[38]

Once yeast has overgrown and infected other areas of the body, bowel toxemia and deficiency problems must be corrected. Yeast proliferates in an alkaline environment. Attempting to kill the yeast using drugs is only working on the symptom. In women especially, a yeast infection can be temporarily controlled in two or three days by drinking unsweetened cranberry juice or water to which a tablespoon of unpasteurized apple cider vinegar has been added. This can be done three or four times a day along with douching with a stronger solution of water and apple cider vinegar. This way, the pH of the urinary tract and vagina become slightly acid, killing the yeast.

To effectively control candida, a person must also be careful with their diet. All foods and drinks containing sugar, or carbohydrates that convert to sugar in the body, must be avoided. In addition, a high-grade probiotic such as acidophilus should be taken two or three times per day for a period of time, thereby repopulating the colon with a healthy colony of friendly flora. In addition, increasing the oxygen content of water you drink by adding a product such as Aerobic Oxygen is very helpful since candida cannot tolerate oxygen. During the correction period, supplementing with natural food-based trace minerals and enzymes will help to correct nutritional deficiencies and digestive inadequacies. In a healthy body, the intestinal flora population is constantly rebuilding itself.

For detailed information on correcting a candida problem, I recommend the brief but excellent book titled *Candida: Treating it Successfully*, written by Dr. B. R. Blinzler. He has worked with thousands of patients, effectively eliminating their candida problems in 30 to 40 days through the means of strict diet and glandular support, plus a supplement containing undecenoic acid from the castor bean. In his book, Dr. Blinzler lists several symptoms in the form of questions as a "good home screening test" to help a person determine the possible presence of candida overgrowth in their body. They are repeated here with his permission for your information and consideration:

Answer *YES* or *NO* to the following questions:

1   Do you fatigue more easily now than in the past?
2   Are you troubled with depression, memory loss or confusion?
3   Do you crave sweets?
4   Have you taken antibiotics within a year or two before you started feeling the way you do now?
5   Have you ever taken birth control pills?
6   Have you ever taken cortisone, prednisone or any other steroid drug?
7   Have you any digestive troubles such as constipation/diarrhea, bloating, heartburn or indigestion?
8   Have you any PMS symptoms?
9   Has your sex drive decreased?
10  Have you had, or do you now have recurring bladder/kidney, vaginal or prostate infections?
11  Are you sensitive to perfumes, smoke or chemical odors?
12  Are you troubled with skin problems, such as rashes or hives, for example?
13  Do you have any joint or muscular aches?
14  Do you now have any allergies causing sinus or bronchial troubles that you did not have in the past?

If there are more YES answers than NO answers, the probability of a candida overgrowth is very high. If there are about 25% YES's, there is a good possibility of a mild candida problem. And if there are 75% or more YES's, then you can count on a moderate to severe case of candidiasis. The symptoms of candidiasis are diverse and will affect the individual from mild to moderate to severe. Candida can be anything from an annoying pest to a serious life-threatening condition. Diagnosis of candida can be very elusive, especially through traditional laboratory testing, but through my experience, using the above method has proven to be fairly accurate and much less costly than complicated laboratory tests.[39]

When a person does embark on a candida elimination program, their body will likely go through some reactions. As the candida die-off happens, toxins released by the dying candida can cause a worsening of the previous symptoms, including fatigue, concentration and memory problems, and muscle and joint pains. Reactions usually begin during the first week of the program and may continue for one or two weeks. Staying with the control diet and program is important and the reward is worth working for.

### Candida's Mixed Blessing

According to Drs. Hal Huggins and Thomas Levy[40], candida does have its positive side, if that's a consolation.

As we learned in the last chapter, one of the worst poisons our bodies are subjected to is mercury, which has a strong link to candida. Mercury's most usual source of entry into our bodies is from so-called "silver" amalgam tooth fillings. As this mercury enters the body, it is inorganic. Bacteria within the body then convert the inorganic mercury to organic mercury, called methyl mercury, which is extremely toxic and deadly because of its ability to pass through cell barriers in the body. Methyl mercury triggers an increase in Candida albicans in the body.

Here again, it is impressive and amazing how the innate wisdom of the human body works. Even though candida causes many other problems in the body, the body tries to limit damage to the lesser of two evils. The positive benefit is that candida converts methyl mercury back to its inorganic state, which is less toxic. But, other bacteria then go right back to work attempting to balance the candida population, leaving inorganic mercury to convert back to methyl mercury. This vicious cycle repeats itself until the immune system becomes too weak and the body gives in to disease or until a removal of mercury from the mouth and body tissues occurs. In the case of mercury poisoning, the appearance of candida is a coping mechanism by the body and a signal for assistance to rid it of the heavy metal that is wreaking havoc within all its systems.

There are so many factors that can cause chemical imbalances within the body and work against its ability to deliver health. This can be very confusing. But is there a common denominator? That is the subject of the next chapter, where we examine the body's one critical chemistry requirement for health.

# 10 | THE CRITICAL CHEMISTRY OF HEALTH

≈

*The best and most efficient pharmacy is within your own system.*

ROBERT C. PEALE

≈

## A BASIC CLUE

WE ALL KNOW we can live many days without food, a few days without water, but without oxygen, we die within a few minutes. This most important nutrient of the body should give us a big clue to the secret of health.

When the oxygen content in and around the cells of our bodies is optimum, disease symptoms do not manifest. As oxygen content decreases, the various aliments and diseases that plague us increase. Viruses, parasites, and fungi thrive in an oxygen-deficient environment. These facts lead us to understand a basic key to health and disease.

As the body's acid/alkaline ratio becomes more acidic, oxygen levels decrease. When it is balanced, oxygen levels are optimized, and that is how vital health is established.

## THE BODY'S ACID-ALKALINE BALANCE

Without acid-alkaline balance we cannot achieve true health. It is that fundamental. The human body was designed to function best in a slightly alkaline state, and it has awesome innate intelligence to be healthy. Still, it depends on us to supply its requirements of good food and positive attitudes. It always seeks balance or homeostasis, and works to produce optimum health. It never makes a mistake, and always does what is necessary given the circumstances it is dealing with.

### pH Is "Potential for Health"

Technically, pH means potential of hydrogen. But, because it is so critical to health, Dr. M. T. Morter calls it "potential for health."[1] I also refer to it as your passport to health, because when you get it right, that is where your body goes.

### Understanding pH

The pH scale is used to measure acid and alkaline strength. pH, or hydrogen ion concentration measures, are from 0 to 14. Zero is the most acidic and 14 the most alkaline; 7 is neutral. Balanced liquids have a pH of 7. The body *must* maintain a blood pH as close as possible to an alkaline level of 7.4. If blood pH moves 0.2 either way, the body dies.[2] The body does whatever it must in order to keep blood pH healthy. A small change in pH has a large effect in the body.

The pH scale for acid-alkaline is similar to the Richter scale for measuring the intensity of earthquakes; they are both measures of exponential change. Each one-point change in the scale results in a tenfold change in strength. For example, a reading of pH 6.0 indicates an effective acid strength of ten (10), while an acid at pH 5.0 would be ten times as strong again, with a strength of one hundred (10 × 10). A pH of 4.0 compared to a pH of 7.0 would have a strength of one thousand (10 × 10 × 10). Similarly, as a fluid pH moves upward on the scale, it increases exponentially in alkaline strength.

When healthy, cells of the body are slightly alkaline. In disease, cellular pH is below 6.8. The more acidic cells become, the sicker we are and feel. Cells do not die until their pH falls to approximately 3.5, but in the process of getting there, all kinds of disease symptoms can manifest.

The pH of saliva and urine, upon waking, are reliable indicators of the acidity or alkalinity of body fluids and tissues. Saliva pH indicates the effect that emotions are having on body chemistry. It can also be an indication of the strength of the body's alkaline reserve. The pH of the first urine of the day is the main reflector of the level of acidity or alkalinity within the body. It provides a picture of what the kidneys are attempting to eliminate. Minerals that the body voids through urine are mainly the excess of either acid or alkaline water soluble minerals. It gives us an indication of whether we fed our body an acidifying diet or an alkalizing diet. When alkaline reserves have been exhausted, however, the urine pH will always indicate acidity, except in cases of more serious illness when pH appears to be normal, but actually is not. More on this later.

During the day, the pH of both saliva and urine is influenced by what we eat and drink; therefore, they will fluctuate. Saliva pH is also affected by our emotions. Stress and tension from negative emotions such as anger, worry, fear, resentment, and jealousy are significant body acidifiers, causing a drain on our alkaline mineral reserves.

### Healthy pH Balance

In perfect balance and health, both saliva and urine, upon waking, should be in the 6.8–7.2 range. The objective is to have them both at about 7.0. Just as water in a swimming pool develops problems when its acid-alkaline ratio becomes unbalanced, so does the human body. If swimming pool water is allowed to become too acid or too alkaline, cloudiness in the water or problems with algae become evident; the water environment becomes a medium for unhealthy organisms. To achieve the proper balance for clear water again, the pH must be adjusted by adding the required acid or alkaline chemicals. The same thing happens within our bodies, except that we don't notice it unless we test for it. The problems are still there regardless, preparing a medium for disease conditions.

### Research Findings

The maintenance of a proper acid-alkaline balance is critical to all functions in the body. Aging is the result of accumulation of acid waste products.[3] Research has shown that when the pH of the first urine of the day is under 6.4, the body cannot optimally assimilate vitamins or minerals,[4] and that digestion and assimilation processes are severely handicapped. Digestive difficulties begin even before this level of acidity is reached:

> Clinical research by Dr. M. T. Morter (Arkansas, U.S.A.) has shown that if the anabolic urinary and saliva pH (measured immediately upon awakening) is below 6.8, we can be relatively certain that digestive support must be provided. Controlled clinical studies by Dr. Paul Yanick (Pasadena, U.S.A.) have confirmed Dr. Morter's findings and recorded that intracellular assimilation of nutrients is significantly decreased when the anabolic pH is below 6.8. [5]

## ACIDITY

As the body moves into an acid condition, called acidosis, this sets the stage for cellular changes. Cells start adapting to the changing environment, and as a result begin to change form and function. When this process has continued long enough, symptoms of dis-ease begin to develop in the body.

### Symptoms of Body Acidosis[6]
Beginning symptoms include:

- Acne
- Agitation
- Bloating
- Chemical sensitivities to odors
- Cold hands and feet
- Constant throat clearing
- Constipation
- Dizziness
- Excess head mucus (stuffiness)
- Fatigue
- Food allergies

- Morning lethargy
- Heartburn
- Hot urine
- Hyperactivity
- Indigestion
- Irregular heartbeat
- Joint pains that travel
- Lack of sex drive
- Low energy
- Metallic taste in the mouth
- Mild headaches
- Muscular pain
- Panic attacks
- Premenstrual and menstrual cramping
- Premenstrual anxiety and depression
- Rapid heartbeat
- Rapid panting breath
- Slow circulation
- Strong smelling urine
- Weight problems
- White coated tongue
- Plus more …

Intermediate symptoms include:

- Acid reflux
- Asthma
- Bacterial infections
- Bowel disorders
- Bronchitis
- Cold sores (Herpes I & II)
- Colitis
- Cystitis
- Depression

- Diarrhea
- Disturbances in smell, taste,
- Earaches, vision, hearing
- Endometriosis
- Excessive falling hair
- Fungal infections (candida, athlete's foot, vaginal)
- Gallstones
- Gastritis
- Hayfever
- Hives
- Impotence
- Insomnia
- Loss of concentration
- Loss of memory
- Migraine headaches
- Numbness and tingling
- Psoriasis
- Sinusitis
- Stuttering
- Swelling
- Urethritis
- Urinary infections
- Viral infections (colds, flu)
- Weight problems
- Plus more …

Advanced symptoms include:

- Arthritis
- Crohn's disease
- Diabetes
- Excess weight gain
- Fibromyalgia
- Heart disease

- Hodgkin's disease
- Learning disabilities
- Leukemia
- Lou Gehrig's disease
- Lupus
- Multiple sclerosis
- Muscular dystrophy
- Myasthenia gravis
- Parkinson's disease
- Sarcoidosis
- Schizophrenia
- Scleroderma
- Tuberculosis
- All other forms of cancer

### How the Body Becomes Acidic

Acid conditions within the body are produced by certain foods and beverages we eat and drink, physical exercise, stress, negative emotions, contaminated air, and by thousands of chemicals in processed food products, personal and household soaps, cleaners, and skin treatments we use.

A diet of overcooked foods, junk foods, foods devoid of live enzymes, and foods that leave an acid residue place an increasing amount of stress on our bodies.

The main offenders are:

- Protein, especially animal
- Shellfish
- Caffeine
- Dairy products, especially pasteurized, processed
- Nicotine
- Sugar and artificial sweeteners
- Carbonated beverages, soft drinks
- Table salt
- Margarine, commercial cooking oils

- Processed flour products, pasta, pastries
- Grains
- Alcohol

The normal waste products of cellular metabolism are acidic. The body has to neutralize the acids because a healthy blood pH must be maintained at all costs. It does this with alkaline minerals. The only sources of alkaline minerals for the body are from the foods we consume, the supplements we may be taking, or from its own tissue stores. As alkaline minerals are used to neutralize acids, they are then excreted in urine and lost. This is how the body's alkaline reserve becomes depleted if it is not replenished through proper nutrition. A diet that is predominated by animal and dairy protein produces excess acids, which depletes the body's vital stores of alkaline minerals.

### How the Body Neutralizes Acids

In a healthy state, the fluid in and around the cells of the body is neutral to slightly alkaline. The by-products from a diet of fruit and vegetables, normal cellular wastes, and exercise are weak acids that the body easily eliminates via the lungs. However, acid by-products from the metabolism of other foods, especially animal proteins, are very strong. The body needs to neutralize the acid minerals from such foods with alkaline minerals from its own reserves. As indicated previously, the more acidic our cellular chemistry is, the harder our bodies have to work to combat the acidity. This process is called buffering, and the body uses several minerals to do this.

When strong acids are produced from the metabolization of food, organic sodium is used first, to bring intracellular fluid pH up to 6.1. Next, organic potassium reacts with the now weaker acids to bring pH back to a near neutral 6.8. When the intake of acid-forming foods continues to be more than the intake of alkaline-forming foods, the alkaline reserves of sodium and potassium become depleted. The body is then forced to move to its backup buffer system, which requires the withdrawal of calcium from its bones.[7] If the body is forced to continue this backup buffer process due to a lack of sufficient alkaline foods in the diet, serious bone loss can result. According to Dr. M. T. Morter:

> Anyone who eats more than 47 grams of protein a day—no matter what the source of the protein—will eventually develop osteoporosis.[8]

Although calcium and its supplement forms can act as effective acid buffers, calcium is not meant to do this on a permanent basis. The primary alkaline buffer minerals of sodium and potassium need to be restored to the body. They are vital to continued health.

In the absence of sufficient reserves of sodium, or in the presence of excess protein, the kidneys can produce ammonia to eliminate nitrogen, an acid mineral, via the urine. This ammonia has a pH of 9.23, which would give urine a neutral or slightly alkaline pH. However, this system can only be utilized on a short-term basis.[9] The alkaline urine pH in this situation is misleading—the body is actually in extreme acidosis. The acidic condition has not been neutralized throughout the body. The positive result represents a short-term gain from what amounts to damage control. One sometimes detects this odor of ammonia in homes or hospitals for the seriously ill.

## CELLULAR OXYGEN

The most important nourishment for the body is oxygen, since all functions require this element to operate efficiently. The body always tries to maintain an alkaline blood pH near 7.4. Research has shown that the maximum amount of oxygen is transported to cells at this specific pH.[10] Blood pH is influenced by cellular pH throughout the body, and the pH of the body's cellular and intracellular fluids is determined by the quantity of acids in the system. As cellular pH becomes more acid, it has an acidifying influence on the blood, causing it to carry less oxygen.

Cells normally produce energy by using oxygen. As acidification increases, and less oxygen is available, the energy production in cells must

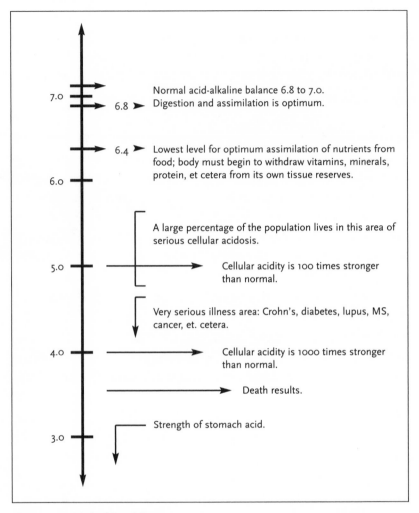

**Figure 10.1 pH in health and disease**

shift from an aerobic (oxygen) process, to an anaerobic (lack of oxygen) process, which utilizes fermentation. This results in a ten-fold decrease in efficiency of energy production.[11]

Disease organisms thrive in an anaerobic environment; the more acidic a body becomes, the faster disease organisms multiply. Dr. Otto Warburg, mentioned in chapter 3, discovered that cancer cannot live in the presence of oxygen. He stated that: "The fundamental cause of all degenerative disease is hypoxia; oxygen starvation at the cellular level."[12] Scientists and researchers have added to this discovery and it now appears that no disease causing organism, bacteria, virus, fungus, yeast, parasite, amoeboid, or cancer cell can live and reproduce in a high oxygen, increased electron, alkaline body environment.[13]

As cellular oxygen increases, fermentation in cells decreases, and cellular metabolism improves. Food is "burned" more efficiently. Obnoxious bacteria and parasites are killed, and excess fat storage is reduced. If the body was overweight, it begins to lose weight. Daily energy also increases. Figure 10.1 shows, in summary format, the main relationships of cellular pH to health and disease in the human body.

In summary, when the body's pH is out of balance (below 6.8), we cannot digest and assimilate food and supplements effectively. This means we do not benefit from their essential nutrients; most of them pass right through us. Our cells gradually begin to metabolize at a lower rate and body mineral reserves start to deplete. But when the body is in an acid-alkaline balance, cellular oxygenation is optimized, and the body is able to function efficiently, heal faster, and return to health. Additional information on how to check, monitor, and correct the body's pH can be found in chapter 21.

### Healthy Diet

A healthy diet should consist of approximately 80% alkaline-forming foods and 20% acid-forming foods. Most raw fruits and vegetables are alkaline foods. These must be regularly supplied to the body to maintain a healthy balance between acid and alkaline. The factor that determines the alkali in a food is its content of alkaline minerals, mainly, sodium, calcium, magnesium, potassium, and iron.

*Caution:* When switching from a very acidic, predominantly cooked food diet, the transition to a healthier diet should be done gradually to allow the body time to adjust its production of enzymes required to process more raw food. Otherwise, considerable discomfort could be experienced.

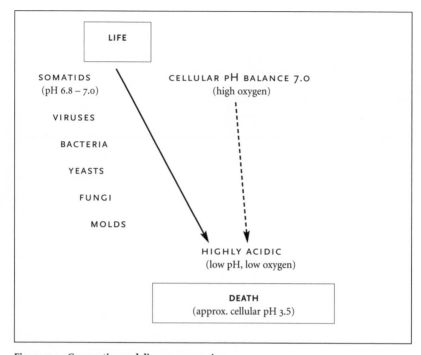

**Figure 10.2  Composting and disease progression**

## COMPOSTING AND DISEASE

Some disease-causing bacteria, viruses, and parasites thrive and multiply in an anaerobic environment. They actually perform an important function in nature by appearing in toxic and rotting areas to consume waste. This is what happens in our garden compost pile; microorganisms convert dead plant and animal matter back to soil.

This process happens in us too. Because of our typical diets, most of us are acidic and therefore have less than optimum levels of oxygen in our systems. This allows microform bacteria to grow and proliferate, and in the process, drain our energy reserves. When we die, these little creatures really go to work and are able to compost the dead body back to the soil. While living, the body is meant to be slightly alkaline. After we die, the body, the corpse, becomes fully acidic, which allows the microorganisms to multiply without restriction in order to complete their composting work.

### Pleomorphic Life Forms

The smallest living units within us, much smaller than our cells, have been called microzymes, and more recently are referred to as protits or somatids.[14] They are in the cells, in extracellular fluid, lymph, and blood. What is interesting about somatids is that when the body terrain has become too acidic and natural fermentation has accelerated, they have the ability to "pleomorph," or change form and function, to become viruses, bacteria, yeast, fungus, and eventually, mold, as oxygen levels continue to decrease.[15]

Because these organisms are part of nature, when they experience an acidic body environment, they "think" the body is in the process of dying, so they proceed with their composting job. By allowing acid to build up in our bodies, we are actually initiating this process ourselves. The process of chronic disease is activated when a person is toxic enough to push the "composting button." An example of this is fermentation that triggers cancer.[16]

### Microform Bacteria

Microorganisms, also called microform bacteria, are always present in our bodies to some degree. The strength of their populations depends upon how much toxic debris has been allowed to build up in the body and how acidic the body's terrain has become. The problem is that, as parasites, these microforms live off the energy that is meant to be utilized by us. In addition, they produce mycotoxin acids in their excrement, which further reduces the body's pH as well as cellular oxygen levels. Essentially, they work to compost our toxic bodies toward death while we are alive; but they can only advance their cause if they have the right environment.

### Turning the Composting Button Off

Our objective is to stop the fermentation that allows microform bacteria to multiply and pleomorph. The key to reducing or eliminating microform bacteria is to remove their food sources. Their main food sources are acid-producing foods, especially meats and dairy, acid beverages, sugar in all its forms, plus foods that convert into sugars, for example, potatoes, rice, pasta, and pastries. (See appendices 1 to 4 for a more complete listing.) If we keep our digestive tracts clean and our acid-alkaline ratios balanced, cellular oxygen levels will remain high and microform bacteria will not be able to change into their composting varieties.

Up to this point, we have considered most of the main elements that can work against our bodies. We will now shift our focus to the conditions our bodies require to be able to produce health.

# 11 | WHAT THE BODY NEEDS FOR HEALTH

*I believe the doctor of the future will be a teacher as well as a physician. His real job will be to teach people how to be healthy.*

Dr. D.C. Jarvis

## COOPERATING WITH THE BODY

IF WE WANT the body to serve us well, we must take care of it. The human body is a cooperative working enterprise with great intelligence and capabilities. It was created to serve us, but it also has requirements of us. We need to honor, respect and cooperate with it as a valued friend if we want it to perform at its best and serve us a long time.

All parts of the body are interdependent. They depend on each other to carry out their functions so that the whole body benefits. If one area is overloaded, other parts have to take on extra tasks to accomplish the collective job; this causes increased stress and energy loss. The body depends on us to supply its basic needs so that it can produce health.

We usually try to avoid injuring the tissues of our bodies through trauma or exposure to temperature extremes. When we are injured, or are too hot or too cold, we experience pain and the loss of certain body functions and mobility almost immediately, so we tend to take corrective action quite quickly. However, we cannot feel the effects of nutritional deficiencies immediately because they happen so slowly.

## NUTRITION

Nutrition is the most important overall consideration we have to make. Any farmer knows that without proper nutrition, his livestock will not grow to be at their marketable and performing best; it is the same with our own bodies. All living organisms require a regular supply of the full range of nutrients to survive and thrive. Those nutrients must include live enzymes that help provide working energy for a long and healthy life. If we do not put quality nutrition in, we cannot expect to get quality performance out. If we put dirty gasoline into the fuel tank of a car, we know it will not be able to function properly, perform smoothly, and provide trouble-free service for us. However, we regularly do something similar with our bodies. Why?

We do not seem to realize that junk, processed, and chemically-enriched foods are very harmful to our bodies. We have not educated ourselves nor have we been educated about the true nutritional requirements our bodies have. We have been conditioned by our family upbringing, advertising, and busy lifestyles to eat foods that have been prepared in certain ways. We have grown to like the taste of particular foods and are reluctant to give them up. Nevertheless, after a time of switching to healthy eating, our tastes can change. The unhealthy foods that used to taste good will no longer appeal to us as much. Healthy foods that satisfy the body's requirements will become more and more appealing as time goes on. The flavors of quality foods are more satisfying to our taste buds than the tantalizing tastes of denatured and poor quality foods.

As the body becomes cleaner and more efficient, it becomes easier to feel its reactions when we eat unhealthy foods. We can sense and understand its system of communication with us. A simple example of this is indigestion, or heartburn. The body is trying to tell us that the food or combination of foods we have eaten is wrong and is causing stress, or that the digestive system is weak. But, do we listen and then work with the body? Typically, we do not. We take antacids, and because they are advertised everywhere and are used by so many people, we think of it as normal. Using antacids is harmful to the body in the long term. As long as we continue to ignore the body's symptoms, we continue to stress it. And, as mentioned earlier, it is stress in its various forms that causes disease and the breakdown of our bodies.

The U.S. Surgeon General's report on health and nutrition, published back in 1988, concluded that 8 out of the top 10 causes of death in America were directly related to diet.[1] The number one cause of death, heart disease, has been directly linked to trans fats from hydrogenated oils.[2] Chronic degenerative diseases in general are higher where diets are richer in animal products and in total fat.[3] Our personal choices concerning what we eat appear to have the most influence on our long-term health prospects.

We have been conditioned to eat mostly cooked foods, meat, dairy, sugar, salt, caffeine, junk foods, fried foods, processed foods, and canned foods. These may seem as if they satisfy our hunger, but they do not satisfy our nutritional needs. Industries, which control the eating habits and conditioned beliefs of the populace, desire a continuous market for their processed food. The unhealthy foods we consume make us sick. But when we do become ill, we tend to blame it on a germ or virus. The germ or virus would not have been able to get a foothold in us if the body had not been burdened with toxic and metabolic wastes, and if our immune system had been strong.

To illustrate this further, consider the environment of the mouth. At any given time, several disease-causing germs such as streptococcus, staphylococcus, tuberculosis, and pneumonia can be found in the average mouth. Why don't we have these diseases? The answer is that the body's vitality and immune system are strong enough to keep these bacteria out of the tissues. Only after the continued lowering of the body's vitality, as a result of burdening it with harmful food and starving it of the nutrients essential to building defenses, does our immune system weaken.

Because of toxic storage buildup, germs or viruses are able to germinate and grow in our bodies. All germs and viruses are scavengers. They can only feed on, survive, and multiply in toxic and decaying matter. They cannot live in healthy tissue. If we keep our bodies cleansed and free of toxic acid debris, there is no suitable environment for germs and viruses to live in. We remain in health even when others around us may be developing illnesses.

If we want to have a healthy body and vitality for a lifetime, we must take responsibility for educating ourselves, and from that, exercising personal discipline to change our lifestyles. Proper, mostly alkaline, nutrition is fundamental for building healthy cells.

## WATER

Clean water, and enough of it, is an absolute requirement for health. Everything that happens in the body happens in a medium of water. It is our second most critical requirement, after oxygen. Because the body is approximately 75% water, and the brain about 90% water, it is easy to see how even a small degree of dehydration can hinder body processes. We must consume sufficient water from raw fruits and vegetables and drinking water, every day. If we wait until we are feeling thirsty, we are already beginning to dehydrate. The subject of water will be covered in further detail in chapter 13.

## EXERCISE

Our bodies need regular exercise. Many of us shortchange this area of helping the body function properly. We do this partly through ignorance; we do not really understand how important exercise is to the body. And many of us neglect exercise because of laziness. It is hard work, takes effort and discipline, and utilizes time that we may want to devote to other things.

As far as efficient bodily function is concerned, the old saying of "move it or lose it" is very true. When the entire body is exercised, the circulation of blood is increased and the removal of metabolic wastes from cells via the lymphatic system is more efficient. Rapid muscle contractions and expansions create a pumping action on the lymphatic channels, the body's cellular elimination conduits. This action pumps toxins and wastes to the liver for filtration, and subsequent deposit into the colon for elimination from the body.

Walking, swimming, and any other activity that increases heart rate for a sustained period of twenty to forty minutes is good exercise. The best and most efficient overall exercise is five to fifteen minutes each day on a rebounder or mini-trampoline. Because it utilizes the rapid reversal of gravity, every cell in the body is exercised, thereby improving the oxygenation of cells for energy production, and lymphatic movement for the elimination of cellular wastes. Another great exercise which only requires a piece of rope is skipping. Be sure to breathe deeply during exercise and periodically throughout the day.

## WOMEN AND BRASSIERES

As a special note to women, breasts should not be bound tightly with bras all the time. Remember that the lymphatic system must move lymph fluids through connective tissues, and the only way it has of doing this is through the movement of tissue. The body needs our help in exercising each area. The continuous restriction of movement causes a constriction of fluids and obstructs lymphatic circulation. In women, the long-term restriction of the lymphatic drainage system in breasts blocks natural energy flow and can be a factor in the development of breast cancer. This can be avoided by exercising each day wearing loose apparel that allows the breasts to move.

## FRESH AIR

Breathing is very important. In one day the average person inhales about 2,880 gallons (10,901 liters) of air, which weighs more than the food and water we consume, and eliminates carbon dioxide, equivalent to eight ounces (236 ml) of charcoal, via the lungs.[4] Complete breathing is fundamental to health. When we do not breathe properly, or only practice shallow breathing, we are allowing too much carbon dioxide, a metabolic waste product, to accumulate in the body. Proper breathing is promoted by inhaling full but comfortable breaths. Shallow breathing restricts the intake of oxygen and therefore the elimination of metabolic wastes, making the blood more acidic.

Fresh air, unpolluted by fumes, car exhausts, smoke, and other particles and gases, promotes good health. Pollutants in the air we breathe are absorbed by our lungs and carried to body tissues for storage and future removal. When the pollutants are not able to be eliminated, they contribute to degenerating health and disease.

We should work and rest in well-ventilated areas; spend time in fresh outdoor air; allow our skin to "breathe" by wearing loose-fitting non-synthetic clothing; and exercise enough to cause full deep breathing every day.

A healthy regimen would include five to ten minutes of slow, deep, rhythmic breathing at the beginning and end of each day. This involves inhaling through the nose and expanding the diaphragm, and pushing out the stomach area until it is fully expanded before filling the lungs; and finally, exhaling through the mouth to empty the chest first, then the diaphragm, until it is completely deflated as far as it can go. This method of breathing maximizes oxygen intake and expels stale air from the bottom of the lungs. Diaphragm breathing has the added benefit of exercising the liver, promoting more efficient circulation and function. The benefits of deep breathing, on a regular basis, are tremendous for the entire body.

## REST

The opposite of exercise is rest. The body needs regular, proper, and sufficient rest, so it can "catch up" from the day's activities and address its job of restoring energy and health. This is when energy can be redirected to manufacturing a new supply to get us through the next day, to detoxify, and to repair and build new tissue. We cannot continually go short on quality sleep and expect to regain vibrant health.

Research on sleep done by Kacper M. Postawski has found that the main factors contributing to quality sleep are going to bed at a regular time, sleeping in a darkened room, exposing our eyes to bright daylight upon waking, being outdoors in sunlight during the day, exercising moderately each day, and eating a healthy diet. In addition, daily naps of between ten and forty-five minutes are noted to be very beneficial to health. However, napping longer than forty-five minutes can induce states of deep sleep that may be difficult to wake from; long naps can also interfere with the regular night sleep cycle. By adopting these habits, a person will have more restful sleep, feel more energized, and actually, may require one or two hours less sleep each night.[5]

## ADEQUATE TIME TO ELIMINATE WASTES

The body needs adequate time to eliminate metabolic wastes. It can do this properly only when it is not being required to digest and assimilate food. It counts on having sufficient time between the evening meal and the next day's first meal to do this. When it is not given this time, the body stores the wastes, which reduces cell function efficiency and sets the stage for degenerative disease conditions. The habit of eating late in the evening places an extra load on the body and works against the elimination cycle. We assist the body when we do not eat solid food in the evening, and when we extend the body's time for elimination by eating fresh, ripe, raw fruit for breakfast, since such foods are cleansing and do not halt the elimination process.

## SKIN CARE

Skin is much more than an outer covering for the body; it also protects the more sensitive tissues beneath. It is the largest organ of the body and a major organ for the elimination of metabolic wastes. Waste products are disposed of through the skin as we perspire. The skin also plays important roles in regulating body temperature and manufacturing vitamin D from sunshine.

Considering the skin's many roles, we should appreciate the importance of keeping it free of soaps and chemicals, allowing it to breathe and perform its functions unencumbered. All these substances, many of which are toxic, clog the pores, which then forces toxins and waste products to accumulate in the skin and in the deeper layers of the body. This reduces the body's ability to eliminate metabolic wastes, which can lead to disease as well as discomfort and loss of self-esteem when the skin doesn't look and feel healthy. Using soap on the body washes natural protective oils out of the skin and causes dryness. Moisturizing lotions clog the pores, which further hinders the elimination of wastes.

A skin problem is never a problem by itself. It is an indication that the entire body is suffering. When a skin problem is evident, it is due to the body's attempt to dump toxic wastes. Unhealthy skin is a prime indication that there are more serious malfunctions within the body. When the skin has difficulties, there is always a problem in the colon, and probably in other areas as well.

Fingernails and toenails are actually skin. If they are dry, cracked, brittle, or ridged, it is a sign that all is not right with the health of the rest of the body, and with the nutrition being supplied to it.

As an aside, why and how do antiperspirants work? The skin is a sensitive and vital organ designed to protect the body from harmful substances. Antiperspirants work because aluminum chlorhydrate, found in most underarm deodorants, is so toxic to the body the pores immediately close in an attempt to keep it out of the body. Nevertheless, some of the chemical is inevitably absorbed through the skin. It is thought that there is a strong link between aluminum and the development of Alzheimer's disease.

An excellent exercise for the skin is brushing it vigorously and regularly with a soft, natural fiber brush, which can be purchased from a healthfood store. A good time to brush the skin is just before a shower. This helps remove dead skin, unclog the pores, and improve blood and lymph circulation. The skin is naturally acidic. Rubbing the body all over after a shower with a dilute solution of unpasteurized apple cider vinegar will help keep the skin healthy and vital.

Moderate exposure of skin to the sun promotes health in many ways, but must not be overdone. Gathering sun should be done for its general revitalizing benefits to the entire body, but not to tan for the sake of appearance. Suntan oils and lotions are harmful and should not be used because they are toxic. In addition, they reduce the efficiency of the skin's oil-producing glands and block the absorption of ultraviolet rays as a source of energy for the body. Hemp oil, which has a natural sun protection factor of 15, may be used.

The body produces healthy, good looking skin in response to a healthy diet that is rich in enzymes, vitamins, minerals, oils and fiber, and adequate quantities of pure water. It also requires exercise, rest, moderate exposure to the sun, and efficient elimination. The same factors also apply to healthy hair and a scalp that is free of dandruff. One should avoid harsh or medicated shampoos, hair treatments, dyes, hot temperatures from hair dryers and curlers, and too frequent washing of hair, as these are all stressful to the hair and scalp. In a like manner, commercial toothpastes, breath fresheners, and gargles should be avoided, because they contain toxic chemicals that are absorbed in the mouth and taken into the body. Ideally, we should use a minimum of skin, hair, and toothpaste products. Acceptable alternatives can be obtained from healthfood stores.

## EMOTIONAL ENVIRONMENT
## RELATIVELY FREE OF STRESS

Emotional stress can have a profoundly negative influence on the health of the body. This can be due to circumstances such as a difficult or unsatisfying job, unhappy relationship, and financial difficulties. The effect of negative attitudes and the emotions of anger, fear, guilt, grief, apathy, rebellion, selfishness, bitterness, and resentment is extremely significant, and unfortunately, somewhat less understood. Such attitudes are termed negative because they have depressive and destructive effects on various organs and glands in the body. They are very acid-producing.

When the body's functional balance is impaired for long periods by an overly acidic internal environment, dysfunction begins to develop and early aging sets in, along with feelings of decreased energy. Keeping energy reserves high is key to staying young and healthy. Understanding energy is the subject of the next chapter.

# 1 2 | ENERGY

∾

*We don't live off the food that we eat;*
*we live off the energy in the food we eat!*
DR. CAREY REAMS

∾

WHEN WE HAVE energy, we feel great. We are usually "upbeat," and feel anything is possible. That's the way we are supposed to feel. Traditional Chinese medicine calls this concept of internal energy "Chi." It is also known as "Ki," "Qi," or "Vital Life Force." Oriental medicine has known for thousands of years that a subtle energy field exists in the body, and that when the energy pathways are open, a person is in superior physical, mental, emotional, and spiritual health.

## ENERGY IS EVERYWHERE

As explained in chapter 2, the energy in our bodies is actually electricity, or polarized energy. We learn from quantum physics that everything in the universe is an expression of energy. Solid objects are actually composed of spinning and vibrating energy vortices. This invisible energy is everywhere and composes itself into different combinations of atomic structure to form matter. Energy vortices that are not physical matter are free to move and are available to be accessed and directed for our use. Western medicine has yet to incorporate this concept into its understanding and practice.

In a healthy state, life force circulates freely throughout the body. Chinese medicine places a great focus on opening up energy pathways, or meridians, so the body is better able to return to health. In an unhealthy body, our natural energy can be lowered by stress, a buildup of toxins, and illness. When energy is flowing freely throughout, the body is able to regenerate and detoxify itself, and is better able to cope with the stresses and strains of life. Health is directly dependent on energy flow.

## ENERGY IS ALL ABOUT ELECTRICITY

The human body runs on electrical energy. When we are low on energy, we do not feel strong, and cannot accomplish much work. We all know what it is like to feel tired. Most of us have probably said: "I feel pooped," or "I feel drained"; and we were. When we have lots of energy, life seems to take on a new brightness. We feel better physically, mentally, and emotionally. But when we don't have energy, we feel older than we actually are. This makes sense because aging is the result of a general loss of electrical vitality in the body.

Our bodily energy is electrical. When we say, "I feel drained," we are stating an electrical truth. It simply means our reserves of electrical energy are down; our batteries are getting low. Remember that each cell in the body functions as a little electrical battery. The body depends on living, electrically active food that is suitable for conversion into electrical matrices to recharge its own cells.

All processes that take place in the body are electrical in nature. Healing, getting stronger, and overcoming disease all depend on adequate reserves of energy being available. Most of the energy we feel during the day is manufactured the night before, while we are asleep. That is why getting adequate rest is so important. Digestion, for example, requires a tremendous amount of energy. When the general energy reserve in the body is low, digestive processes are inefficient. A person may be eating the best of foods as well as taking nutritional supplements, but their body may not have enough energy to properly break down the nutrition and convert it into a useful energy form. The food just passes through without the person receiving much benefit.

## BIOELECTRICAL ENERGY

Vital force energy, or bioelectricity as it is known in the West, can actually be measured. Dr. Timothy Ray[1] speaks of amperage measurements to indicate the strength of this bioenergy field. The body's normal electrical strength, measured at the end points of acupuncture meridians, is between 400 and 800nA (nano-amps). (Nano means one-billionth.) When the body's electrical strength is below 400 nA, it is operating on a weak charge. This "low battery" reading, so to speak, means the body has a lowered potential for efficient functioning. In electrical terms, we might say there is resistance in the body interfering with the generation and smooth flow of energy currents. When the body's electrical strength is too low, it cannot properly digest, process, and assimilate foods, supplements, and herbs.

## HOW OUR ENERGY IS CREATED

Energy is produced within the cells, specifically in the mitochondria, which are the cells' power sources. The main fuels used are glucose, produced in the liver, and oxygen. The end result of the process is energy in the form of high-energy electrons and ATP (adenosine triphosphate). ATP is the main source of usable energy for cells. The food we eat is processed through many metabolic steps in order to arrive at this ultimate energy form. The production of sufficient ATP depends on a properly functioning body that is receiving adequate nutrients through food and liquid intake, as well as essential fatty acids and alkaline minerals, which optimize the oxygen-carrying capacity of hemoglobin.

## INCREASING OUR ENERGY

### Areas to Focus on

There are seven main areas we can focus on to maximize energy production within our bodies.

1 *Maximize Oxygen Generation.* Oxygen is the most vital nutrient requirement of the body. The less acidic the cells of our bodies are, the more oxygen they can hold. (Chapter 10).

2 *Detoxification.* Cooperate with the body by helping it reduce its load of toxic wastes. (Chapter 13).

3 *Nutrition.* The human body requires a healthy, predominantly alkaline, whole live food diet to manufacture health. (Chapter 15).

4 *Rest.* The body can only create energy during sleep or rest.

5 *Water.* Ideal water for our body is structured and contains natural biophotonic energy. (Chapter 14).

6 *Reduce Emotional Stress.* Negative emotions place a great strain on energy resources. (Chapters 17, 18).

7 *Minimize or Neutralize Noxious External Energies.* Electromagnetic fields and geopathic radiations may be interfering with the natural flow of energy within in our bodies. (Chapter 8).

### B Vitamins

The B complex vitamins warrant a special mention here because they are vital to an energetic life. This complex comprises a group of eight vitamins: thiamine (B1), riboflavin (B2), niacin (B3), pyridoxine (B6), folic acid (B9), cyanocobalamin (B12), biotin, and pantothenic acid.

I have not gone into deep discussion about individual vitamins in this book because on a well-balanced diet they should be adequately supplied. Nevertheless, on a continual diet of processed food, or one that is mostly vegetarian, a deficiency in one or more of the B vitamins can develop. In earlier times, vitamin B was amply obtained from diets that included organ meats and whole grains, but few diets still include such foods. By

1970, Adelle Davis had already stated that, "the 15 or more B vitamins are so meagerly supplied in our American diet that almost every person lacks them."[2]

Vitamins in the B complex are required for metabolism in every cell in the body; they are central to the cellular production and release of energy. The main sources of B vitamins are liver, brewer's yeast, wheat germ, and rice polishings. When supplementing, we should always look to food sources that supply the whole complex of vitamin B rather than taking the chemical versions of individual, or combination, vitamins. The body only recognizes nutrition from whole, living foods and herbs as complete vitamin sources.

### Iron

Closely related to the B vitamins for energy production is iron. A deficiency of this mineral can lead to anemia, with symptoms such as fatigue, short attention span, weight loss, and irritability. Iron is needed in red blood cells to form hemoglobin, whose primary role is to collect oxygen from the lungs and carry it to every cell in the body.

The main sources of iron are red meat, liver, dried fruit, egg yolks, sardines, spinach, broccoli, wheat germ, and brown barley. Vegetarians especially can become iron deficient due to an insufficient intake of foods that contain iron. Attention should be given to ensure sufficient iron is being obtained from several different food sources or from whole food mineral supplements.

## RAISING OUR ELECTRICAL POTENTIAL

Our magnificent human body has a tremendous ability to draw on and enhance the universal energy that is freely accessible to us all. This potential lies dormant and untapped in most people, even though Oriental cultures have been accessing it for ages.

## Qigong

Qi, pronounced "chi," in Chinese means internal energy; "gong" means exercise. Qigong is a gentle physical training practice which combines breathing with various physical movements of the body, mostly hand and arm. Qigong and another form of exercise, Tai Chi, have been practiced in many forms for thousands of years. They are mostly taught for the benefit of increasing energy flow in the body, and achieving and maintaining good health and a youthful appearance through stress reduction and exercise. Body movements, coordinated with breathing, enhance energy to such an extent that one can actually feel it, at first in the hands, and then throughout the body, as a gentle electric current or tingling magnetism. Even beginners can feel these sensations in their bodies quite easily.

Qigong teachers explain that, besides taking in oxygen, we are also collecting life force, or Qi, to store in the body. We can then move the energy to the direct benefit of organs and for the healing and rejuvenation of the whole body. A little time spent on the Internet will reveal many sources about Qigong as well as testimonies of illness recoveries.

## Quantum Touch

Quantum touch, or hands-on healing, is an easily-learned skill that can provide comfort, balance, healing, and even postural alignment to the body. Richard Gordon explains in his book *Quantum-Touch*, that love is the universal "foundation of all healing and the core-essence of life-force."[3] Through breathing techniques, body awareness, and intention, a person is able to raise the life-force energy vibrations in their hands. With a little practice, these vibrations are clearly evident and can become very strong. The body draws on its innate intelligence to access universal chi, or prana, as it is called in India. Chi is then intensified and transferred through the hands to promote healing in other living things. Quantum touch works on the principle that areas of illness, vibrating as they do at lower frequencies, will naturally move to harmonize with the higher vibrations being held by the quantum touch practitioner. It is the loving intent and focused attention that allows quantum touch to work. Energy follows thought.

Quantum touch gives us the ability to connect with our latent spiritual power to energize and heal ourselves and others.

## Chiropractic Adjustment

Chiropractic is a drug-free, non-surgical science that focuses on total body wellness including fitness, nutrition, and psychology. Its objective is to restore efficient energy flow in the body. When people think of chiropractic treatment, most think "back pain relief," but that is only a part of what chiropractic focuses on.

The muscular structure that holds our spines and other body parts in proper alignment can become weakened due to various stresses, improper nutrition, and lack of fitness. As this happens, the spinal vertebrae, and discs between them, can slip out of place. This "subluxation" creates pressure on, or irritates, spinal nerves. The nervous system provides pathways for energy and command signals to flow from one part of the body to another. Since nerves from the spine go to all parts of the body, subluxations can cause malfunctions throughout the body (most significantly, in internal organs) because of insufficient electrical communication from the brain.

True chiropractic treatment focuses on restoring health to the entire spinal column and balancing the nervous system to restore life force to an optimum level, so energy can flow freely from the head down, and from inside to the outside. There is strong logic to support the practice of regular, gentle spinal adjustment as part of an ongoing personal health program to promote the efficient flow of energy within the body.

When seeking the services of a chiropractor, it is important to ask what the doctor's philosophy is. Does he or she work to restore neurological function (life force), or mainly focus on the manipulation of the vertebrae for the purpose of restoring spinal function to relieve pain? The former practitioner is concerned with assisting the innate intelligence of the body to restore its optimum function, and the latter with just reducing pain or discomfort.

## ELECTRONICS AND ENERGY ASSISTANCE

Some inventors in the field of electronics have used their knowledge of quantum physics to develop instruments that can work with the body to enhance its bioenergy. These instruments can be a helpful addition to natural modes of energy enhancement.

It is my opinion that, over a period of time, boosts of energy and improvement in energy flow from technology can help the body recharge, detoxify, and rebuild itself to a certain extent. Understand clearly though, these devices don't in themselves do anything *to* the body. They make energy available to the body, which the body then uses according to its own capability and need. Any positive changes will only be temporary, unless and until proper pH, nutrient, and mineral stores are balanced in the body.

### Chi Machine

Dr. Shizuo Inoue, Chairman of Japan's Oxygen Health Association, spent many years researching the relationship between oxygen levels and the quality of health in the human body. After watching goldfish swim, and noting how healthy and well toned they were, he surmised that the steady undulating movement of their spines showed how their bodies were exercised and oxygenated. This concept was then engineered into a machine that replicated this pattern of motion in the human body. He called the machine a "Chi Machine" because it actually increases chi or life force within the body.

A person lies on their back on a firm floor and places their ankles on the Chi Machine. When the machine is turned on, it moves the ankles from side to side, stimulating a body response through gentle figure-eight oscillations of the body. Over time, many benefits can be achieved. The main ones are as follows: optimization of oxygen intake; activation of the lymph system; movement of spinal fluid; increased energy; strengthened immune and respiratory systems; and exercising and strengthening of the spine. The Chi Machine actually provides an aerobic workout for the whole body. Its developers claim that five minutes on one of these units is equivalent to walking more than a mile, without expending the energy that walking requires.

Chi machines come in various models. While the original was the "Chi Machine," clones of varying quality are now available. Before deciding which model to buy, ask suppliers of health equipment, and search the Internet. In my view, using one of these machines once or twice a day is a good health investment.

### Pulsed Electromagnetic Therapy

The use of pulsed electromagnetic fields is a relatively new form of physical thereapy in North America, although it has been used in Europe for many years. Pulsed magnetic fields are different than permanent magnetic fields and are reported to produce much superior physical health benefits, without negative side effects. When the body is exposed to a pulsating bio-energetic field within its own healthy electrical frequency range, it is able to free itself from inharmonious electrical interference at the cellular level and reestablish "normal biological rhythms."[4]

Benefits claimed and reported from the influence of pulsed electromagnetic field devices include: increased energy, increased oxygenation and blood circulation, improved nourishment of cells, stronger immune function, better removal of toxins from cells, reduction of stress, improved sleep, and improvement of many disease symptoms, including relief from chronic pain.

Pulsating electromagnetic therapy devices such as matress pads for home use can be found on the Internet. As with all health aids, one should conduct their own due diligence before purchasing and using such devices.

### SCENAR

The SCENAR (Self-Controlled Energetic Neuro Adaptive Regulator), was invented in Russia for the Russian cosmonaut program. Because they didn't want the cosmonauts taking medications while flying, their scientists developed this device to enhance the body's own healing resources. Using direct biofeedback, the SCENAR identifies and works to remove energy blockages in the body. The device has been widely used in Russia since the 1980s but remained a secret until perestroika. It is starting to be used in the West, and appears to be quite effective for improving many disorders. An advanced version of the SCENAR is now available as the Tennant Biomodulator.

## VIBRATIONAL ENERGY MEDICINE

Homeopathy is energy medicine. It is based on the principle of "like curing like." When a very dilute concentration of an illness-causing substance is administered (usually under the tongue) repeatedly over time, the body's own defense system is mobilized to overcome the offending problem, and the result is normalized energy pathways and healthy functioning.

Homeopathy was widely practiced in the 1800s, with successes greatly exceeding allopathic medicine, which used combative drug therapy. The pharmaceutical industry and the American Medical Association squeezed homeopathy out of the health practice picture in the early 1900s by discrediting it and providing financial support to only those medical colleges that offered instruction based on pharmaceuticals. In the last decade, however, homeopathy has made a comeback, especially among naturopathic physicians. It continues to gain more recognition because of its non-invasive nature and because the dosages used are very dilute and non-stressful to the body, and quite simply, because it works!

Dr. Herbert DeloRey is a researcher and practitioner in the field of energy medicine.[5] What is interesting about his work is that he has taken computerized electronic analysis technology, like the "Interro" and the "Quantum Xrroid" systems, and married them to homeopathy. This involves studies in quantum physics and advanced computer programming that lead to a "complete unconscious interface with the right hemisphere of the client's brain."[6] Working through the modality of homeopathy, he is able to assist the body to deal with issues on the physical, mental, and emotional levels. The goal is to help the brain stimulate its own acupuncture points without needles or probes. In this way, the brain can perform its own self-adjustment requirements, re-establishing the energy pathways of the spine through miniscule muscular manipulations within the body. The polarity of every cell and system within the body is re-established, thereby allowing the body to conduct its own healing. The technology is able to reflect back to the patient the deep and often hidden reasons for their health challenges. While the technology itself does not do any diagnosis or prognosis, it does highlight the precise correcting home-opathic requirements for assisting the body in effecting self-cure.

As shown by Dr. Herbert DeloRey, this type of vibrational energy medicine is a combination of electro-analysis and bioenergetic therapy. Here is how he describes it:

> The body is a highly complex electrical-chemical entity and is depend-ent upon the smooth functioning of both systems. The body's electri-cal energy is distributed throughout in a logical and sensible way, such that it interacts with its own very sophisticated and exquisitely precise chemical system. Electro-analysis is an objective method for the meas-urement of functional disorders before they become pathological. It is based on analysis of the paths of energy flow in the body.
>
> At the atomic level, every substance is composed of like matter. Each specific substance, whether metal, wood, plastic, skin or bone is governed by the amount and rotational speed of its atoms. This speed of rotation determines the electromagnetic frequency of each specific substance. Keeping this in mind, it follows that in our bodies, each specific tissue and organ has its own unique pattern of electromag-netic frequencies. When a body tissue has had an abnormal frequency for a protracted period, unnatural changes will begin to appear in the tissues' biochemistry. This translates into tissue damage and patholog-ical or degenerative conditions. Electro-analysis assesses the body functioning on the electromagnetic level. This revolutionary health breakthrough is remarkable because, not only does it give an accurate early assessment, but it also indicates to the practitioner what fre-quency that medications or supplements, specifically individualized to the client, are required to correct the condition.[7] There is no guess-work. In treatment, the most recent problems are taken care of first

and as they are removed other more chronic problems, that have been hidden but are still doing damage, will show up and can be addressed.[8]

## ADVANCED ENERGY CONCEPTS

The energy of the universe is polarized energy. It is electrical in nature, and magnetic in expression. Our thoughts are also energies that have creative abilities, which can be positive or negative, depending on the thoughts and beliefs behind them. It is one thing to say, understand, and accept this, but the further question is: "What is the power or energy behind this electricity?"

Scientists know that the universe pulsates with energy; there is a constant energy exchange of receiving and emitting going on between objects, both organic and inorganic. They also know that energy is never lost, it just changes form. Further, the universe is forever expanding; new matter is continually being created. But if new matter is being created, where is the energy source for that creation coming from? What is the ultimate, or primary, or universal, energy source?

On Earth, it is thought that our energy source is our sun. What about the rest of the universe? There has to be a greater and more universal energy that everything can, and does draw from, for its creation and sustenance. For that, we have to look to the power behind all creation, the creative universal intelligence.

What we have learned to date is that the original source energy is actually vibrating light particles, called photons. All life forms are composed of condensed energy of biophotons. Biophoton means "life-light;" it is a term that refers to light emitted in some fashion from all biological systems.[9] Our bodies and the energy we feel are a manifestation of light that is directed by the creative universal intelligence and the innate intelligence within our own cells. As science, research, and experimentation in the area of water reveals, this is where things get interesting.

**Water Has Memory**

Dr. Masaru Emoto is a Japanese researcher who began investigating the properties of water from different locations on earth to discover how it is affected by various conditions. In 1991, he and his staff began freezing water samples and observing the resultant ice crystals under a microscope. He published the results of his work in several books, one of which is *Messages from Water*. He was able to photograph and demonstrate how pollution affects the health of water. This in itself is not too surprising. However, the astounding discovery he made was that water picks up the consciousness of people around it; it has a capacity for memory.

Pure natural water, when frozen, has beautiful and completely formed ice crystals similar to those of a snowflake. As it becomes polluted, the ice crystals become increasingly deformed and fractured. They look unhealthy. Dr. Emoto found that environmental pollution is not the only thing that affects the structure of water. He has proven, through thousands of photographs, that words spoken to water, or even written and placed on a water container, clearly change the structure of water as reflected by the ice crystals formed from it. Harsh words like, "You fool," or, "You make me sick," or, "I will kill you," render the ice crystals incapable of forming in any organized manner. On the other hand, positive uplifting words such as "Love" and "Thank you" result in crystals as beautiful as the finest pieces of jewelry. Opposite words such as "Angel" and "Devil," "Soul" and "Demon," "Let's do it" and "Do it" showed the same results of organization versus disorganization. Similarly, sounds from different music selections of folk and classical versus heavy metal did the same.

The researchers then experimented with prayer. Water that was spoken to consciously in prayer, blessing, or appreciation invariably resulted in organized, healthy and alive-looking ice crystals. Is it any wonder that most religions of the world have practices of blessing their food before eating it? We may have thought of this as simply a religious ritual, but the positive effects of giving thanks and blessing food (expressing love to it) are now clearly observable from a scientific viewpoint. It also explains why plants that are spoken to with words of love, encouragement, and appreciation, grow better.

Since our own bodies are about 70 to 75% water, and the air around us contains water vapor, this would mean that our thoughts and words determine the quality of the water molecules making up our bodies, food, and air. The emotions we choose to have and to express, plus those of others around us, are picked up by water molecules and become part of us for either harmony or disharmony, psychologically and physiologically.

As Dr. Emoto put it, "Water is a mirror reflecting our mind." It takes on the consciousness of individuals as well as that of groups around it, and ultimately, that of the world population. As we ingest the resulting waters through eating, drinking, and breathing, we are affected either positively or negatively.

What we learn from Dr. Emoto's work:

- Our thoughts, words (sounds), color, and emotions have an influence on water.
- Love and gratitude are the emotions that cause water to structure itself most perfectly.
- Love is more than a sweet feeling; it is energy, and it is the ultimate creative power.

### Water Contains Light

Scientists, such as Dr. David Schweitzer in England, are able to photograph light particles that are present in water by using a special high-magnification microscope. The particles are also emitted from the cells of living biological organisms. The German physicist, Fritz-Albert Popp, is a researcher of light particles and is most well known for his discovery of the "biophoton mechanism of cell communication." He found that photonic light, which he called biophotons, emanates from the DNA of every living cell.[10] These biophotons act as information transmitters and are the means through which cells communicate with each other. The brighter the photonic light is (indicating more biophotons), the healthier and more vibrant the cells are.

Building on this research, scientists and various companies are inventing devices to restructure water and increase its biophotonic content.

According to microscope photographs of water samples treated by these devices, many are apparently successful. But to what extent?

## VIBRATIONS—THE NEXT STEP

Different things in the universe vibrate at different frequencies. When we speak of something as vibrant, we are referring to its vibratory energy, or aliveness; the higher the vibration, the more life energy it has.

In November 2001, I heard an interesting presentation given by Dana Young of the Brain Garden company. He was speaking on the ability of essential oils to increase the electrical vibratory frequency within the body. During the lecture he explained that the electrical energy, or vibratory activity, of atoms in our bodies is measured in megahertz. (A megahertz—MHz—is one million cycles per second.) If the electrons, protons, and neutrons of an atom revolve in their orbits one million times per second, we would classify this as 1 MHz of electrical energy.

Disease symptoms begin to appear at 58 MHz when the body's normal healthy frequency of 62 to 72 MHz has been reduced due to poor nutrition, lack of exercise, increased acidity, and toxicity in the body. Progressive deterioration indicates when disease conditions would start to manifest:

| Symptom | Body Freqency |
| --- | --- |
| Cold | 58 MHz |
| Flu | 57 MHz |
| Candida | 55 MHz |
| Chronic Fatigue | 52 MHz |
| Cancer | 42 MHz |

Table 12.1 Body electrical energy and disease symptoms

Mr. Young made a summary statement that, "We are energy beings in search of a recharge." The main point of his lecture was to illustrate that most essential oils vibrate at higher frequencies than the human body or the disease conditions that the body may be suffering from. When we ingest a substance with higher vibrations, these vibrations naturally work to raise the frequencies of the body, alleviating ailments of lower frequencies. For example, the essential oil with the highest vibratory frequency is Rose Oil, with an electrical activity of 320 MHz. When we work with essential oils to restore health, we are using natural vibrational medicine.

Raw foods also carry natural energy vibrations, with green vegetables having the highest. Cooked and heat processed food has zero MHz. When it is eaten, it actually depletes the body's electrical charge. Similarly, positive thoughts raise frequency vibrations, while negative thoughts lower them. Prayer and meditation have been found to be among the most effective mental activities for raising the body's electrical frequency vibrations.[11]

## LINKING LIGHT AND ENERGY

The point of the previous discussion is to make a link between energy as electricity, composed of light particles (biophotons), and energy as a frequency vibration. From a health perspective, when our energy reserve is low, our body vibrations are also low because the living light in our cells is dimmer. The food and water we consume affects us vibrationally according to the amount of biophoton light particles they contain.

Let us now move to the discoveries made by a man and woman who go by the name of Excelex. For six years they lived quietly in harmony with nature in a pristine country environment where they raised much of their own produce. They concentrated on learning about primal energies, how to access them for growing and living as nature intended, and how to develop products and technologies that contain and enhance living energy. Their focus was to first improve their own health, then to share their findings with others. The following concepts are those of Mr. E. Excelex, although the explanations presented here were written by me, with his assistance.

## General Vitality and White Light

First, we need to be open to the idea that all creations originate from Love and Light, which are then condensed into: sound vibration, electrically manifested shapes or forms, new life, such as human babies and seed sprouts. All new life is bursting with vitality, or life in action. Each has its own General Vitality (GV) at that stage. As it grows toward maturity, vitality begins to decrease. Compare, for instance, the energy exhibited by a two or three-year-old to that of a typical seventy- or eighty-year-old human.

Next, individuals have a White Light (WL) potential, which can be measured with a biophoton amplifier. Imagine or visualize that the body emits, for the average person, between 80 and 120 biophoton units/sec/sq. cm. Multiplying this by the surface area of the body in square centimeters gives an estimate of the magnitude of the bio-life force the body is generating every second. Healthy newborns can have as many as 150 biophoton units/sec/sq. cm; whereas elderly people near the end of their lives emit 50-units/sec/sq. cm, or less. Whereas a healthy newborn's biophoton light is bright, the older person's light is dim. Similarly, a healthy newborn's vibrations are high, while the older person's vibrations are low.

All life forms have their own individual GV and WL potentials, and Kirlian photography is a method of capturing pictures of these electromagnetic energy fields. A Kirlian photograph of a human body clearly shows these energy emanations as varying colors surrounding the individual, relevant to their vitality and mental/emotional states. What is important to understand is that General Vitality comes from the level of White Light that one has. Therefore, when we ingest any food or liquid, in order for it to be regenerating to our health, it needs to have a WL potential that is higher than its GV. This is because it is the WL that provides vitality.

## Energy in Fruit and Vegetables

The energy (GV) that raw fruit and vegetables contain varies according to how far or advanced the produce is in terms of age and growth cycle. When healthy fruit and vegetables are in the first half of their growing life cycle, they have the highest vitality and vibrations. This is when their regenerative properties for our bodies are at a maximum. A good example would be half-grown raw carrots. They are succulent, sweet, and brimming with new-growth energy, whereas large, mature carrots harvested several months ago will have passed their prime. They are on the second half of their energy cycle, moving towards decay.

For maximum health benefits, we should choose produce that is in the first-half of its life cycle, is freshly picked, tender, and not overripe or aged.

### The Source of Energy

The power or energy that feeds and sustains everything in the universe is Universal Love Life Force or ULLF. This is the primal energy, the living light that all things seek on a daily basis. Biophotons, in their primal and pure form, are particles of that love light. Primal energy is a magnetic expression of love.

Everything originates from love and light, including our bodies. It is the biophotonic light in the chromosomes of our cells that provides the silent language of the DNA. Further, it is minerals in cells that enable memory inside DNA to be retained, just as minerals on an audiotape allow the recording and retaining of sound.

In order for rejuvenation and longevity to manifest in a body, above all, there must be an increase in biophoton emissions. In other words, there must be an increase in the brightness of the telomeres (chromosomal tips). Without these biophoton emissions, any product or supplement is useless, because it requires life to regenerate and sustain life. Love is all there is. Life is love in action.

### Collecting Primal Energy

Certain primary source (unrefined) minerals, especially quartz crystals, are natural concentrators of the primal ULLF (biophotons). Crystals can be programmed, just like microchips, to hold and radiate the magnetic love energy frequency. We can utilize this knowledge to produce structured water that is alive, active, and high in energy. This is an example of the application of the Universal Love Energy that all organisms seek.

### Biophotons and Derivative Energy Devices

It was suggested earlier that the quantity of biophotonic light does not necessarily equate to quality. Any electrical or magnetic energy device that is man-made is secondary to the primal energy; it is derived from it. Electricity, magnets, and electromagnets are derivative energy sources and, as yet, cannot duplicate original life force energy. They can only produce copies, with outputs that are much lower in General Vitality and White Light. GV and WL potentials can be measured and demonstrated. They can be measured by a radionics instrument such as the SE-5 and most convincingly, they can be demonstrated by observing the growth of plants, fruits, and vegetables that have been fed vibrant primal energy water, as you will read about in chapter 14.

Man-made electronic and magnetic energy devices, and water treatment units, can definitely have a positive effect on some health problems by helping the body raise its General Vitality, or frequency vibrations. A body of lower GV and WL has the potential of rising to the level of that produced by the electronic or magnetic device. The downside is that, once the body has raised its vitality to the White Light potential of the device being used, it will be held at that level of energy output. In other words, the device can only help to improve vitality up to a certain level but no further. After that it becomes a drain or a limiting factor on one's vitality.

### Energy Sources and Rejuvenation

As a result of its own level of energy, every food and liquid that we take into our bodies has a positive or negative effect on our energy stores. It can either add significantly, marginally, or take away from the body's level and store of vitality. That is, food and liquids either contribute to rejuvenation or cause degeneration in the body.

Excelex describes it this way. We have three types of waters and foods:

- Regenero-active or Life ++        (Significantly rejuvenating)
- Genero-active or Life +          (Marginally rejuvenating)
- Degenero-active or Life –        (Degenerating)

In order to be classified Regenero-active, a water or food must have a minimal reading of GV=5000, WL=5100, a biophotonic (BP) activity of 3 units/sec/sq cm, and a Level of Structural Organization (LSO) equal to 8 out of 10. A Genero-active classification must have a reading of at least GV=1700, WL=1750, BP activity of 1 unit/sec/sq. cm and an LSO of 2 out of 10. Degenero-active substances have readings below a GV of 850. Substances with a GV between 850 and 1700 can sustain but not regenerate life.

When we consider that the average population has GV and WL levels of 400 to 700, we can appreciate the effect that the above classifications of foods have on our bodies. What we eat and drink either makes us stronger, weaker, or maintains our present level of vitality. Consuming Regenero-active foods and water contributes WL energy and rejuvenates cells.

From this understanding, whatever we eat can be viewed as Life$^+$ or Life$^-$. It either adds to our life energy or draws from it.

### Regenero-Active Substances

These include:

- Yellow sprouts (before exposure to light), grown with TLC and/or structured water producing Photo Reactive Enzymes (PRE™), which, as a result of their synthesis by the body, become Regenero-active.
- Garden produce watered with structured water, starting with heritage seeds (i.e. Genetically modified organism/terminator-free seeds), yielding structured produce that is Regenero-active.
- Highly structured waters rating above 8 on a scale of 0 to 10.
- Restructured energized waters with a GV above 5000 and a WL above 5100.
- Generally, all food preparations done with love. The magnetic expression of love infuses primal energy. There is no structure which cannot be rearranged by the magnetic infusion of love.
- Good quality gem elixirs.
- Some good quality essential oils.

Don't be fooled by "organic" labels, because genetically modified organism (GMO) and terminator seeds can be grown organically. Since the body becomes what we feed it, genetically modified foods and produce will have a negative influence on one's cellular structure.

### Genero-Active Substances

These include:

- All heritage seed produce in the first half cycle of life. For example, young carrots, potatoes, smaller cabbages, fruits before they are overly mature, that is up to a few weeks old or so, according to the nature of the fruit and vegetable.
- Generally, all sprouts, including green sprouts. The quality of the water used will reflect the GV and WL potential.
- Most clean brook, well, and spring water.
- Re-energized water with a WL higher than the GV; GV above 1700 and WL above 1750.
- Most fresh herbal teas naturally grown from heritage seeds.
- All good-quality herbal tinctures infused with the magnetic of love.
- Good quality essential oils.

### Degenero-Active or 'Life-less' Substances

These include:

- All demineralized water.
- Reverse osmosis, deionized, UV, ozonated, and distilled water.
- Electrically reionized water.
- All microwaved beverages and foods; even at two seconds, the damage is done.
- All commercially prepared, canned, and fast foods.
- All commercial alcohols—wines, beers, liquor.
- Soda pop.
- All second-half life cycle food produce.

- All *white*—salt, sugar, vinegar, bread, pasta, rice, pasteurized and homogenized milk.

### Garden Produce

When garden produce is grown commercially to be large-sized through the use of chemical fertilizers, herbicides, mineral-depleted soil, and poor quality water, it is lacking in GV and WL. Likewise, if it is harvested in its second half life cycle, it is deficient in GV and WL. The same can be said for average garden produce that reaches large sizes after months of growth.

There is a net dual benefit from growing produce with structured water where it can reach large sizes and still be in its first half life cycle, without producing seed. Generally, before a plant is engaged in making seeds, it is in the first half of its life cycle. For example, when a potato plant has its flower open, during the following four weeks or so, the potatoes are in the first half of their life cycle. They are small to medium, depending on the quality of water used. Some of the potatoes may be quite large if the plant has been fed structured water.

Structured water makes structured plants, which yield structured foods, which in turn, help us in the structuring of our body cells.

## BOTTOM LINE ON VITALITY

Simply put, as far as our health is concerned, the foods and liquids we consume either add to the body's vitality, or they subtract from it. Foods that are dead, acidic, or poor in life and nutrition have lower General Vitality levels than our bodies do. The body has to give up valuable energy to process them. On the other hand, live fruits and vegetables in their first half life cycle, and energized water, have higher General Vitality levels than those of our bodies. This allows our bodies to gain in vitality from them, resulting in an increase in energy stores. We should think about this each time we eat or drink something.

We all want to be healthy, feel good, and have energy. Is it any wonder that these three states are connected to each other? When the body is unable to generate sufficient energy to meet its needs for daily operation, detoxification, and repair, it ages. It is that simple. If we want health and all that it implies, we must pay attention to optimizing nutrition, water quality, rest, detoxification, and oxygen intake to maximize energy generation.

Now that we have laid a foundation for understanding what health and disease are and how the body works, let us look at how we can detoxify the body to help it operate more efficiently. This is a critical key to reversing existing health problems, and getting back on the road to health.

SECOND KEY

# CLEANSING

# 13 | DETOXIFYING AND HEALING

∿

*He who has health, has hope;*
*and he who has hope, has everything.*
ARABIAN PROVERB

∿

LOUIS PASTEUR promoted the theory that microbes, or bacteria, are the cause of disease. However, he amended his position just before he died by stating that "the microbe is nothing; the terrain is everything."[1] That is, the environment that surrounds our cells determines their health. Harmful bacteria and viruses cannot thrive in a body that has a healthy terrain.

## TERRAIN IS EVERYTHING

The word "terrain" usually refers to soil, but where the human body is concerned, it means biological terrain. Just as farmers need to be concerned about healthy nutrients and the condition of the soil to produce viable crops, we also need to be concerned about the healthy electrical and chemical condition of the body's biological terrain. The main factor in the weakening of our biological terrain is the gradual acidification of body tissues, which consequently reduces oxygen content throughout the body.

An acidic body is a body in which conditions of disease have begun to take over. All the signs of aging—gray hair, loss of muscle tone and mass, wrinkles, thinning of the skin and discoloration, weakened eyesight, lack of energy, and digestion problems—are related to excess acidity in the body. Aging problems can be reversed, but only by reinstating conditions of a healthy terrain in the body.

The process starts with detoxifying the body to make it less acidic. It requires the elimination of all foods, drinks, harmful practices, negative attitudes, stresses, and environmental contaminants that have a deleterious effect on the pH, oxidative, and electrical conditions of the body. It also depends on introducing into our diet and lifestyle those foods, drinks, and practices that promote a healthy acid/alkaline balance and reduce oxidative stresses in the body. Our success in slowing and reversing the aging process will be directly related to our diligence in doing whatever is necessary to re-establish a healthy terrain.

## GIVING UP STIMULANTS

In chapter 6 we discovered that stimulants are substances that cause the body to increase its metabolism. Stimulants trigger an abnormal speeding-up reaction in the body as it attempts to remove the toxins that the stimulants introduce. In this process, we can be fooled into thinking that the stimulant is giving us more energy. The stimulant contains no energy. It only causes the body to use its own stored nutrients to increase metabolism. This results in depleted nutrient reserves and an early "burnout" for the body. The main food stimulants used in our society are caffeine, nicotine, red meat, sugar, and salt. They are toxic and very acid-producing.

When we stop introducing stimulants into our bodies and start eating alkaline, mineral-rich foods, our bodies can begin to replenish their reserves and move toward improved health. But, there is a temporary price to pay. The body may have become dependent on stimulation from these foods for such a long time that it may be addicted. When these foods are discontinued, the adrenaline rush is absent and consequently the feelings of energy are immediately reduced. This is because it was actually false energy that did not come from nutrition. It came from a drug-like reaction, from a substance that caused the body to react.

Consider the example of the person who drinks several cups of coffee throughout the day. When they go off coffee suddenly and completely, by mid-morning of the next day they feel tired and irritable, and shortly after, begin to experience a headache. The tiredness is due to a lack of energy stimulation from adrenaline. The headache is from stored toxins entering the bloodstream for elimination from the body, thereby irritating nerves in the brain. As soon as the input of caffeine is discontinued, the body uses this opportunity to eliminate the poisons that had to be stored when the intake was continuous. In its wisdom, the body knows it must clean house because these poisons are detrimental to its long-term survival.

The bottom line on what we can expect when we discontinue the use of stimulants is some discomfort during the period of withdrawal. It may be preferable to eliminate the number and quantity of stimulants from our diet and lifestyle gradually. Over time, as stimulants are replaced with wholesome food, clean water, fresh air, exercise, positive attitudes, and health-restoring supplements, the body will cleanse itself and begin to produce increasing energy. We will experience new feelings of vitality that are genuine and lasting.

## FOOD ADDICTIONS

We all become addicted to certain foods for various payoffs, be they physical (more energy), psychological/emotional (feel better, calmer, happier), or chemical (satisfy a craving). A diseased or unhealthy part of the body is in control. It is relatively easy to understand addictions to caffeine, nicotine, alcohol, and drugs, but it is a little harder to consider foods such as bread, pasta, meat, and desserts as addictive.

The ultimate, but not so obvious, addiction that virtually all of us have is to cooked food. This is what causes our diseases; consider the Pottenger cats experiment. Addiction to cooked food is so ingrained and set in from thousands of years of custom, tradition, and practice that we accept it as normal. But, for the way we were designed physically, it is not normal; it destroys our health. Newborn babies still have innate intelligence within them that finds cooked food repulsive. Babies usually try to spit out cooked and canned food preparations when they are first introduced to solid food. After the mother's persistence and coaxing, they finally give in and accept it. It is not long before they too become addicted to sugar, salt, and cooked food. Humans are the only species that cooks its food.

While we are removing stimulants from our diet, we should also begin eating more raw fruits and vegetables, and reducing the amount of cooked food we eat.

## SMOKING

If you are a smoker, the first and most important step you can take in your health program, without exception, is to quit smoking. Easy to say, but for most people, very hard to do.

Nicotine was discussed briefly in chapter 8, *"What Are We Doing Wrong?"* It is extremely toxic to the body and, as any smoker or former smoker will tell you, very addictive. I have been told that it is even more addictive than hard drugs. If you are serious about reclaiming and improving your health, there is no doubt that you need to quit! "Oh," you might say, "I've tried many times but it's so hard to do. How can I quit and stay off cigarettes without driving myself half crazy?" This is a good question. As a non-smoker, I do not claim to be an authority on the subject. Aside from the nicotine patch, nicotine gum, and various other drugs and herbs to help one kick the habit, I have heard of one other program that may be of assistance.

Dr. Herbert DeloRey has had a great deal of success helping people quit smoking by using the following technique. It takes considerable time to accomplish depending on the degree to which one smokes. It is simply this: Start with the number of cigarettes you are presently using each day and keep this as the absolute maximum ration for the day; no exceptions! Do this for 21 days. Each three-week period thereafter, reduce the ration by one cigarette, until finally you are down to one cigarette for the final three-week period, and then none.

Dr. DeloRey explained how this works. By adopting this very gradual reduction in the amount of nicotine intake every three weeks, it fools the body into adjusting to a gradual reduction of its addictive requirement. In addition, part of the program calls for taking a teaspoon of cream of tartar powder in a glass of freshly squeezed orange juice (not concentrated or processed) each evening before going to bed. This helps to remove nicotine from the body. He said that since nicotine tends to accumulate around two glands in the brain called the hypothalamus and amygdala, the mix of cream of tartar and orange juice helps to drain nicotine from the glands during sleep. When nicotine is removed from the body, it normally sets up a craving for the nicotine to be replenished. However, since this is done during sleep, the craving goes largely unnoticed, and the body adjusts to the new level. By instituting this slow and steady approach to quitting smoking, Dr. DeloRey said that many people have been successful, where prior to using this method, nothing else had worked for them.

If all else has failed for you, this method may be worth trying because your health program depends on your being able to eliminate nicotine from your lifestyle.

## TURNING THE DISEASE BUS AROUND

To become consciously healthy, we must understand what is involved. We need to be aware of what the body is doing when it is going through various stages, and why. When we are consciously aware, we can cooperate with it and be patient during the process.

### Bumps Along the Way

It can come as a shock to people, after they have started to do all the right things and begun to feel much better, that there have to be downtimes of illness again. But, our body corrects and builds toward health in stages. The road to normal vitality is not without its challenging times. True healing is not just the removal of symptoms, it is the complete and thorough reversal of the disease process.

Figures 13.1 and 13.2 illustrate the disease and healing processes. The diagrams and explanations were created by Mr. V. E. Irons and are reprinted here with the permission of V. E. Irons Inc.

### The Downward Road to Ill Health

In the early part of life we don't go straight from good health to ill health, it usually happens in stages. Toxic accumulations from our lifestyle choices gradually reduce the body's detoxification and energy generation capabilities. Over time, the body's general immunity is weakened. The

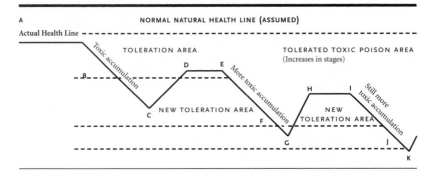

**Figure 13.1  Downward road to ill health**

A.  The health line nature intended, with no aches or pains—vibrant health.

B.  The point where toxic poisons break through the physical tolerance area, meaning you are sick enough to call in a doctor.

C.  Crisis of illness. The point where toxicity starts to recede, and you start to feel better.

D.  Nearest you get back to Line A. You feel "OK," but lack the original vibrant, buoyant vitality.

E.  The point where, again, you start to accumulate toxic poisons faster than they can be eliminated.

F.  Breakthrough to new and lower toleration point, producing a new acute illness that is intolerable, necessitating a call for the doctor.

G.  End of crisis. You start to feel better.

H.  Nearest point you can now get to Nature's Health Line A. You feel fair, but lack nature's vibrant vitality because you have still more toxic poisons which your body has learned to tolerate.

I.  Again, you start to accumulate poisons faster than they are eliminated.

J.  Breakthrough of new and lower toleration point, thus presenting a new crisis, necessitating another call for the doctor.

K.  End of latest crisis and start of temporary recovery and so on and on, until each new crisis brings a lowering of the reserve vitality and a greater permanent accumulation of toxicity with its chronic symptoms.[2]

body fights through each illness crisis by attempting detoxification and repair. But as poisons continue to overload the system, each return to a healthy-feeling state is achieved with a lower level of vitality. This is the movement toward degenerative disease.

## The Upward Road to Health

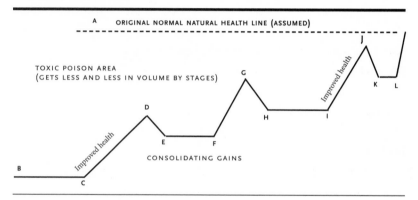

**Figure 13.2 Upward road to health**

A. Your original Natural Health line.

B. Line representing your state of poor health with its many symptoms, aches, complaints, and toxic poisons, after years of consuming civilized, demineralized, devitalized, empty-calorie foods.

C. The point at which you decide to do something about it. The point where you decide that nature's way is the only way with which to rebuild.

D. The point in your road back to health where you experience a reaction—where some glands have recuperated as much as they can, while others still lag or take longer to get into condition. Your renewed vigor has caused you to be more active, and you have carried your new-born activity a little too far for some of the lagging glands, muscles, et cetera, so you suffer a relapse or reaction.

E. You start to lose faith in nature's way.

F. Gives time for body reserves to stabilize and let lagging units catch up with advance units. This is your Danger Point. Have you got what it takes? Will you say to yourself: "This is not for me, it may be all right for others, but it is not for me!" Or will you still stick to nature's way?

G. Your body is now ready for a new spurt toward better and more wholesome vitality.

H. Again, advance units get too far ahead of more devitalized glands, organs or muscles. Over-exuberance causes a strain on more advanced units, hence, a setback to I. Stick to it!

I. To J. Stabilization of ground gained.

J. Start of another spurt toward health.[3]

Just as the road to ill health is not straight, the road back to energetic health is also traveled in stages. We go back to health gradually with periods of detoxification and repair, first feeling much better, then having a recession, then up, then slipping back; but each time, the reactions UP go farther than the reactions DOWN. The body is gaining vitality and immunity as it cleans and rebuilds itself.

Complete healing takes time. The body cannot restore everything simultaneously. Some parts, some organs, some muscles are usually more deteriorated than others. We must be prepared for reactions and upsets on the road back to health. If we are doing everything right, these are simply healing corrections. The relapses of illness are natural times of thorough healing when strength and vitality are being rebuilt into our bodies.

### Healing Reversals

When practices that lead to disease are discontinued, in order to move toward health the body starts by correcting and removing disease conditions. This is called the "reversal process." There is no way that the body can overcome or overlook the disease conditions that have become established within it without retracing them; they must be corrected. What went in must come out. A condition that built up must be broken down. Conditions that have been treated with drugs or antibiotics, for instance, have been put on hold; a complete natural healing has not taken place, only the symptom has been removed. Disease conditions must be re-entered and reversed for damage to be undone.

Constantine Hering, born in Germany in 1800, made many contributions to the study of homeopathy. He is still known today for his observations of the healing process, now known as, "Hering's Law of Cure." It states that during a healing and reversal process, the body heals from the inside out; from the head down; and, in the reverse order that diseases developed.

The body follows a clear pattern in the process of healing itself. The most serious and most recent disease conditions are given first attention. As progress is made on these, the body works backwards in time, so to speak, retracing and correcting other conditions in reverse order to when they appeared. Remember that this is all conditional on the body continuing to receive regular nutrition and rest, over and above that which is required to carry on daily activities, so it doesn't have to borrow from its own nutrient reserves to accomplish the process.

This is what healing is. There is no magic pill. The body only builds from a firm foundation and does it step by step. The only way out of the problem is through it.

**Healing Crises**

A healing reversal is also a healing crisis. It is a turning point in the course of a disease, a period of intense but necessary housecleaning as the body prepares to heal.

The body cannot accomplish the tasks of serious detoxification and healing and still be able to provide energy for everyday activities. Rest is required. That is why we feel we have less energy during a cold or flu. These are times of intense internal cleansing. The body doesn't have less energy, it is redirecting the energy it does have for healing purposes.

We may continue to experience periods of illness and low energy. However, during a healing crisis, there is one very large difference. This time, under the influence of a healthy lifestyle, the body experiences symptoms related to a disease healing crisis, as opposed to a disease survival crisis. At the completion of such a crisis, the body will have gained vitality, not lost vitality. The body is getting stronger, not weaker.

> *A healing crisis is an accelerated period of symptom reversal in a person who has grown strong enough to throw off accumulated toxic wastes from the past.*

The healthier we become, the less intense the healing crises will be. This is logical, since the amount of toxins to be eliminated from the body is decreasing, while the organs and tissues are getting stronger. Not every healing done by the body slows us down completely. We may note a little less energy for a period of time, when the body is working on

243

some internal condition before returning to a feeling of renewed and increased vitality.

The body not only heals itself in areas that display symptoms that we clearly notice and can identify, such as allergies, asthma, and arthritis, but it also works on internal physical problems and emotional aspects as well. While internal conditions are being corrected, we may notice a period of low energy and not know the reason why. As long as we are practicing a healthy lifestyle, we can be fairly certain the body is healing and requires extra energy for the process. As the physical body is cleansed, it will also bring emotional crises to the surface for correction. Old feelings of inferiority, sadness, depression, anger, and emotional conflicts can manifest. These also need to be eliminated, because in one way or another, they are connected to the development of a disease. We need to be patient and work through these periods. The body is working to return us to a complete, "wholistic" health of body, mind, and spirit.

A healing crisis usually lasts three or seven days. However, if there is adequate healing energy available, the body may run several healing crises consecutively.[4] One should try not to interfere with the process by taking medication to ease pain or discomfort. If this is done, it will slow down and can even stop the natural corrective process. Likewise, it is not wise to stimulate the body to cleanse or focus healing on a part that has not been selected as a priority at any given time. If this is done, the body is forced to refocus and expend energy and nutrients dealing with the medication. It has to change priority. Remember that the body uses its innate intelligence to heal on a priority basis that is best for healing and survival. We must work with the body, not against it. Let your body dictate what and when things will be worked on. It knows best!

### The Body Starts Healing When It Is Ready

The body will not begin a healing crisis until it has stored enough energy and nutrients to carry out the healing process it intends. The stronger the body is, and the more vitality it has, the greater or more intense a healing crisis can be. A very ill body with low vitality will tend to have less intense and shorter healing crises at first. The body knows what it is capable of handling. However, it attempts to detoxify whenever it has the opportunity.

When the intake of healthy food is greater than the intake of unhealthy food, the balance is tipped in favor of the body. It is able to divert some of its efforts away from survival toward healing, and begin to detoxify. Toxins are moved from areas of cellular storage via lymphatic fluid to the bloodstream for transport to the liver where they are separated from other blood components. From here, they are sent onto the colon for elimination. During this process, circulating blood passes though the brain. Toxins being carried in the blood at that time irritate sensitive nerves in the brain, causing a headache. In my personal case, when I know that my diet and lifestyle are healthy, the classic sign my body periodically sends me, which indicates that is it detoxifying, is a mild to medium headache across my forehead. This kind of headache, although unpleasant, is always tolerable and will pass when the detoxification cycle is concluded. We can assist the body during these times by increasing our intake of healthy water.

### Cooperating With Our Healing

During a serious healing crisis, one should rest to conserve energy, and eat sparingly, if at all. All animals, when they are not feeling well, fast and rest quietly. This is the quickest and most efficient way to heal. The body does not need food for energy at this time because it has already stored the energy required for the healing being undertaken. If it needed the energy from food, it would not have begun the healing crisis. Continuing to eat regular meals during the healing crisis requires a lot of energy for digestion, which the body is then forced to withdraw from healing activities. It also interferes with the focused detoxification and elimination processes. Drinking good water and diluted fresh fruit and vegetable juices is best, or consuming a little broth made from an assortment of vegetables. In this way, the body is supplied with vitamins and minerals in non-solid form, which it can readily use without expending excessive amounts of energy for digestion. A fresh juice diet requires only about 10% of the energy needed to digest solid food.

When nausea is evident, it is the result of a concentration of toxins in the intestine. This can happen due to overeating, or eating overly toxic or spoiled food. When there is a toxic overload being eliminated from the body, the liver, which normally metabolizes waste products, may be forced to expel toxins directly into the intestines, where they cause irritation and nausea. When this happens, the last thing the body needs is more food. The body brings on nausea as an attempt to eliminate the toxins through vomiting and perhaps diarrhea, or at least, to signal that it wants us to fast, that is, abstain from eating until it has re-established digestive equilibrium.

To work with the body during a healing crisis, we should consume healthful liquids, sleep and rest as much as possible, and stay warm. The whole intent is to conserve energy, so that it can be directed to healing. Also, as this is a time of increased dumping of toxic wastes, it is helpful to clear the bowel with a warm water enema once or twice daily, or to have a colonic irrigation. This assists with the elimination of toxins so they are not reabsorbed into circulation.

If, for some reason, it becomes necessary to stop a healing crisis, this can usually be done by consuming cooked vegetables, grains, meats, potatoes, or by drinking coffee.

## HOW LONG BACK TO HEALTH?

How long does it take for the body to heal itself once we have started to eat properly and have adopted healthy lifestyle practices? The answer to this question varies for each person. Dr. Robbins teaches that, as a general rule, it takes one year for every seven years that you did it wrong. But don't become discouraged. Let us understand why it can take this long, and how the time can be shortened.

The actual time required depends on how sick the body is in the first place, and on how willing the person is to give the body what it needs to heal itself. It also depends on the disease present; the vitality and digestive ability of the body; the person's attitudes; the environment the person lives and works in; how quickly the person changes to a healthy diet; what supplements are consumed; and on lifestyle practices.

It takes a long time for our bodily conditions to develop. The body needs to go back chronologically through the disease conditions to reverse and heal them. Serious problems take a long time to develop and are deeply seated. They cannot be corrected and replaced with totally healthy tissue immediately.

The sooner and more completely a healthy lifestyle is adopted, the sooner our return to health will be. For example, consuming fresh raw fruit and vegetable juices daily can achieve in one month what might normally take six months for a healthy diet of only solid food to achieve.[5] Restoring digestive enzymes and friendly bacteria, and consuming complete foods that contain alkaline minerals can shorten recovery time considerably.

Quantum physics has now proven that in three years we don't have one old cell left. Ninety-eight percent of the body can be totally regenerated in one year on a good program of enzymes, complete foods, and proper detoxification.[6] So the answer to the question, "How long to health?" is that it depends on the age, present health, attitudes and beliefs, determination, circumstances, and capability of each individual. It also depends on our willingness to change our lifestyles and spend the money required to restore enzymes, nutrients, and healthy pH balance to the body. It can take a year or two, or it can take ten. For the average middle-aged person who undertakes a serious lifestyle change and does all the helpful things, it is reasonable to expect some positive changes in a matter of weeks or months. Significant changes can be expected in one to two years and a return to full health in as little as two to five years.

## DETOXIFICATION

The process of removing wastes and toxic acid stores from the body is fundamental and absolutely necessary in our pursuit of improved health and vitality. When the body's needs are being adequately supplied on a continual basis, it detoxifies naturally, as a matter of course. However, when there is a buildup of toxins from years of depriving the body of what it requires, and from abusing it with toxic foods, drinks, chemicals, drugs, smoke, and other stressors, it needs assistance to clean out and reverse degenerating disease conditions.

In the detoxification process, we can work directly to remove toxins from the colon and liver. Once these organs have become less congested, other organs begin to release their congestion as well.

## Benefits of Detoxification

The benefits of effective and regular detoxification are improved health. When hard fecal matter, mucoid plaque, which has built up on the walls of the colon over years is removed, the body begins to function more efficiently. Poisons and toxins are removed efficiently and good nutrients from foods are readily absorbed as the cellular pH moves closer to 7.0. Digestion is improved. Immune function is enhanced. The endocrine system works more harmoniously. The lymphatic system becomes more fluid for effective drainage and elimination of cellular debris. We begin to notice the difference because we have more energy and feel better.

## Colon Cleansing

As long as the colon remains toxic, the liver and other organs will remain congested. Once we clear out the pollution at the "bottom end," the pressure is relieved, and the rest of the body is able to start dumping its toxins. This will be an ongoing program for quite some time, because it can take several years to fully clean a body that has been toxic all its life. A diet that includes adequate fiber from raw fruits and vegetables is the best and most natural colon cleanser and should always be the first priority for colon health. There are also several herbal or oxygen-inducing colon-cleansing and rejuvenating products available in healthfood stores, as well as advertised on the Internet.

While cleansing the colon of impacted debris, we should be increasing our stores of probiotics (friendly flora), to restore the symbiotic bacteria for this part of the body.

## Colon Therapy—A Shortcut to Health

Every ailment, sickness, or disease will respond to treatment quicker and more effectively after the administration of a series of colon irrigations.[7]

The detoxification of body organs and tissues will happen under a good program of raw fruits, vegetables, good water, and exercise. However, to really speed the process up, to assist the body toward health, and reverse aging, nothing is more immediately effective than thorough colon therapy. This means the use of colonics, also called colonic irrigations, hydrotherapy, and high enemas. Ordinary enemas only reach the last eight to twelve inches of the bowel; whereas colonics reach the entire five to six feet of the colon.

Colonics are essentially large-volume enemas, using many gallons (or liters) of water at each session to gently and thoroughly cleanse the entire large intestine. Water is injected through a tube that has been inserted into the rectum, several ounces (100 ml or so) at a time, and then allowed to be expelled, carrying wastes from the colon with it. This procedure is usually carried out by a colon therapist and lasts from 30–60 minutes. During that time, up to 4–8 gallons (15–30 liters) of filtered water passes into and out of the colon. The subject lies on their side and back and relaxes while the therapist performs the procedure. The process is not uncomfortable. After two or three colonics, the rejuvenation benefits are usually quite evident. In addition to removing poisons, colonics exercise colon muscles, help to reshape the colon, and stimulate colon reflex points that relate to other organs and parts of the body.

Colonic irrigations are safe and have been practiced for hundreds of years. Present-day fears about colon therapy are based on misinformation. Records of the use of enemas date back to about 1500 BC in Egypt. In the 1800s and early 1900s in North America, enemas were in common use as a means of maintaining health. Colon irrigation machines were commonly used in hospitals and doctors' offices up to the 1930s, until the widespread introduction of chemical laxatives and drugs.[8] Colon hydrotherapy, even when done frequently, does not wash out friendly bowel flora. Healthy bacteria are constantly being introduced into the colon from the small intestine. Colon walls, just like the lining in our mouths, are composed of soft tissue and are not harmed by the introduction of water any more than our mouths are. It is the practices of wrong eating, the use of drugs and antibiotics, exposure to insecticides and chemicals, as well as toxins and organisms picked up during travel that change the chemical balance in the colon, depleting friendly flora and promoting an increase of unfriendly bacteria.

Some people who are serious about staying young and healthy have colon therapy units in their homes, and perform them two or three times every week. By doing this, and by eating properly, acid conditions never have a chance of building up in their systems. The resulting benefits are increased energy, better skin, less wrinkles, improved digestion, and improved bowel function. The benefits are systemic, meaning all functions in the body are improved.

There are two types of home colonic devices that can be purchased. The more reasonably priced one employs the use of a "colema board"; the other is more expensive but more automatic and less messy.[9] Information on both devices can be found by searching the Internet.

Dr. Norman Walker, who lived an active life until he died at the age of 109, was a strong proponent of colon cleansing. He recommended using colonics on a regular basis to keep the colon clean. As a preventative measure, he suggested that at least six colon irrigations per year should be taken throughout life.[10]

If we want to rejuvenate our health, and maintain our ability to stay on top of it for the rest of our lives, we should consider introducing colon therapy into our health regimens.

### Liver Cleansing

The liver is the master organ and gland in the body; it performs over 600 functions. If the liver is not a clean environment, it cannot operate efficiently. It would be like a car radiator that cannot cool the engine water because it is clogged and corroded; it needs to be flushed. Similarly, the liver may need to be cleansed several times to increase its overall efficiency. Acid wastes that are stored in tissues, joints, and fat layers cannot be disposed of as long as the colon and liver are congested and under-functioning. As liver function improves, toxins from the rest of the body can also be released and eliminated. This is how the detoxification process happens.

One of the liver's main functions is to produce quantities of bile to alkalize and break down foods in the small intestine. Adequate amounts of bile cannot be made when the liver is congested with toxins, cholesterol crystals, and stones. Digestion suffers accordingly. This partly explains why people who may be consuming the best foods and supplements do not receive full benefits from them. This is because digestion is key to health, and bile is key to digestion in the small intestine.

Going through the process of removing stones from the liver and gall-bladder may be the most difficult and "not fun" procedure we will undertake on the road to improved health, yet it is necessary if we want to hold and reverse the aging process. As we get used to the routine, it isn't all that bad. According to many practitioners, although it may be somewhat unpleasant, it is absolutely safe. However, one must not attempt this cleanse when they are seriously ill because the body does use a significant amount of energy in the process.

There are several different approaches to cleansing the liver. Essentially, what is involved is reducing the strain on the liver by eliminating red meats, concentrated fats, and refined foods, as well as consuming liquids and herbs to soften deposits in the liver for a few days. Then, on the evening before the flush, drinking a mixture of fresh lemon juice and olive oil and going directly to bed and lying as still as possible for the night. In the morning, stones of various sizes should be eliminated in several bowel movements. An example of a gentle cleanse formula may be found on Dr. Linda Page's website, and a more aggressive recipe for liver and gallbladder flushes may be found under the name of Dr. Hulda Clark on the Internet.

According to Dr. Clark, one should repeat the cleanses until, by estimated count, nearly 2,000 stones of varying size, plus numerous cholesterol crystals and toxins that appear as "chaff," have been eliminated.[11] Most of the toxins are eliminated from the body in liquid form. Only after thoroughly completing this process can we expect to overcome allergies, serious digestion problems, bowel conditions such as leaky gut syndrome, and persistent aches and pains.

**Detoxification Summary** [12]

- Detoxification is the body's process of eliminating toxins.
- Detoxification of the body has many names including: healing crisis, healing reversal, reactivation, and cleansing crisis.
- Detoxification will initially cause your symptoms to feel worse.
- Detoxification occurs in cycles of 3 days, 7 days, 14 days, or 21 days or a combination of these days.
- Detoxification may cause your pH to become more acid at first, as you release the stored toxins that have to be eliminated by your body. (Keep your alkalizing regimen the same; your pH will come back up as your body rids itself of toxins.)
- You may go through many detoxification cycles before complete health is regained.


## OTHER MEANS OF DETOXIFICATION

There are other ways of helping the body detoxify. Some of the main ones are highlighted below.

### Water
Water is critical to all life processes. The efficient removal of body wastes and toxins simply cannot happen in the absence of adequate clean water. We must drink enough water regularly. If we wait until we are thirsty before drinking, we are already dehydrated.

### Fasting
Fasting is the deliberate creation of conditions that allow the body an opportunity to restore itself to its original state of excellence. Giving our digestive systems and organs a rest from having to process a continual load of food is a great benefit. We cannot eat and detoxify at the same time. Taking solid foods during days of fasting is counter-productive. Food

intake hampers toxin elimination. Fresh raw fruit and vegetable juices are the exception.

Fasting is often the only way our bodies can detoxify quickly enough in cases of chronic disease. It is also useful as a means of preventing illness or serious consequences to the body's integrity and its ability to maintain health. There are several good books listed in the bibliography of this book that discuss programs of detoxification, fasting, and colon health.

In my opinion, a good regimen of body detoxification is one that rests the organs of digestion and assimilation. During this resting time we abstain from eating solid food and take a few natural food source supplements to ensure the body is getting required minerals, enzymes, and bowel flora. It is also necessary to have at least one good bowel movement daily while on a detoxification program. Bowel stagnation increases toxicity, blocks healing, and defeats the purpose of fasting. During fasting, it is also helpful to have an enema each day to remove toxins and prevent their resorption into the blood, organs, and tissues. The use of colonic irrigations would be even more effective. (See Appendix 5: How to Use a Water Enema.)

### Fresh Fruit and Vegetable Juices

Excellent results can be achieved by combining fasting with the consumption of raw, freshly made fruit and vegetable juices, while keeping citrus juices, except for lemon first thing in the morning, to a minimum. (See the section on juicing in chapter 21).

### The Master Cleanser

Stanley Burroughs developed a cleansing fast, also called "the lemonade diet," and published the booklet *The Master Cleanser* in 1976. It is a very effective whole body cleanser used by many people today. The diet consists of combining 2 tablespoons of fresh lemon or lime juice, 2 tablespoons of genuine maple syrup, and $1/10$ (more or less) of a teaspoon of cayenne pepper in 10 ounces (300 ml) of cold to medium hot water. Drinking six to twelve glasses each day is recommended. When you feel hungry you just have another glass. This fast is convenient and comfortable as there is no loss of energy. Some detoxification symptoms such as mild to moderate headaches may be experienced. Regular coffee drinkers, for example, can experience fairly strong headaches for two or more days as their bodies quickly eliminate stored toxins. During any cleansing fast, headaches are a clear sign that detoxification is happening in the body. The best way to end this fast is to taper it off with two days of fresh orange juice, then fresh fruit for a day or so, and finally, a normal diet.

In my opinion, the reason this fast is so effective is because it is alkaline-based, it supplies requisite vitamins and minerals in the lemon juice and maple syrup, and takes the load off the organs of digestion. This allows the body to concentrate on eliminating toxins and restoring a balanced acid-alkaline environment in the body. Mr. Burroughs suggests using the cleansing diet for 10 days or more, depending on the seriousness of health problems. Further instructions, as well as special instructions for diabetics, are contained in his booklet.

### Watermelon Fast

A cleansing fast that is easy to do is based on a watermelon diet. Watermelon is very pleasant to eat, satisfies the urge to chew something, consists mostly of water, provides simple sugars, contains enzymes and minerals, and requires very little energy from the body for digestion. Watermelon is also very alkaline. A side benefit is that watermelon is a natural diuretic. For a fast longer than three or four days on watermelon, it may be a good idea to also consume a green phytonutrient product, plus cold-pressed oil, enzymes, and probiotic supplements, depending on individual needs. The body needs these food source minerals and will utilize them directly, without interfering with the detoxification process that is underway.

### Breaking a Fast

It is very important to break a fast properly while moving on to eating solid foods. During a fast, especially water-type fasts, the organs of digestion and assimilation are at rest. They are not producing and secreting digestive chemicals and enzymes. If solid food (especially cooked food) is taken soon after the fast, it is quite a shock to the body and can cause serious problems with digestion. The body's system needs to be gently encouraged back into action. Starting with diluted fruit juices and vegetable broth soups does this best. Thereafter, small amounts of solid foods can be reintroduced, starting with the more easily digested ones. Protein foods, especially meats, should be reintroduced last and in small quantities, until the system has adapted and feels normal again. During this transition phase, the addition of digestive enzyme supplements with meals can be helpful. The longer the length of fast, the more gradually one should end it.

### Infrared Saunas

Saunas have a history dating back to the bath houses of ancient Rome and the Turkish Empire.[13] The Finns and Russians have revered the health, beauty, relaxation, and social benefits of saunas for over two thousand years. Throughout their history in North America, native tribes have utilized sweat lodges.

A traditional sauna is a small room, typically heated to approximately 140 to 230°F (60 to 110°C), in which one or more persons disrobe and sit or lie down for a period of time while their body temperatures rise and perspiration is induced. During this process, the body relaxes and metabolism and circulation speed up, enabling cells to eliminate toxins, such as chemicals and heavy metals, more efficiently.[14] Raised body temperature, also called hyperthermia, emulates the conditions of a fever, normally created by the body to combat infections and viruses. Under these conditions immune responses are enhanced, and healing of many conditions, including infections and tumors, is achieved more rapidly.[15]

Infrared heat is the warmth we feel when our bodies are exposed to sunlight. When a cloud shades us from the sun, we immediately feel cooler even though the air temperature has not changed because we are no longer receiving the sun's infrared radiation. The human body receives and also emits infrared energy.[16]

Dr. Tadashi Ishikawa of Japan received a patent in 1965 for a zirconia ceramic infrared heater used in the first healing infrared thermal systems. This led to the development of the far infrared (FIR) sauna, or more simply, infrared sauna, which can maintain lower and more easily toler-ated air temperatures between 100 and 120°F (38 and 49°C).

Whereas traditional saunas heat the air and skin surfaces, the FIR waves of infrared saunas penetrate beneath skin layers, creating a deep heating effect on tissues, muscles, and fat. As blood flow increases to cool the body, a cardiovascular conditioning and calorie-burning effect occurs and sweat is produced. Since many toxins are stored in body fat, as fat cells are heated they release toxins into the sweat which is then eliminated via the skin. And because internal organs are largely unaffected by the sauna's direct hyper-thermic effects, detoxification can be achieved without placing stress on the liver or kidneys.[17] Dr. Zane Gard has reported "significant reductions in body toxin levels and improvements in a wide array of medical condi-tions" resulting from sauna therapy.[18] Dr. Sherry Rogers, in her article "The Ultimate Solution to Disease," recommends the infrared sauna as the best way of removing heavy metals and pesticide residues from the body.[19]

All saunas provide health benefits and the regular use of one makes sense in our modern world where it is becoming difficult to avoid ingest-ing toxins that are now present in much of our food and air. However, as one infrared sauna manufacturer explained to me, there is a great deal of unsubstantiated and misleading information in the marketplace regard-ing toxin sweat analysis as well as which sauna features are superior. Do your own research before deciding to buy one. Some concern is being expressed that cheaper imported units are made of inferior materials and components which do not meet North American safety standards. When purchasing an infrared sauna, look for one that is well-built, contains a genuine ceramic heater, does not use plywood in its construction, and meets North American safety standards.

## DETOXIFICATION AS A LIFESTYLE

Whatever modes of detoxification are adopted, they should become part of a lifestyle if one is to regain vibrant health. Be patient. Don't rush the detoxification process, because it requires energy and time for the body to heal. We all have enough toxins in us to keep us working at it for years. The objective is to help the body move to a neutral acid-alkaline balance.

Up to this point, we have gained knowledge about how the body functions, how disease develops, what the body needs for health, and how to detoxify toxins and wastes. We will now focus on feeding the body the nutrition it needs to do its job. Water is the subject of the next chapter. We will explore different types of water, including ones that are in the marketplace, and how they have a bearing on our health.

THIRD KEY

# FEEDING

# 14 | WATER FOR LIFE

*The molecular structure of water
is the essence of all life.*

DR. ALBERT SZENT-GYORGY, NOBEL PRIZE WINNER

## OUR NEED FOR WATER

OUR NEED FOR water is second only to oxygen for sustaining life. Without enough water, we die; with water of the best kind, we can thrive. Before I began studying water, I had no idea how special and complex it is.

Our bodies are composed of almost three-fourths water, and every cell is dependent on an efficient supply. The brain is nearly 90% water. Messages in brain cells are transported through water to the nerve endings, and all nutrients for the body are transported via water. Water maintains the body's equilibrium and temperature, lubricates tissues, dilutes the concentration of poisons in the body, flushes wastes and toxins, hydrates the skin, and acts as a shock absorber for joints, bones, and muscles. Water is a very powerful healing force. Normal physical activity can use at least three quarts (2.84 liters) of replacement water each day. Strenuous activity, a hot climate, or a high table salt diet increases this requirement.

When the body gets enough water it is able to work efficiently. Lack of proper hydration in body tissues is now recognized as a substantial factor in the aging process. Even dehydration of 1% to 2% can affect all functions of the body. Symptoms of dehydration can include: headaches, irritability, impatience, restlessness, insomnia, dry skin, loss of appetite, constipation, unexplained weight gain, and swollen hands and/or feet from water retention. The gradual loss of water in the body is one factor of aging which contributes significantly to wrinkles.

Water requirements vary according to body size, physical activity, air temperature, and sweating. It is generally recognized that a normal body requires about eight glasses of water each day, or about one half ounce for every pound (33 ml per kilogram) of body weight. The raw fruits and vegetables we eat supply some of the water in our diet, and the rest is made up in what we drink. If we feel thirsty often, this is an indication that we are dehydrated.

Both the color and the amount of urine produced are good indicators of whether we are drinking enough water or not. We should urinate every few hours. Urine should be a pale straw color; if the urine is dark yellow, we need to drink more water.

### Water Quality

The quality of water we consume is an important consideration. It should be as pure as possible, free of chlorine, fluoride, bacteria, viruses, and parasites. Pure natural spring water is very good, but not always available. Most city tap water should be purified by some method that removes chemicals and disease-causing toxins. Once this is done, the water may be clean and will better sustain life; however, it is still not the best kind of water for promoting health.

Have you noticed that when you drink more water, the number of times you have to run to the bathroom increases? Is this natural? Actually, it is not. The situation is that most of the water is running through us because it is not being absorbed at the cellular level where it is needed. It is not in a form that can easily hydrate the body. The result is that we slowly become dehydrated, which causes toxins to concentrate at the cellular level because there is insufficient water to flush them out. Toxic storage causes cells to change normal function and causes disease to develop. By the time we notice the skin becoming wrinkled, our cells are already dehydrated, toxic, and undernourished. Why does this happen?

## RESEARCH ON WATER

In 1912, Dr. Alexis Carrel, a medical researcher at the Rockefeller Institute, immersed some heart tissue from a chicken embryo in sea water containing food nutrients. He discovered that, as these cells were nourished and flushed daily with slightly alkaline water, they continued to live. In fact, the very same cells were still alive 32 years later when Dr. Carrel died. He predicted that the cells could be kept alive indefinitely. In his words: "The cell is immortal. It is merely the fluid in which it floats that degenerates. Renew this fluid at regular intervals, give the cells what they require for nutrition, and as far as we know, the pulsation of life may go on forever."[1]

This is quite amazing, considering the fact that a chicken's normal lifespan is about seven years. What we learn from this is that if cells are cleansed and fed on a continuous basis, they can live for a very, very long time. The trick is to get good water into and around the cells.

### Water Structure Is the Key

Dr. Mu Shik Jhon was considered an expert in the field of statistical liquid mechanics. He researched the qualities of water for over 40 years. Dr. Jhon concluded that the healthiest water for humans to consume is water that has a high content of individual molecules in the shape of a hexagon, because it has the best hydrating and detoxifying properties. It naturally promotes efficient metabolic function, enhanced immune function, better health, and slower aging.[2] This is due to the greater hydrogen bonding of hexagonally structured water, which creates a higher surface tension, enhancing its ability to rise within capillaries.[3]

Healthy bodies contain high percentages of hexagonally-structured water. Dr. Jhon's research also revealed that water that contains predominantly pentagonal molecules is energetically inferior to hexagonal water, and is less healthy for consumption because of its accelerated aging effect on the body.[4] Magnetic resonance imaging (MRI) has shown that aging is due to a loss of hexagonally-structured water from organs, tissues, and cells, not just a loss of water.[5]

Melted snow water from pristine mountain areas contains a high percentage of hexagonal molecules,[6] but this kind of water is not available to many people. As you will read later, there are water structuring devices that can enhance the structure of ordinary tap water.

### Thoughts Change Water Structure

In chapter 12, you were introduced to the work of Dr. Masaru Emoto. By observing ice crystals, he discovered that water has a capacity for memory. He was able to demonstrate that many things in and around water affect its structure. Pure natural water, when frozen, has beautiful well-formed ice crystals similar to those of a snowflake. He discovered that, as water becomes more polluted, its ice crystals become increasingly deformed and fractured. Similarly, water that has been distilled loses its inner structural organization. It is unable to form organized crystals.

Most revealing was Dr. Emoto's discovery that our thoughts, words, and emotions can significantly change the structure of water. The conclusions from this research indicate that water has the ability to take on and store information, and once it has obtained it, transfer it to other living organisms.

Water takes on the consciousness of individuals or groups around it, and ultimately, that of the world population. Our thoughts and words change the structure of water. In turn, as we ingest the resulting water through eating, drinking, and breathing, we are affected positively or negatively. Knowing this, what kind of qualities do you think the water in your life is taking on? How are you affecting it? How is it affecting you? Personally, I will never take water for granted again as just something my body requires to stay fluid. I have a new and profound respect for it and the role it can play in helping my body stay healthy.

### Water Gets Its Energy from Light

As indicated in chapter 12, biophotons are tiny energy bodies found in the cellular fluids of all living organisms.[7] They are the energizers and information transmitters for and between cells. Light particles, which biophotons are, are the energy of the universe. They pulsate in constant energy exchange with the Universal Love Life Force for all living organisms. This is where the pure or primal energy comes from. It is never lost; it just changes form. Water is alive in direct proportion to its content and quality of biophotons. Water that lacks primal source biophotons also lacks optimal energy.

### The Best Water for Drinking

The research of Drs. Jhon and Emoto lead us to a clear conclusion that the molecular structure of pure, vital water is hexagonal in shape. How well-organized water crystals are, as evidenced by Dr. Emoto's photographs, is also very significant. Any pollution, or change in the water's purity, results in a breakdown of this hexagonal crystalline structure, with a consequent reduction in life force qualities.

The best water for drinking is water that has hexagon-shaped molecules, and maximum activity of biophoton particles.

## DIFFERENT TYPES OF WATER

Let us examine some of the water products that are presently available in the marketplace, as well as treatment methods.

### Bottled Water

Most bottled water in North America is of a good quality. It is clean, because U.S. and Canadian laws require producers to meet strict standards. In my opinion, however, the health claims made by some water marketing companies are greatly overblown because water naturally seeks a neutral balance. Special water qualities, even if they were there, would change over a period of time. In addition, chemicals from some of the plastic bottles and pipes can leach into the water, which would pollute it.

### Carbonated Water

Bottled carbonated water is a popular drink that many people view as good water. It is made by infusing water with carbon dioxide. However, the result is acidic water. Water combines with carbon dioxide to form carbonic acid ($H_2O + CO_2 \rightarrow H_2CO_3$). The pH of bottled carbonated water typically ranges from 4.2 to 4.7. This works against our efforts to alkalize towards greater health.

### Spring and Artesian Well Water

Most spring and artesian water bears natural life force and is of good quality.

### Purified Water—Distilled and Reverse Osmosis

Purifying water removes chemical and bacterial contaminants, as well as minerals. That's the good news. However, in my opinion, purified water is not recommended for drinking over the long term. Purifying processes destabilize its molecular structure. In addition, distilled and reverse osmosis waters are not neutral, as is commonly thought; they are acidic, with a pH of approximately 5.7 to 6.0. When consumed over time, these waters can represent a considerable drain on the body's alkaline resources.

Dr. Emoto's work with different samples of distilled water found that although their frozen samples showed different formations, none had an organized crystalline structure. It is the structure of water that allows it to hold the essence of life force, or biophotonic energy. Both distilled and reverse osmosis waters have very little biophotonic activity.

The concept of "purified water" is a controversial subject. Some sources, even medical, maintain that distilled water is exactly what the body needs since the liver filters out the unusable minerals in ordinary water. Unfortunately, what they are overlooking is its acidic nature, lack of biophotonic energy, and molecular structure.

Distilled water is not found in nature; it is an unnatural and foreign substance for the body. It does have the one advantage of being able to remove unusable minerals from the body. Because distilled water is "empty" of minerals, it naturally seeks to balance this deficiency, as Dr. M. T. Morter explains:

When distilled water is taken into the body, some of the unusable, inorganic minerals that have been stored in the body will fill the available spaces in the distilled water and will be eliminated.[8]

What is important to understand is that the body is always looking for an energy recharge. When energy-deficient foods and liquids are consumed, the body has to use its own energy reserves to process them, which results in a net energy loss. Drinking distilled or reverse osmosis water may be suitable during short periods of detoxification, but they can have a degenerative, depleting effect on the body's energy reserves in the long term.

### Ionized Water

Proponents of ionized water emphasize its antioxidant properties—its ability to neutralize millions of free radicals (unpaired, unstable electrons) in the body and thus slow down the aging process. Think of "antioxidant" as an anti-rusting agent. Ionized water is also alkaline. However, ionized water lacks biophotonic activity and cannot hold its molecular structure for long. It does not meet the definition of structured and energized water.

While I can see the advantage of helping the body to neutralize free radicals by drinking ionized water, this is still like taking a medicine to eliminate a symptom. The main reason why free radicals get the upper hand in the body in the first place is because of the intake of unhealthy air, food, and water. We still need to address the *cause*. What the body is really seeking from any food or water, is *energy*—it requires biophotons and minerals. The body is always in search of an electrical recharge. When it comes to electrical activity, ionized water comes up short.

### Magnetic Conditioning Devices

These devices polarize existing minerals in water, thereby solving mineral scaling problems in water pipes. Running water past magnets also reduces the water's surface tension. But, as we learned in chapter 12, magnets are derivative energy devices and as such, they cannot produce true rejuvenating primal energies. They will energize water up to the energy frequency of the magnets used, but that is their limit. Consequently, when we drink water derived from these devices, we are limiting our potential energy intake.

### Other Water Invigoration Devices

There are many other water devices on the market that claim to be energy enhancers, and even some that show an increase in biophotons under the microscope. But are they legitimate? Does using water from these devices actually result in increased benefits? Does water from these devices produce structured plants and produce? The developers of these units should be doing tests with living organisms to demonstrate this.

## ENERGIZED LIVING WATER

Living water is water that has energy, is naturally structured, and therefore promotes life in everything that consumes it, be it plant, animal, or human.

In its pristine form in nature, water trickles down mountain streams over sand, pebbles, and rocks, collecting minerals as it travels. It is charged with electrical energy from the earth's magnetism and from cosmic energy; it also collects infrared waves from the sun, and ideally, has a pH that is slightly alkaline.

The energy in water is light energy, or biophotons, which are molecular light emissions that regulate cell growth and regeneration, and control all biochemical processes.[9]

### Accessing the Primary Energy Source

The energy work of Mr. and Mrs. E. Excelex was introduced in chapter 12. They have been researching and developing methods of clearing stale energies and raising pure vibrational energies in the human body. Key in this process have been their discoveries of how to access the primal energy of biophotons, what they call Universal Love Life Force energy, and how to create hexagonally-structured water.

Led by Spirit to a greater and continuing understanding, Mr. Excelex has developed various products to assist in the raising of the "White Light" and "General Vitality" of living organisms. Central in this has been his use of quartz crystals, certain minerals, a device to break water's surface tension membrane, plus conscious love vibrations, to develop a primary source water energizer.

For six years, Mr. and Mrs. E. Excelex grew vegetables and fruit in their gardens and greenhouse. Everything was grown naturally. Their water came from a clear, unpolluted mountain stream. The produce was good, both in quality and taste. But a very interesting development occurred in the sixth year after they began watering some of the plants and trees with structured water that was run through one of their primal source energy units, which they call Hexahedron999.[10] The produce grew faster and virtually doubled in size! Further, they said that the taste of the produce was superb.

### Proof Is in the Produce

There are many water invigoration devices on the market. All of them claim they impart more energy or health properties to water. But, how do we separate theory from proof, fact from fiction? That is the important question. What difference do these various waters make to the energy and growth of living organisms? If they make little or no difference to vitality, they are merely theory and perhaps good marketing promotion. What really should get our attention is results!

### Energy Comparisons of Different Waters

Listed below are some average energy comparisons for different kinds of water from the research done by Mr. and Mrs. Excelex.

Note that values vary somewhat according to the source water used, and the length and size of piping in the house through which energized water must travel. An arbitrary value of 100 was used for distilled water as an evaluation baseline.

| Water | General Vitality | White Light |
|---|---|---|
| Distilled | 100 | 90 |
| Reverse osmosis | 130 | 110 |
| Ionized | 150 | 140 |
| City | 150–400 | 130–350 |
| Brook (Excelex property) | 3600 | 3800 |
| Structured by small unit Hexahedron 999 | 15,000* | 15,000* |
| Structured by large unit Hexahedron 999 | 50,000* | 55,000* |

**Table 14.1 Water energy comparisons**
*These readings are minimums as the restructured and revitalized water leaves the unit.*

If these numbers do not appear accurate, we can clearly see by viewing the photographs in Figures 14.2, 14.3, and 14.4, how plants and trees respond to restructured water. The photographs were taken by the Excelexes to illustrate the differences between using ordinary brook water and hexahedron-structured water.

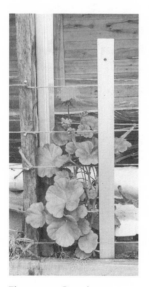 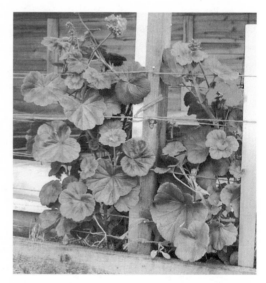

**Figure 14.1 Geraniums**
*The geranium on the left was fed ordinary brook water. The one on the right was given structured Hexadron water.*

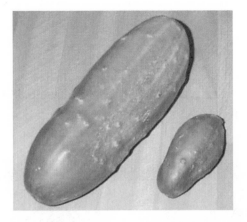

**Figure 14.2  Cucumbers**

*On the right is a normal size pickling cucumber that is usually the optimum size for eating. The one on the left was fed structured Hexahedron water, with average sizes reaching a pound or more. According to Mr. Excelex: "At this size one would expect them to be filled with large seeds and be a bit dry, but they were not. They had a sweet melon taste."*

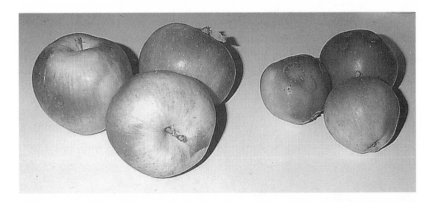

**Figure 14.3  Apples**

*The property on which the Excelexes lived for five years had some abandoned apple trees, which produced small scabby fruit. In 2002, they watered one tree occasionally with structured Hexahedron water. The resulting fruit was up to twice the normal size, and 90% of it was completely free of the blemishes and scabs which the trees normally produced (right). The larger apples were plentiful and delicious.*

271

### Biophotons in Water

When water molecules are structured in the shape of a hexagon, they naturally contain an abundance of biophotons. The following images of biophotons in a drop of water were captured with a somatoscope at 30,000 magnification. To the knowledge of researchers Mr. and Mrs. Excelex and the author, the biophoton detail shown in figure 14.5 is being published in book format here, for the first time.

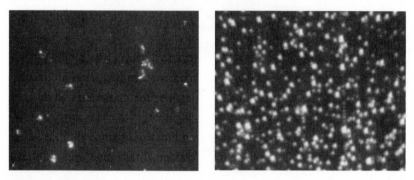

**Figure 14.4  Bio-photons in city tap water and city water after structuring with a Hexahedron999**

*Left: Chlorinated water, Kildare, Quebec. Right: Same city water after passing through a Hexadedron 999 filtering and restructuring unit.*

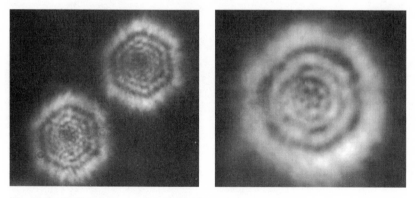

**Figure 14.5  Two biophotons and single biophoton**

*Left: Two biophotons showing hexagonal structures and light energy emanating from them; Right: Single, bright biophoton showing concentric hexagonal structures with a six-pointed star at the centre.*

In recent years, water system manufacturers have begun to talk about hexagonally-structured water, but all such water is not the same. Mr. and Mrs. Excelex have discovered that there are different kinds of hexagon structures in water depending on its source. With the aid of a somato-scope, they have found that there can be many levels of hexagonally struc-tured biophotons in water. Readily-observable examples of hexagon levels in water can be seen in Dr. Masaru Emoto's book *the Hidden Messages in Water.*[11] Glacial water crystals show one to three levels of hexagon struc-tures, whereas the New Zealand groundwater crystals show seven or more hexagonal layers.

Another observation made by Mr. and Mrs. Excelex was that biopho-tons composed of several levels of hexagonal structures have a brighter radiating light (energy field) surrounding them than a single-hexagon level biophoton. This brighter light is a clear indication of higher energy within the water, which explains why Mr. and Mrs. Excelex's plants that were fed structured water grew so well compared to others given different water.

The conclusion from these biophoton studies is that: the greater the number of highly-structured biophotons is in foods and water we con-sume, the greater is the amount of energy available to our bodies for its use. This brings clear understanding to Dr. Carey Reams' quote at the beginning of chapter 12: "We don't live off the food that we eat; we live off the energy in the food we eat."

### The Healthiest Water to Consume

After viewing the results of using well-structured energy water with plants, and observing the images of biophotons in water, there is no doubt about the best kind of water to drink for health and vitality. It should be water that is structured and charged with the primal source biophotons. This is truly a breakthrough in the understanding, application, and health potential of energy in water. The implications for human health and agriculture are enormous. Central to the realization of Mr. and Mrs. Excelex would be the understanding that "life produces life!"

## GUIDELINES FOR DRINKING WATER

Raw fruits and vegetables naturally contain 75% to 90% water. They should be the main sources of fulfilling the body's requirement for water. Because of their high fiber content, these foods also contribute greatly to the efficiency of the body's elimination cycle. They contain the organic minerals that the body needs and can readily assimilate. The water in raw fruits and vegetables is "living water." Depending on the amount of raw fruits and vegetables we eat, our activity level, and the air temperature we live and work in, our bodies require the equivalent of 6 to 8 full glasses of water, or about one half ounce per pound (33 ml per kilogram) of body weight, each day. Other liquids such as coffee, tea, soft drinks, and alcohol do not qualify as fluids that meet our daily water requirement.

While the body needs an adequate amount of good water for health each day, too much can also be stressful. When consumed with meals, water interferes with digestion. Drinking excessive amounts of water overworks the kidneys. As noted earlier, too much distilled and reverse osmosis water can actually contribute to nutritional imbalances and acidity in the body. Drinking one or two glasses of water with fresh squeezed lemon juice upon rising in the morning provides a healthy flushing and liquid replenishment for the body to start the day.

Generally, thirst should be our guide for drinking more liquids other than raw fruit and vegetable juices. If one is drinking lots of water in an attempt to keep bowel contents moist, the basics of the constipation problem also need to be addressed. On a healthy diet, which avoids stimulating and toxic foods and includes ample quantities of fresh raw fruit and vegetables, there is very little natural thirst or need for large amounts of water.

Water is of critical importance to life. We should keep the following guidelines in mind when drinking water:

1   Drink enough of it every day to satisfy the body's hydration needs.
2   Any kind of water is better than no water.

3   Water should be filtered to remove pollutants and chemicals, then remineralized with ionic minerals or sea salt for optimum results.

4   Energized water is better.

5   Filtered and hexagonally structured, primal-source energized water provides maximum life force that is far superior to other waters, unless one has access to pristine, alkaline, alive, natural spring water or melted snow water.

We all have to eat food and we usually look forward to mealtimes. Most people select their meals based solely on what tastes good and what satisfies their hunger at the moment. But do we understand what food our bodies actually need in order to be healthy? Next, we will take a close look at the various qualities and ingredients that must be in food to build health.

# 15 | REAL FOOD
#      FOR THE BODY

∾

*Let food be your medicine ...*

HIPPOCRATES (460 BC)

∾

WE WOULD not need medicines or food supplements if our bodies were supplied with the essential nutrition they require. Unfortunately, that is not the case for most of us. We have lost conscious awareness of what we should be eating for health. Commercial food processing and marketing interests have added to our confusion. We have lost touch with the simplicity and purity of nature's provision. We alter our food and add chemicals to it and wonder why our health deteriorates. We try to prod our bodies back to health with medicines. All the time, the simple solution is readily available.

In his 1952 book *The Elixir of Life*, Arnold Devries said:

> The elixir of life is so very common, so easily available, that it has constantly been forgotten in the search for more elusive and mysterious substances. ... In natural foods, unchanged by the hand of man, are the life-giving factors which determine the state of human health.[1]

Not all foods and supplements have these essential life-giving factors. We need to understand the difference between foods that contribute to our health, and foods that weaken it.

## THE ESSENTIALS OF FOOD

### Real Food Versus Junk Food

Real food contributes to health. Junk food contributes to disease. It is denatured and contains little or no health-producing properties.

Our bodies are always looking for food that contains usable components.[2]

- Glucose—for energy.
- Protein—(amino acids) for building and repairing tissue.
- Fatty Acids—to construct membranes and move electrical currents.
- Ionic, food-form minerals—as catalysts and building components.
- Enzymes (vitamins)—as catalysts.
- Water—the medium for chemical processes.

Real foods:[3]

- Are edible, and grown by nature.
- Can be eaten without processing in any way.
- Can be eaten as an entire meal and be thoroughly enjoyed.

Real foods come to us from nature as "complete packages." They have everything in them that is necessary for the body to process and assimilate for use.[4] Food that does not contain such elements or that contains toxic additives can safely be considered junk.

Real foods have an alkaline effect in the body; junk foods have an acidic effect. Cooked food is incomplete because, at the very least, such cooking destroys its enzymes, some of the nutrition, and binds the amino acid lysine making the protein unusable by the liver to make amino acid building blocks and hormones. Cooking is a form of processing; the food is no longer natural.

Processed and packaged foods such as sugar and refined white flour, and the products made from them, such as candy, soft drinks, desserts, breakfast cereals, and breads, are almost totally lacking in fatty acids, minerals, and enzymes. In addition, they form acids and contain toxic chemicals which are added as preservatives to prolong shelf life and enhance flavor.

When food lacks one or more of the six essential ingredients listed above, the body has to borrow resources from its own tissues to process it. Toxins present the added burden of elimination because of their harmful and hazardous nature for health. The body attempts to eliminate toxins through stimulation, which "revs up" the metabolism and costs the body energy and nutrition in the process.

The simple code for nutritional digestion in the body is: it takes enzymes to get protein; it takes protein to get minerals; and, it takes minerals to get vitamins.[5] Each item is dependent on the one before it for complete digestion to take place.

When food contains all of its live ingredients, digestion can proceed to completion; bowel movements are easy, and produce very little odor.

### Raw Organic Food

Organically grown raw plant food is the most natural and nutritious available to us. It is living, if not irradiated, and is predominantly alkaline. Organic fruits and vegetables contain the most vitamins and minerals and are free of herbicides and pesticides. Raw food still has all its enzymes and is in the best form to be eaten. When we combine the two aspects, raw and organic, we have the best food we can give to our bodies. Such food is not only superior for health, it is superior in flavor.

If you think raw is boring, think again. A book by Juliano Brotman, entitled *RAW: The Uncook Book,* is a delight and an inspiration to read and use. Juliano operates an entirely raw cuisine restaurant in San Francisco that, when it opened, almost immediately won attention in the *San Francisco Chronicle, USA Today, People* magazine, *The New York Times,* and the *Vegetarian Times.* He and his food creations were reportedly, "the toast of Hollywood." The fare was billed as "Uncooked, Unadulterated, Unbelievably Delicious Living Food." Although this hardback volume is somewhat expensive, it is worth the price for the interest, variety, and enjoyment it can add to raw food eating. Its table of contents lists a wide array of items such as: soups, salads, breads, snacks, sushi, pizza, main courses, desserts, drinks, dressings, and sauces. The items are vegan cuisine with nothing heated above 100°F (38°C).

A second recipe book is *The Raw Gourmet* by Nomi Shannon. Another book that fully explains the wisdom of eating raw is *Nature's First Law: The Raw-Food Diet*, by Arlin, Dini, and Wolfe.

Interest in raw food is increasing, and more information on the benefits of preparing and eating it is gradually becoming available. A good source to start looking on the Internet is at www.rawfood.com.

## The Green Breakthrough

The Boutenko family of Ashland Oregon overcame serious degenerative disease problems by converting to eating only raw foods. However, after several years on this diet, they reached a point where their heath progress came to a plateau, and they began to lack energy and some of the vibrancy they had previously enjoyed.[6] In her search for a solution to this problem, Mrs. Victoria Boutenko began to study the diets of chimpanzees, who share 99.4% of the DNA sequence of humans.[7] Most of them have blood type A, while a minimal number have blood type O.[8] Her research led to the discovery that chimpanzees are remarkably healthy and disease-resistant on their natural diet that includes 50% fruit and 25–50% green vegetation, depending on the season. They only eat roots in time of drought or when fruits and greens are unavailable.[9] This is very interesting because we typically eat the roots of carrots, turnips, and beets, and discard the tops.

As Victoria continued her search for understanding, she discovered that green leaf vegetable tops provide superior health benefits compared to the roots. The advantages are mainly twofold: the first is nutrition and the second is fiber. The green leaf tops of root vegetables such as carrots, beets, parsnips, and turnips, contain a far greater abundance of chlorophyll, vitamins, alkaline minerals,[10] and essential amino acids.[11] The reason why humans prefer to eat the roots is because they contain "significantly more sugar and water. The tops are bitter from the abundant amount of nutrients in them."[12] Greens also contain both soluble and insoluble fiber, which is needed for colon health.

Although she tried to eat the way chimps do, Victoria could not chew and eat anywhere near the quantity of greens required. And when they are juiced, the pulp and fiber are lost. So she turned to blending leaves of spinach and kale with water. But this had an offensive odor and an unpleasant taste. Then from the notes of Jane Goodall, the famous researcher of chimpanzees, she noted that chimpanzees eat mostly fruit in the morning and turn to eating green leaves in the afternoon—but they often combine them with fruit. When Victoria blended her organic greens and water mixture with organic, sweet ripe fruit, she was amazed at the difference. The result was smooth, tasty, and enjoyable to consume. This is how her "green smoothie" was born.

As Victoria made and consumed green smoothies, in a very short time her energy, vibrancy, and feelings of well-being returned, and her cravings for less-healthy foods disappeared. Her family took note and soon joined with her in this addition to their diet, and they too started to experience renewed health benefits.

Extending her research, Victoria teamed up with Dr. Paul Faber of Roseburg, Oregon to do a 30-day study with 27 volunteers who were experiencing symptoms of low stomach acid. The results were remarkable, with 66.7% of participants showing "vast improvement" in their hypochlorhydria symptoms. In addition, all participants experienced health improvements, some of which were dramatic.[13]

The reason why inclusion of green smoothies produces such positive health changes appears to be due to the high-speed blending of whole green leaves. A blender thoroughly ruptures the plants' cellular structures, making all nutients available in significant quantity and in readily usable form for digestion. Chewing alone cannot achieve this level of efficiency.

The Roseburg experiment demonstrated that regular consumption of green smoothies can significantly improve health in a relatively short period of time. The health gains appear to be associated with improved levels of hydrochloric acid in the stomach, which results in more complete digestion and absorption of nutrients from all food consumed.

### Feeding Babies and Children

Everything in this book is relevant for children. If we want to have healthy children, we should feed them healthy food. Mothers should prepare their bodies nutritionally, well ahead of becoming pregnant, by detoxifying, drinking lots of fresh juices, eating raw foods, getting essential fatty acids such as hemp and flax oils, breathing fresh air, exercising, and resting.

When babies are changed over from breast milk to a cooked, solid food diet, they try to spit the food out. They intuitively know it is dead food. However, after repeated persistence and coaxing by mom or dad, they give in and accept the substandard cooked nutrition. Their natural instincts for healthy food are gradually suppressed.

Several unhealthy processes begin to happen in a baby's body as a result of eating cooked food. First, cooked food digestion is incomplete and stools take on an offensive odor. The undigested matter is literally, rotting food. Second, the body starts to use its stored nutritional reserves to maintain life-sustaining activities. If the feeding pattern continues, nutritional deficiencies start to develop. Third, toxins from the incompletely digested and assimilated food begin to accumulate in the organs of elimination. Fourth, retained toxins begin to be stored in various tissues throughout the body, thereby reducing its overall efficiency. When the combination of organ congestion, toxin storage, and nutritional deficiencies reach the point where the body can no longer maintain homeostasis—usually later in life—disease symptoms begin to manifest.

Babies should be fed breast milk—with the mother eating correctly—until they have teeth for chewing. Breast milk is natural food. It contains everything needed in the correct proportions for the proper growth and development of a baby. Babies do not begin producing digestive enzymes in their bodies until their teeth have begun to erupt, meaning they have great difficulty handling solid food. If for some reason, the mother is unable to breast feed the infant for long, the next best substitute is raw goat's milk mixed with equal parts of fresh carrot juice, juice from a stick of celery, and pure water. Cow milk is not recommended, even raw, because it is too high in calcium and protein, in addition to its acid-alkaline balance being wrong. Pasteurized products should not be fed to babies, while canned formulas should only be used as a last resort. These are dead, mucus-producing foods; they precipitate sinus problems, ear infections, allergies, and lung disorders.[14]

Infants and children thrive on raw, whole foods. When weaning babies, introduce raw fruit first, then after a while, vegetables, both of which can be pulverized and broken down in a blender, food processor, or juicer. As they grow, babies are gradually able to handle a greater variety of whole fruits and vegetables. Make this type of food a major portion of their intake, and watch the results.

Further information about feeding babies and children is available in Dr. Robbins' booklet, *Pregnancy, Childbirth and Children's Diet.*[15]

### Enzymes

An enzyme is "a protein molecule that catalyzes chemical reactions of other substances without itself being destroyed or altered upon completion of the reactions."[16] Enzymes are so essential to health that they deserve a special focus. They are the living catalysts that activate all biochemical reactions within our bodies. Without sufficient enzymes, the body degenerates into disease.

Other than traumatic physical injuries, there is no disease that can maintain its existence in our bodies if our enzyme resources are complete and functioning perfectly. It is important for us to understand both the scope and necessity of enzymes in our bodies:

> About 5,000 individual enzymes have so far been isolated and identified, but some authorities estimate that it takes about 100,000 enzymes to run the body, each with a specific job to do. ...
>
> Even though there are thousands of different enzymes, there are basically only three types: digestive enzymes that digest food, metabolic enzymes that run the body, and food enzymes that are found in raw food.[17]

Enzymes make things happen in our bodies. It is estimated that there are in excess of 20 billion new cells created in the body each day. Within each one of these cells there are numerous biochemical actions taking place, all initiated and accelerated by enzymes.

Dr. Edward Howell discovered the principle of enzyme nutrition in 1932. He did extensive research and teaching on the role of enzymes in nutrition, human health, and disease. He found that a full complement of digestive enzymes must be consumed, in or with food, for its complete nutritional value to be delivered to the cells of the body. When food is incompletely digested, it becomes toxic and a burden to the body. The body produces an elevated white blood cell count in response to the lack of enzymes in cooked food in an attempt to clear the additional toxins from incompletely-digested food. Dr. Howell made this discovery while observing that his leukemia patients all had elevated white blood cell counts. When he fasted his patients so that their bodies would not require enzymes to digest cooked food, the white blood cell counts lowered. As the patients gained strength, he worked on replenishing their enzyme reserves by feeding them raw food, resulting in considerable improvements in the health of his patients.

Dr. Howell concluded that, since cooking routinely destroys enzymes in food, a diet devoid of enzymes would result in enlargement of the pancreas, leading to an increase in chronic degenerative diseases and cancer. The pancreas is the master gland of digestion. It increases in size in an attempt to produce more enzymes in the absence of a healthy food source. Eventually, it gives in to deficiencies and exhaustion, and succumbs to disease.

Enzymes create and support all bodily functions. Staying young and healthy depends on keeping enzyme activity in our bodies at an optimum level.[18]

### What Kills Enzymes?

All raw foods contain enzymes; it is what we do to food that destroys them. Chemical additives, radiation, and exposure to oxygen kills enzymes. Fluorides and nicotine are two of the strongest killers of enzymes. However, the main enzyme killer is heat from cooking. Enzymes are destroyed when food is heated above 112–120°F (44–49°FC). When we eat cooked food, the body needs to draw nutrients from its own tissue reserves to manufacture digestive enzymes. The greater the load we put on the body to produce digestive enzymes, the less energy and nutrients it has to produce the other metabolic enzymes needed throughout the body. Over time, this leads to enzyme, vitamin, and mineral deficiencies, and eventually, to degenerative diseases.

In a healthy diet, enzymes must be part of all food. They must be part of every supplement. No food or supplement has healing and normalizing abilities except when it is functioning in combination with specific enzymes.

### Enzymes Are Part of a Team

Although enzymes perform important functions on their own in the body, other nutritional building blocks must have the assistance of enzymes to be able to contribute to health.

Proteins, minerals, and vitamins provide little permanent or nutritional benefit unless they work together as parts of a team, along with enzymes. The absence of any one member of this team reduces the efficiency of the whole team by as much as 95 to 99%.[19]

### Our Enzyme Bank

We start life with a healthy stock of enzymes in our bodies. Dr. Howell called this reserve our "enzyme bank account."[20] When we were young, most of us could eat almost any kind of food or combination of foods. However, after our eating habits have been unhealthy for many years, our enzyme reserves become depleted, and our body's metabolic functions become less efficient; they begin to slow down. If the exact combination of required enzymes is lacking in our stomachs, food is incompletely digested, becomes toxic, and putrefies; we are unable to benefit from the full nourishment of the food. The digestive enzymes we use are supposed to be continuously replenished from an outside source, namely raw food.

One of the first indications that enzyme activity is diminishing in our bodies, especially as we grow older, is the appearance of digestive problems.

Tests have shown the enzyme count in the saliva of young adults to be thirty times stronger than in people over sixty-nine years of age.[21] Fortunately, we are able to supplement our diet with live enzymes to assist with digestion as well as make deposits to our enzyme bank account. Every time we eat cooked or processed food we should supplement with good quality plant-source enzymes to assist the digestive process. Enzymes taken on an empty stomach are also helpful because they go straight to the liver and on into the body where they are used for detoxification and repair. The most important thing we can do to help a flagging enzyme reserve is to supplement with digestive enzymes. Enzymes are so valuable to the body that any excess is added to the body's enzyme pool for later use.[22]

Over time, as we improve our diet with enzyme-rich foods and enzyme supplements, we can replenish our enzyme bank account. This means making steady deposits into our enzyme account rather than steady withdrawals. With a good enzyme reserve and a regular supply of active enzymes in raw, alkaline-producing food, disease conditions can be reversed and eliminated; the effects of aging can be reversed. Not only can we live longer, but our quality of life will be much improved. Energy, strength, health, and longevity are directly proportional to enzyme resources.[23] Every enzyme we consume in food or in supplement form means one less enzyme the body must deplete from its resources.

### The Main Digestive Enzymes

There are four main kinds of digestive enzymes—amylase, lipase, protease, and cellulase. The body is able to manufacture the first three of these in the pancreas. But, there is a catch; pancreatic enzymes only work in the small intestine, which is alkaline, and not in the stomach, which is acid. They work in a pH range of 7.8–8.3. Although pancreatic enzymes are very powerful, their areas of work and influence are restricted. In comparison, plant enzymes are much more versatile and work in both the stomach and small intestine.[24] Plant enzymes work in a pH range of 2 to 12.

The purpose of the four main digestive enzymes for supplementation purposes, are:

1  Amylase—to break down carbohydrates.
2  Lipase—to break down fats.
3  Protease—to break down proteins.
4  Cellulase—to break down soluble parts of fiber.


The body cannot manufacture cellulase; it must be obtained from foods that are high in fiber, or from supplements. Cellulase plays the very important role of transporting nutrients into the body through the gut wall and moving heavy metal toxins out, which can alleviate multiple chemical sensitivities.

### Amino Acids

There are twenty-two known amino acids in protein, of which eight (or nine, depending on sources consulted) are considered essential for human health. The value of protein depends on its amino acid profile. The body cannot make protein tissues from the foods we eat *unless* all eight essential amino acids are present *at the same time, at the same meal.*[25] Lysine is one of the eight essential amino acids. It is considered a *limiting* amino acid because, if it is not present, it can "make practically worthless the other seven amino acids at the site of protein formation."[26] One characteristic of lysine is that it can be inactivated by heat.[27] This is an important point to remember since active lysine must be present for complete digestion to take place.[28] It means that whenever we eat cooked protein, it cannot be completely digested. This causes the body to be starved of essential amino acid building blocks; our hunger is satisfied, even as our nutritional reserves are being depleted.

Complete amino acids are absolutely necessary for health. When active lysine is not available during digestion, the other amino acids cannot be broken down sufficiently enough to pass through the walls of the small intestine, and from there, on to the liver. The liver gradually becomes lacking in the complete amino acids it requires to manufacture and supply metabolic enzymes and hormones to the rest of the body.[29,30] Undigested matter proceeds to the colon where it putrefies, produces toxins, and causes foul bathroom odors. A lack of essential amino acids in the diet leads to hormonal imbalances and degenerative diseases.

## Bowel Flora

Bowel flora are friendly bacteria, or probiotics, that live and work in the intestinal tract. After enzymes, friendly bacteria in the intestinal tract comprise the only other group of organisms that perform healthy transactions in our bodies. They are a necessary part of the biological process because they produce enzymes, vitamins, and antibiotics, and create electrical matrices that can inhibit cancers, deactivate viruses, reduce cholesterol, and enhance the immune system. Due to our modern diets, processed foods, chlorinated and fluoridated water, pharmaceutical antibiotics, and intestinal toxemia, friendly bacteria populations are greatly reduced in the human intestinal tract. Because of this, they should be reintroduced on a regular basis by supplementing the diet with a probiotic product that is a synergistic formulation of natural and requisite live bacteria. There are many strains of probiotics. Acidophilus and bifidus are the more commonly recognized strains available in healthfood stores. Others, such as L. Salivarius and L. Plantarum are more powerful.[31]

## Fiber—the Colon's Friend

Fiber is vital to the body's detoxification process. The colon depends on it for efficient elimination. Fiber absorbs and holds toxins from chemical pollutants, dead cells, and waste matter in the colon for elimination. Without adequate fiber, complete elimination is almost impossible. Fiber is the broom and sponge of the intestinal tract. It prevents constipation, hemorrhoids, and diverticulitis, and may play a role in controlling weight, regulating blood sugars, and reducing the risk of heart disease and some cancers. Fiber absorbs many times its weight in water, resulting in softer, bulkier stools. When extra fiber is added to the diet, the intake of water should be increased also.

There are two kinds of fiber: soluble and insoluble—neither of which is broken-down for nutritional purposes. Soluble fiber forms a gel when mixed with a liquid and functions to keep the stools soft for easy passage through the colon. Insoluble fiber acts as a sponge to hold toxins and sweep the walls of the colon during elimination. Cellulose, hemicellulose, and lignin are types of insoluble fiber found in apples, beets, broccoli, pears, and whole grains. Foods such as oats, oat bran, psyllium husks, and flax seeds are rich in both soluble and insoluble fiber.

If we do not consume adequate fiber, waste matter accumulates in the body, reducing its efficiency and setting the stage for degenerative diseases.

### Minerals

Minerals are used by the body in virtually all its functions and they are an intricate part of its building structure. They are classified as major and trace. The major minerals, by decreasing percentage of body weight, are calcium, phosphorus, potassium, sulfur, chlorine, sodium, fluorine, magnesium, iron, manganese, silicon, copper, and iodine. Trace minerals are those found only in minute, though nonetheless necessary, amounts in the body. They include: zinc, cobalt, molybdenum, aluminum, chromium, lead, neodymium, selenium, titanium, tin, silver, rubidium, nickel, neon, strontium, argon, beryllium, boron, cerium, helium, lanthanum, scandium, vanadium, and others.

The body needs a full spectrum and balanced array of the minerals nature provides in foods grown in mineral-rich soil. When soil has become depleted of some of its minerals, foods grown in such soil will also be mineral-deficient. Relative sweetness is one test of determining whether raw foods have an adequate mineral content. The sweeter-tasting the fruit or vegetable, the higher the concentration of minerals.[32] Generally speaking, mass-produced vegetables sold in grocery stores are grown in mineral deficient soils. When consuming these, we should supplement our diet with food-form or herbal-form mineral preparations, as well as natural sea salt, to ensure we are getting all of the minerals required by the body.

### Good Oils and Bad Fats

First, we need to understand that the body requires oils from our diets. It cannot produce certain fatty and essential fatty acids (EFAs) which are present in good cold-processed oils. Staying on a low fat diet for too long can lead to degenerative diseases and death.

We need to know the difference between good oils, which our bodies require, and bad oils and bad fats that lead to degenerative disease. An excellent reference on this subject is the book *Fats that Heal, Fats that Kill* by Udo Erasmus. In his book Erasmus states:

> Degenerative diseases that involve fats prematurely kill over two-thirds of the people currently living in affluent, industrialized nations.[33]

By correctly addressing malnutrition and pollution, many degenerative conditions such as cardiovascular disease, cancer, type II diabetes, arthritis, multiple sclerosis, asthma, and hypoglycemia can often be completely reversed. Changing the kinds and quantities of fats we eat, as well as how we process and use them is part of addressing both malnutrition and internal pollution.[34]

Essential fatty acids and unsaturated fats are good oils for the body. Trans fatty acids and hydrogenated oils are harmful oils.

Essential fatty acids are utilized by the body to build cell structure, to help generate electrical energy, and produce hormones. They are required for nerve impulses, brain development and function, healthy skin, digestion, inner organ function, the cardiovascular system, and immune system. They are critically important for health. Most people are oil deficient because good oils are lacking in their diets.

All the essential fatty acids are obtained from a diet of real food. A deficiency of one or more of the essential fatty acids is usually evident in degenerative disease conditions. On the road to recovering health, supplementing with hemp oil, olive oil, flax oil, or a combination of these oils is a good measure. They are rich in linoleic and alpha-linolenic acids—more commonly known as omega-3 and omega-6 fatty acids—which are the key components of healing oils.

Officials of the World Health Organization, Health Canada, Japan, and Sweden, recommend a 1:4 ratio of omega-3 to omega-6 for oil consumption. Hemp oil is closest to this range among naturally occurring oils with a ratio of at least 1:3. Udo Erasmus indicated that "one can use it for a life-time without ever suffering EFA deficiency."[34]

For therapeutic purposes, Erasmus suggests using a ratio that is higher in omega-3 for correcting degenerative conditions. He has found that flax oil, with a ratio of 4:1, produces good results. After improvement is evident, a lower omega-3 content is recommended for the long term, since the extended use of high omega-3 oil can lead to an omega-6 deficiency. Omega-6 deficiency can produce symptoms such as, dry eyes, skipped heartbeats, painful finger joints, and fragile, thin skin. Erasmus recommends a 2:1 (omega-3 to omega-6) ratio for maintenance after the condition has been corrected or reversed.[35] This can be achieved by mixing approximately three parts flax oil to one part hemp oil. Readers should do further research to determine the best ratio for their own situations.

### Oil Supplementation

A good indicator of the need for oil supplementation is when the skin is dry. If it is dry or flaky when scratched, the body is in need of oil supplementation. Several tablespoons per day may be taken until a smooth skin is achieved again. Good oils for this use may be purchased from health-food stores. They must be kept in the refrigerator and used before their expiry dates. Otherwise, they turn rancid and become toxic to the body. It is preferable to keep oil supplements in the freezer to preserve their freshness. This way, they can be kept for long periods of time and warmed slightly under the tap for immediate use.

### Unsaturated and Saturated Fats

Unsaturated oils, or unsaturated fats as they are sometimes referred to, are liquid at room temperature. They are so named because they lack two or more hydrogen atoms in their molecular structure. Raw vegetables, fruits, grains, nuts, and seeds contain naturally-occurring unsaturated fats.

Saturated fats have no openings in their chemical structure. They are usually solid at room temperature. Naturally-occurring saturated fats are found mainly in animal fats, meats, dairy products, eggs, and tropical oils.

They are also synthesized in the body from carbohydrates. Contrary to popular belief, not all saturated fats are responsible for the many diseases they are accused of contributing to. In fact, saturated fats are very necessary and are utilized by the body—for energy, to build cell membranes, for the incorporation of calcium into bone structure, and to strengthen the immune system. However, long-chain fatty acids, found mostly in animal and dairy products, do have a tendency to aggregate or stick together, causing sticky blood platelets. This is why people who consume large amounts of animal and dairy products suffer from an increased incidence of cardiovascular disease.

Unsaturated EFAS, like those found in seed oils and fish, prevent saturated fats from aggregating by keeping them dispersed. This may explain why Eskimos who consumed traditional diets had a very low incidence of heart disease. The fat of land animals does not contain omega-3 EFAS, whereas the fat of sea mammals and fish does.

### Trans Fats

Trans fats are a major contributing risk factor for developing cardiovascular disease. They are formed when oils have been "trans-formed" by hydrogenation and so are also referred to as hydrogenated oils. The hydrogenation process involves heating oils to a high temperature in the presence of a metal catalyst such as nickel or aluminum, which causes a transfer of hydrogen atoms to the oil molecule. The oil molecule becomes straight, or stiff. When hydrogenated, oils that are liquid at room temperature become solid or spreadable, like margarine. Not surprisingly, the high heat of processing destroys enzymes, vitamins, and nutrients that are present in the natural oil. Removing the life-supporting qualities of edible oils removes their natural ability to spoil, thereby giving the product a longer shelf life.

Oils whose product labels indicate that they have been subjected to hydrogenation should not be consumed because they cause significant lowering of "good" cholesterol (HDL) and a serious increase in "bad" cholesterol (LDL). Hydrogenated oils have been strongly linked to cardiovascular disease, diabetes, and other serious health problems.[36] Hydrogenated oils and trans fats can be found in products such as, margarine, shortening and lard, processed vegetable oils, processed cheese, processed peanut butter, french fries, candies, and cookies.

### Supermarket Oils

Most supermarket oils are made from seeds that have been subjected to many destructive processes to produce products that can stay on shelves for long periods of time without spoiling. These processes include: mechanical cleaning, heating at high temperatures, high pressure extraction, solvent extraction, degumming with phosphoric acid, refining with sodium hydroxide, bleaching, deodorizing, hydrogenation, and often, the addition of synthetic chemical antioxidants.[37] Essentially, nutritious seeds are refined into oils that are devoid of nutrition and contain trans fats and toxic chemicals. The finished product is commercially convenient, but hazardous to the health of the consumer.

### Cooking with Oils or Fats

Oils containing EFAS should not be cooked. Even good quality oils begin to be transformed at temperatures above 320°F (160°C); trans fats begin to form. When one sees oil in a cooking pan "smoking," harmful substances are already being produced.

Polyunsaturated oils, which include vegetable oils like sunflower, safflower, soy, and corn, are the worst to cook with because of the trans fats created during the hydrogenation process. On the other hand, saturated fats such as butter or coconut oil may be used for frying or baking at lower temperatures without harming them. If one must fry food, adding water to the pan or wok keeps the temperature at near 212°F (100°C). Better yet, simmer the food in water and then add a good oil at a later stage.

## Cholesterol

Cholesterol is a subject that is generally misunderstood, and that has come to strike fear in the minds of people. Despite cholesterol's bad reputation, it is vital to the body. The subject has become what Erasmus calls a "cholesterol scare":

> The cholesterol scare is big business for doctors, laboratories, and drug companies. It is also a powerful marketing gimmick for vegetable oil and margarine manufacturers who can advertise their products to be 'cholesterol-free.' The fact is that 999 out of every 1000 people (or 499 out of every 500, depending on which expert source you read) can control their cholesterol level and, more importantly, their cardio-vascular health, by nutritional improvement. Medical professionals that are untrained in nutrition cannot help us reach this objective.[38]

The body manufactures cholesterol in the liver and in skin cells regardless of whether it is consumed in the diet or not. We do not need to obtain it from food. The body utilizes cholesterol to manufacture steroid hormones and vitamin D. Cholesterol is a component of all cells and is found in large amounts in nerve tissues and the brain. It is also required in various bodily tissue structures, is part of the process of fat digestion, and may at times serve as an antioxidant.

When cholesterol has been denatured—for example, through cook-ing—it becomes unusable to the body, and devoid of enzymes, which are required for its metabolism. If it cannot be eliminated, it must be stored, which leads to a narrowing and hardening of the arteries. Only foods from animal sources, such as meat, eggs, pasteurized dairy products, fish, and shellfish contain cholesterol; plant foods do not. When we con-sume excess calories, from cooked and processed foods, unhealthy fats, and sugars, or when we are under stress, our bodies are pressured to make more cholesterol. The prime source of blood impurities and deposits that cause heart disease is a diet composed entirely of denatured and cooked foods.[39]

Once made, or introduced into the body, cholesterol cannot be broken down. It must be eliminated through the stool. Increasing the intake of dietary fiber can facilitate this. In the absence of sufficient dietary fiber, most of the cholesterol is reabsorbed from the bowel and circulated throughout the body again.

In summary, cholesterol serves a vital purpose in the body. This is why the body manufactures it. When cholesterol becomes a problem, it is usually when there is an insufficiency of enzymes and fiber. The intake of abnormal, denatured cholesterol through cooked animal source foods increases the problem. Controlling cholesterol problems involves ensuring our enzyme, mineral, and vitamin intake is adequate by regularly consuming fresh greens, raw fruits and vegetables, and by avoiding the consumption of refined sugars and saturated animal fats. As Erasmus indicates, it requires an adequate healthful diet:

> Neither animal eaters nor plant consumers need fear CVD (cardiovascular disease) if they take their foods from unrefined natural sources, and especially if they supplement with (vitamins) C, B3, W3 (omega-3 oils), and fiber, and the rest of the substances long known to be essential for our health. Refined sugars, refined starches, hard fats, and refined, denatured oils from which vitamins, minerals, fiber, and protein have been removed should be expected to create problems.[40]

## SOME INTERESTING AND BENEFICIAL FOODS

### Aloe Vera

Aloe vera is a cactus-like plant that is a member of the lily family. The alkalizing juice and gel of aloe vera have long been used for their nutritional and healing properties. It is one of the safest and most gentle foods for all manner of intestinal and bowel disorders, mainly because of its healing effect on the villi of the small intestine. As the health of the villi improves, so does the absorption of nutrients.

Some of the healing claims for aloe vera are: healing wounds, burns, and psoriasis lesions; minimizing frostbite damage; reducing arthritic swelling; helping to promote internal tissue function; and aiding in digestion and intestinal health. Studies with animals have shown possible benefits for maintaining normal healthy states for kidney function, heart health, general cell growth, blood sugar levels, and the immune system.

Raw juice from the aloe vera leaf has been found to contain over 200 nutrients and biologically active ingredients, among them vitamins, minerals, trace minerals, enzymes, and eighteen amino acids. It is a good alkalizer.

When purchasing aloe vera juice, one should be aware of the different qualities sold in stores. Cheaper products are watered down, improperly stabilized, or refined to the point of leaving only ten to fifteen percent of the actual beneficial aloe vera extract. Products are made from various parts of the plant. There are three main products. Product #1: aloe vera gel is used as a home remedy to soothe and heal minor burns, abrasions, and insect bites. Product #2: aloe vera juice, which is often watered down or processed to remove any disagreeable taste, and is consumed for its nutritional and healing benefits. Because of the processing, it may contain only a fraction of the nutrients of the original plant. Product #3: whole leaf aloe vera concentrate, is the premium and most expensive of the products. It is made by cold-pressing fresh whole leaves of aloe vera. This pure, whole leaf product contains the maximum healing and nutritional ingredients.

### Apple Cider Vinegar

Unpasteurized apple cider vinegar (ACV) has been called one of nature's most perfect foods. When unfiltered and unpasteurized, it is a live food that still contains its enzymes. Pure unpasteurized ACV has a brownish color and a natural sediment known as "mother," which is usually visible on the bottom of a container. This is what we should look for when buying ACV. It must say "unpasteurized" on the label. Pasteurized ACV or distilled white vinegar have none of the beneficial elements of unprocessed ACV; they acidify the body.

Natural ACV contains many organic vitamins, minerals, enzymes, pectin, and other nutrients found in apples. It has been used since Biblical times as a body-cleansing agent, antiseptic, and for its healing qualities. Although acidic in the stomach, it has an overall alkalizing effect in the body. It helps with production of hydrochloric acid in the stomach, aiding better digestion, as well as contributing a healthy environment in the colon.

Among other minerals found in ACV are potassium, calcium, magnesium, iron, silicon, sulfur, and phosphorus. It is especially noted for its high content of potassium, sometimes called the key mineral, since it is required by every cell in our bodies. Its many functions include building soft tissue and youthful skin; synthesizing toxic wastes for elimination from the body; enabling muscle contraction; helping to balance blood sugar and blood pressure levels; producing energy; aiding digestion; and buffering acids in the body. It is interesting to note that although normally potassium stays mainly inside the cells and is balanced by sodium outside the cells, when potassium is deficient, this allows sodium to enter the cells accompanied by excessive water, which causes many cells to burst. This results in water retention and damage to muscles and connective tissue. Taking diuretics to reduce water retention can actually exacerbate a potassium deficiency, further increasing the problem. When we are deficient in potassium we age prematurely and start to develop loose flesh, lines, and wrinkles in the face and neck. For dietary considerations, note that refined foods lose many of their minerals, including potassium, during the milling and refining process.

There is an interesting discussion of the benefits of ACV in Dr. DeForest Jarvis' book *Folk Medicine*. Dr. Jarvis was a country doctor in Vermont in the first half of the 1900s and recorded his observations on the benefits of including ACV in the diets of both humans and animals. He noted that hunting dogs, when given rations of ACV with their daily feed, had more than twice the endurance, better appetites, as well as an ability to retain their weight during hunting season, compared to dogs that had not received regular ACV rations.

ACV has many other uses besides nutritional ones. Some examples are: as a cleaning agent; removing bacteria, fungi, and pesticide residues from fruit and vegetables; restoring acid balance to the skin after a bath or shower; as an insect repellent; as a natural antibiotic and antiseptic; and as an aid to digestion. ACV does not need to be refrigerated. It can be added to raw salads and soups. One can add one or two teaspoons of ACV to a glass of water along with a little unpasteurized honey as a drink first thing in the morning to cleanse the alimentary tract and to aid in the replenishment of nutrients.

An excellent book devoted entirely to the benefits of ACV is *Apple Cider Vinegar Miracle Health System*, by Paul and Patricia Bragg.

## Bee Pollen

Many people consume bee pollen regularly and swear by its nutritional benefits. It has been referred to as one of nature's most complete foods. However, it should not be confused with pollen from flowers and trees, which can cause allergy symptoms.

Bee pollen is very alkaline. It is approximately 25% protein, and contains at least 18 amino acids. It also has 28 minerals, a full spectrum of vitamins, 11 enzymes or co-enzymes, 11 carbohydrates, and hormones. It has antioxidant properties, making it a scavenger of free radicals caused by exposure to radiation and chemical pollutants.

Bee pollen has been found to enhance energy, stamina, and strength, and to improve the performance levels of athletes. It has also been shown to help reduce symptoms of allergies, hayfever, and asthma. By starting with a small amount, say ⅛ of a teaspoon, and gradually building up to one or several teaspoons per day, most people can enjoy the nutritional and therapeutic benefits of this natural food.

## Chlorella

Chlorella is a relatively unrecognized food even though many people who know of it call it "the most magnificent food in the world." Like spirulina, it is a freshwater micro-alga. It is very nutrient-dense, so much so that the 1989 special edition of the World Health Organization stated that chlorella supplies all the minerals, vitamins, enzymes, amino acids, as well as chlorophyll, that the human body needs for good health. It is noted for a property called Chlorella Growth Factor which gives it the ability to promote tissue repair and growth. It is readily digestible and is a very suitable alkaline food for all ages, from infants to the elderly.

Chlorella is particularly valuable for its ability to remove modern-day toxins from our bodies. It is a powerful, alkaline food-source antioxidant, and detoxifier of heavy metals, chemicals, pesticides, and insecticides.

## Liquid Chlorophyll

Chlorophyll is a potent blood-builder and alkalizer. The chlorophyll molecule is remarkably similar to human blood in composition, except that it carries an atom of magnesium in its molecular center instead of iron. It also has a high content of bio-viable iron. An article in the *Idaho Observer* quotes Ingri Cassel, president of the North Idaho chapter of Vaccination Liberation, regarding chlorophyll substitution for blood. Cassel relates two incidents of people who successfully restored their blood count and platelet levels back to normal by drinking one pint of liquid chlorophyll the night before scheduled blood transfusions.[41]

Chlorophyll helps to build red blood cells, which carry oxygen to every cell of the body. Adding chlorophyll to our diets, especially healing diets, reduces acid in the system, enhances immunity, calms the nervous system, aids the detoxification of organs (particularly the liver), and helps to remove drug deposits and heavy metals.

### Coconut Oil

Coconut oil is one of the healthiest oils we can use for eating and cooking. Unfortunately, it has been given an undeserved and false reputation as a result of the media's campaign against saturated fats. Over one hundred years ago, the many benefits of coconut oil were well known and widely recommended. What happened?

Commercial interests, mainly in the United States, convinced food manufacturers to abandon the use of this tropical oil in favor of processed oils made from various crops, including soy, that were "home grown." Mary Enig points out that poor research practices were also to blame: "The problems for coconut oil started four decades ago when researchers fed animals hydrogenated coconut oil that was purposefully altered to make it completely devoid of any essential fatty acids."[42] As already pointed out, the hydrogenation of oils produces trans fats, which are very unhealthy. Here was another example of deceit for commercial gain at the expense of people's health.

Coconut oil is classed as a medium-chain saturated fatty acid (MCFA). Since the body does not store it as fat, it:

> … metabolizes medium-chain SAFAs the same way it metabolizes short-chain SAFAs: to produce energy. It does not store them as fat. For

this reason, they are used as medium-chain triglycerides (MCTs) in diets of people with digestive and liver problems.[43]

Other research sources have determined that MCFAs are easily broken down by the saliva and gastric juices, and are therefore ready to be absorbed directly from the small intestine into the liver without calling for more digestive enzymes from the pancreas.[44]

Because it is easily digestible, coconut oil has many health benefits for everyone, the young and old, and the healthy and ill. It provides a quick source of energy that promotes healing. In several research articles, it is cited as alleviatory for conditions such as excess weight, heart disease, high cholesterol, bowel conditions of Crohn's disease and irritable bowel syndrome, candida and giardia, diabetes, chronic fatigue, thyroid, and skin problems. Coconut oil has anti-inflammatory and antimicrobial properties. Dr. Joseph Mercola calls coconut oil, "the healthiest oil you can consume ... and one of the most nutritious of all foods."[45]

When purchasing coconut oil for consumption, rather than for cooking purposes, look for extra virgin. This oil is delicious and really tastes and smells like coconut. It is pure white in its solid state below 76°F (24°C). Coconut oil is very stable and can remain at room temperatures for long periods of time without showing signs of rancidity.

### Colostrum

Colostrum is produced in the bodies of all female mammals toward the end of their pregnancies and secreted by the mammary glands during at least the first forty-eight hours after delivery. It is the all-important food that gives a baby its nutritional foundation for life. It contains powerful immune-building and growth factors, antibodies, vitamins, minerals, enzymes, amino acids, plus other substances that fortify the body against harmful microorganisms and environmental toxins. Research has identified at least fifty processes, from immune system development to the growth of all body cells, which are triggered in the newborn by colostrum. Evidence shows that these same immune-system-modulating benefits are also available to adults who supplement with colostrum.[46] Depending on the conditions, it is reported that improvements can occur in periods that vary from one week to over six months, as the body works to rebuild and strengthen.[47]

Colostrum for human use is harvested from dairy cattle because its components are similar to those of human colostrum, except that bovine colostrum is more concentrated. During the first 48 hours after birth, a cow secretes approximately nine gallons (34 liters) of colostrum. The calf needs about four gallons (15 liters), which means the rest can be harvested. To ensure maximum purity and potency, colostrum must be collected in the first 24 hours after the calf is born. A good colostrum product is dried into a powder while avoiding excess heat which would destroy its enzymes and immunoglobulin. It is generally considered that the purest colostrum comes from New Zealand, where farms are organic or near-organic, meaning cows graze on live grass in healthy pastures free of insecticides, herbicides, and antibiotics.

Colostrum was designed by nature as the first kind of food we should consume after birth. It is possibly the one supplement that can help everyone who takes it.

### Flax Seeds

Flax seeds are a high quality food with many benefits. Mahatma Gandhi once stated that: "Wherever flax seed becomes a regular food item among the people, there will be better health."[48] Flax seeds are a rich source of essential fatty acids, lignans (known for their anti-cancer properties), all the amino acids essential to health, as well as soluble fiber and insoluble fiber, both of which are so important for colon health. They also contain an abundance of vitamins and minerals. However, in order to obtain the nutritional benefits that flax seeds offer, they must be ground before they are eaten because their tough outer shells are not digestible. Dry flax seed is easily ground using a coffee grinder or a blender.

### Hemp—Seeds, Oil, and Protein

First of all, let's clear the air about hemp. It is not marijuana! Although both are related to the plant *Cannabis sativa*, industrial hemp, from which food products are produced, is very different. It contains minute (less than 1%) amounts of tetrahydrocannabinol (THC), the main psychoactive ingredient in marijuana. The story of how this confusion came about is interesting, and in retrospect, sad and infuriating for the health of people and for the economy of North America.

Prior to the U.S. Marijuana Tax Act of 1937, hemp was widely grown and used mainly for making rope, cloth, and paper. Hemp is the world's strongest and most durable soft natural fiber. As an example, a typical large frigate from earlier times required over sixty tons of rope for rigging and anchor cable, plus sails, all made from hemp. There is abundant information to be found on the Internet on the history and present uses of hemp products.

Hemp had been cultivated for thousands of years, and by 1937, it was being used to produce over 25,000 products. It has been described as the most useful plant known to man. Various sources state that hemp can be used to make virtually anything that is currently made from cotton, timber, or petroleum. Hemp is an easily and quickly grown annual crop, and therefore a perpetually renewable resource. But, this was a problem, as some interests saw it. It threatened powerful business interests in the emerging nylon industry. It is reported that petrochemical producer DuPont joined forces with Randolph Hearst, the newspaper magnate, whose company was the main user of chemically treated wood pulp and a major holder of forest logging licenses. Together they mounted "an hysterical fear campaign of racism and misinformation" linking industrial hemp to its cousin, Cannabis, which can contain significant amounts of THC.[49] This campaign was so fierce and effective that the word "hemp" became synonymous with the slang word "marijuana," and resulted in the U.S. government prohibition of 1937. The confusion over hemp versus marijuana remains to this day, especially in North America, but it is beginning to change.

While the development of a hemp industry is severely restricted in the United States, today industrial hemp is cultivated in many countries, among them Canada, China, Russia, Hungary, Germany, the Netherlands, France, Spain, England, and Poland.

"So what are the benefits of hemp?" you may ask.

### Hemp Seed

When we speak of hemp as a food source, we are referring to its seed. Technically, hemp seed is a fruit, because, unlike a nut or most seeds, it contains no enzyme inhibitors. It can be eaten immediately and is readily digestible. Hemp seed is a nutritional powerhouse. Shelled or de-hulled hemp seed, often referred to as hemp seed nut or hemp nut, is composed of approximately 34% pure digestible protein, and 31% essential fatty acids (EFAS). It is a rich source of EFAS and pure digestible protein, as well as vitamins, minerals, and antioxidants.

### Hemp Oil

Oil from hemp seeds is an excellent balanced source of the essential fatty acids omega-3 and omega-6. Dr. Johana Budwig, who has been nominated for the Nobel Prize seven times, is a pioneer researcher of EFAS. She has found that when the diet includes adequate amounts of EFAS, cell membranes continue to work properly and are electron-rich. EFAS are also important because they enhance our ability to absorb and utilize energy from the sun's rays. Quantum biologists have discovered that in order for this solar enrichment to take place, cells must contain "like energy"—the kind contained in foods that are rich in the sun's stored energy from solar rays. These electrons (biophotons) are abundant in unprocessed seed oils. Dr. Budwig found that when her ailing patients, who could not tolerate the sun, were given an EFA-rich diet, they were able to tolerate the sun very well.[50]

### Hemp Protein

When whole hemp seeds are cold-pressed to expel the oil, a dry cake is left. This cake can then be milled at low temperatures to produce hemp protein powder that can, depending on the variety of seed and the area it was grown in, produce an average of 48% protein. Hemp protein contains all known amino acids, including the essential amino acids. This makes it a very important source of amino acids. During the digestion process, our bodies chain together various amino acids to make proteins. About 75% of our body tissue is protein. A deficiency of amino acid building materials leads to immune deficiencies and other disease problems. Our bodies must have an adequate regular supply of usable protein in raw form.

Ideally, we should consume amino acids that are similar to those utilized by our human tissues. This is exactly where hemp protein shines:

> The body needs the necessary kinds of amino acids in sufficient quantity in order to make proteins such as the globulins. ... The best way to insure the body has enough amino acid material to make the globulins is to eat foods high in globulin proteins. Since hemp seed protein is 65% globulin edistin, and also includes quantities of albumin, its protein is readily available in a form quite similar to that found in blood plasma. Eating hemp seeds gives the body all the essential amino acids required to maintain health, and provides the necessary kinds and amounts of amino acids the body needs to make human serum albumin and serum globulins like the immune enhancing gamma globulins.[51]

Of all plants in the vegetable kingdom, hemp protein has the closest resemblance to our human protein profile. Hemp seeds contain all the essential amino acids and essential fatty acids necessary to maintain a healthy human life.

Recently, the Canadian government lifted a 50-year ban on the growing of hemp. Farmers, under a special license, are now growing industrial hemp with the proviso that they must not produce plants that have more than 0.3% of the psychoactive ingredient. The seed, from which the protein food and oil comes, does not contain THC, only the flower does.

The development and marketing of foods made from industrial hemp is still in its infancy. More healthfood stores are beginning to learn about and stock these nutritious foods. In my opinion, these products should be a regular part of our diets to ensure that our bodies are getting the best proteins and unsaturated oils. Raw hemp seed supplies both. It has a delicious nutty flavor and can be eaten plain or sprinkled on salads and other foods. Hemp oil can be mixed into smoothies or taken right from the spoon. It has a green color and a pleasant taste. Hemp protein can be added to other foods or mixed into blender drinks or made into bars. None of these should be heated because heat alters their electrical structure and destroys their life-giving properties.

The time is surely coming when this wrongfully-vilified plant will be properly recognized for its many industrial uses, and for its uniqueness as an unparalleled source of nutrition.

### Lemon

Dr. Cary Reams, a scientist in physics, is known for developing the Reams Biological Theory of Ionization in 1976. It centers on the importance of pH balance in the body. During his research on foods, he discovered that electrons in all foods, except one, spin in the same direction. Electrons in lemons spin in the opposite direction. The importance of this discovery was the realization that an overlap of electrons spinning in opposite directions causes resistance to be formed and allows energy to be released.[52]

Dr. Reams treated thousands of terminal patients, achieving greater than a 90% success rate. Especially, he used fresh lemon juice in distilled water to restore balance to the bile.[53] From these impressive results, it is evident that the creation of balanced energy in the body is very important for the efficient functioning of the liver.

Although lemon juice is naturally acidic, it is has a powerful alkalizing effect on the body after being digested. Fresh lemon also works to loosen and remove mucus.

### Natural Sea Salt

In the Middle Ages, salt was traded ounce for ounce for pure gold. Roman Legions were paid in salt. The Latin word for salt is "sal," from which our word "salary" is derived.

Our bodies need salt, but not common table salt (sodium chloride), or any of the other refined salts. Certain elements found in sea salt are essential for life.[54] Without a properly-balanced salt base we run out of electrolytes, and our "batteries die out." Refined table salt, and even many of the processed "sea salts" available from healthfood stores, can promote pathological calcification and a breakdown of cellular tissue.

Our blood requires natural whole salt to function because our cells must be bathed in a sodium-based fluid. Digestion depends on having a sufficient quantity of stomach hydrochloric acid to properly digest food and emulsify fats and oils. Hydrochloric acid can only be produced if chlorine is available in the right ratio. The solution to these requirements can be found in whole natural sea salt. Varieties of unprocessed, crystalline, natural sea salt are available in healthfood stores.

There is a difference between salt from life-sustaining seas and salt from mines or dead seas. Salt crystals from pristine living sea water are gray and contain a full complement of mineral elements, in exact proportions necessary to support and promote life. Such salt still has its life energy. Mined and refined sea salts have lost some of their macro and trace minerals.[55] The sodium chloride content of living sea salt is approximately 84%, whereas the sodium chloride of mined salts is approximately 98%. Mined salts are trace mineral deficient and unbalanced for true health.

Besides sodium and chlorine, natural sea salt contains at least 82 other minerals in trace amounts. The body must have, and can only utilize, minerals that are in trace amounts of parts per million, furnished in ionized form. Natural sea salt recharges cells just like batteries get charged. It also improves digestion by enhancing hydrochloric acid production, stabilizes bodily functions and fluids, and provides natural sodium that is required by the body's acid buffer system.

When salt is processed or even heated by boiling, natural iodine, which is required for many hormonal and metabolic functions in the body, is destroyed.

Technically, sea salt is a complex, balanced mixture of essential minerals the body needs and craves in almost the exact proportions.[56] Chemical analysis of natural sea salt shows an almost identical composition to that of the salty "mini-ocean" of a fetus' amniotic fluid. As an illustration of how natural and critical sea salt is for health and life, recall the experiment conducted by Dr. Alexis Carrel, as described in chapter 14. Dr. Carrel kept a pulsating chicken heart alive for more than 30 years in a solution of sea water. He proved that living cells can remain alive virtually indefinitely when furnished with the nutrients and environment they require for life.

Bodily salt needs to be replenished because as the body sweats, it loses electrolytes as well as salts and fluids. Without a sufficient balanced salt base, every problem in the body for which cell repair and rejuvenation must occur is made worse. Properly balanced salt is the primary cleanser of veins and arteries. It has the ability to clear plaque, as well as oils and cholesterol from artery walls.[57]

Natural sea salt in its raw crystalline form may be added to food in the final stages of cooking, or finely ground and lightly sprinkled on fresh raw fruits and vegetables. A few crystals can also be placed on the tongue after drinking water. We do not need to worry about an accumulation of natural sea salt in the body because, in its balanced and ionic form, the body will use what it needs and excrete the rest.[58] Generally, people find they use about one-third the amount they would use with other types of salt.

For balanced health, the entire body depends on a regular supply of good, natural ocean salt.

### Spirulina

Spirulina is one of the most concentrated and nutritious alkaline foods available. It is one of over 32,000 species of algae on earth. Some of these are very nutrient rich, while others contain deadly poisons. I knew a man who eventually died a miserable death as a result of eating a type of algae he had found high on a mountain, thinking it was a nutritious variety. It was a poisonous variety which unfortunately, attacked his nervous system.

One certified organic micro-algae grown in Hawaii, Spirulina Pacifica, is a superior strain of blue-green algae. It is about 60% protein, packed with enzymes, with 18 of the 22 amino acids, 92 trace minerals, and gamma linolenic acid (GLA). It contains proportionately 58 times more iron than raw spinach and 28 times more than raw beef liver. It is nature's richest source of vitamin B-12 (4 to 6 times more than raw beef liver), has high amounts of the strong antioxidant super oxide dismutase (SOD), vitamins (including all the B vitamins), as well as other nutrients.[59]

Research indicates that spirulina is more digestible than most other foods. It is an alkaline whole food that is also a powerful detoxifier.

Spirulina's only slight drawbacks are its strong seaweed smell and taste. All in all, it is a super food that everyone can benefit from.

### Sprouts

If there were ever a club of "superfoods," then sprouts would certainly be on the membership list. When compared to their parent grains or seeds, they have higher vitamin contents of between three and six, and in some cases, as high as fourteen times. They are an alkaline nutritional storehouse, a raw food goldmine for the body.

Sprouts contain live vitamins, minerals, proteins, phytochemicals, and enzymes in surprising amounts, as well as essential fatty acids. They are low in calories. The enzyme count of sprouts is reported to be ten to one hundred times higher than in vegetables or fruits, depending on the enzyme and the seed being sprouted. There is no other food with higher enzyme content. Sprouts are highly regarded for their detoxification, healing, and rejuvenation qualities.

The sprouting action of a raw seed causes it to be partially predigested, which breaks down concentrated starches into more simple carbohydrates. At the same time, protein is broken down into free amino acids. This predigestion means the sprout requires fewer enzymes from the body to complete the digestion process before use. The digestion and absorption of the food becomes more efficient.

Even though raw nuts, seeds, and grains have high nutritional values, they have limitations. The inhibitors keep the enzymes dormant until they have been activated by water. When dry nuts, seeds, and grains are consumed, the body has to secrete extra enzymes to neutralize the inhibitors before the foods can be digested.

However, when raw nuts, seeds, or grains are soaked in water, the enzymes within them become active. This causes them to start growing, and in the process, increases their nutritional content. Most sprouts are ready to eat in four or five days. At this time, they are at their peak in terms of nutritional and enzyme content. Eating fresh sprouts at that time in their development is an excellent way of introducing a large quantity of enzymes into our diets. After the fifth day, the enzyme content diminishes significantly as the sprout starts to grow longer. Also, after sprouts are harvested, they need to be immediately refrigerated as the enzyme content reduces rapidly at room temperature.

Sprouts sold in the stores are generally displayed at room temperature and may be several days old. In addition, some commercial sprouts are treated with mold inhibitors to keep them fresh-looking while they are displayed. Growing your own sprouts is the best alternative.

Sprouts can be grown very easily at home. This means we can grow nutritious and tasty food for our diets at any time of the year, inexpensively, indoors, and without soil. Furthermore, the whole sprout is consumed; there is no waste in preparation. No wonder sprouts have been called the "ideal supplement" and "the food of the future." There are several good books on sprouts and sprouting. One book is *Sprouts—the Miracle Food: The Complete Guide to Sprouting,* by Steve Meyerowitz.

Typical methods of sprouting, admittedly, can be somewhat tedious with the time that is required for soaking and rinsing of seeds. Fortunately, there is a more convenient alternative. Gene Monson of Lake Mills, Wisconsin has developed a system which requires no rinsing of most seeds and produces sprouts in a shorter period of time. His website, www.sproutamo.com, contains information about his sprouting device and helpful directions on sprouting various seeds, nuts, and grains.

Most of the fruits and vegetables in our supermarkets today do not contain the complete range of nutrients, compared to those of earlier times. Because of overfarming, soils have become depleted of many trace minerals that are required by our bodies for complete health. If we are not able to consume a diet of organically grown food, we can avoid or replenish mineral deficiencies in our bodies by using supplements. In the next chapter, we will examine the criteria for good supplements and also consider some alternative suggestions.

# 16 | SUPPLEMENTS

~

*… and let your medicine be food.*

HIPPOCRATES (460 BC)

~

## THE BUSINESS OF SUPPLEMENTS

THE PURPOSE OF supplements is to compensate for nutritional deficiencies in the food we eat, or to correct deficiency conditions already in the body. True supplements are composed of whole food ingredients; they feed the body with balanced nutrients it can use to heal itself.

It is my belief that when the body has been starved of vital nutrients or has been abused from an intake of improper nutrition and toxic substances, supplements are needed to correct deficiencies.

Many people take supplements of one form or another to ensure they are getting what may be deficient in the food they eat. The business of supplements is a huge, multi-billion dollar industry, but not all supplements supply the life forces that the body needs to regenerate itself. Many vitamins sold in drugstores and even in healthfood stores are chemically derived, synthetic, and therefore do not contain the organic components required by the body to build health. In fact, they may actually contribute to vitamin and mineral imbalances.

When you buy vitamins or minerals, do you really know whether they are good for your body? Assuming that your body is deficient in certain vitamins, minerals, or enzymes, do you know whether your body can utilize the supplements you are buying to build health? Or, are they simply adding to the stress and toxic load the body must handle?

## NATURAL VERSUS SYNTHETIC

Supplements are not created equal! Nature's vitamins heal. Synthetic vitamins stimulate, but do not heal.

Dr. Royal Lee, who founded Standard Process Laboratories, notes that:

> Natural complexes differ from synthetic, crystalline vitamins in many ways:
>
> 1 They are colloidal, protein in nature, in the form of an enzyme or coenzyme.
>
> 2 The crystalline vitamin itself, in the natural product is in a critical combination and cannot be split off without destroying its biological activity. If separated, it must recombine with the other members of the complex before it can function as a nutrient.
>
> 3 The natural complex carries trace mineral activators, without which the vitamin fails as a biochemical catalyst.
>
> 4 If so-called, "HIGH POTENCY" crystalline vitamins are ingested, they must be put into proper combination, as a complex, before the vitamin function can be appreciated. Meanwhile, most (if not all) of the crystalline component is lost through the kidneys.[1]

Natural complexes are ionically active, which is an extremely important factor for the absorbability of a nutrient. The smaller a nutrient is the more capability it has of entering into combination with other elements and forming the electrical matrix required to transfer energy to a cell. Synthetic vitamins, due to their non-ionic structure, do not have this capability, nor are they complete complexes.

Any food or vitamin must contain the appropriate live enzymes to be utilized by cells. Enzymes make transport of nutrients through cell walls

possible. Live food comes complete with enzymes to assist with its digestion and assimilation. Most vitamin and mineral supplements do not contain enzymes. A majority are produced or chemically processed in laboratories. Such mass-produced synthetic products are good for profit and
shelf life, but they are stimulative, toxic, and detrimental to the body. They
are unnatural and cannot be used by the body for health.

An example of a synthetic vitamin which is perpetrated as the real
thing is ascorbic acid. The drug industry calls it vitamin C. Ascorbic acid
is not vitamin C, but rather a fraction, the outside layer of the biologically
utilizable vitamin C complex, as shown in Figure 16.1.

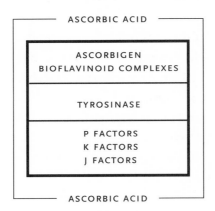

**Figure 16.1  Complete vitamin C complex**

Likewise, alphatocopherol, which is sold as Vitamin E, is only part of the
Vitamin E complex. As Richard Murray points out:

> … synthetic vitamins are not vitamins at all but synthesized FRAC-
> TIONS of a vitamin complex … a mirror image duplication of just a
> portion of the real, biologically active and physiologically precise
> nutritional complex. There is no possible way that a fraction of a vita-
> min can be called a vitamin. The analogy here is essentially the same
> as an automobile salesman handing you a wheel from a car and telling
> you the wheel is an automobile.[2]

## HELPFUL OR HINDERING?

To be useful to the body, a supplement must be of an organic origin and contain enzymes. It must be derived from natural food sources. Vitamins and minerals must be delivered in trace amounts, as they are in whole natural food. This way, the body can utilize them to correct deficiencies without causing other problems. What food on earth can you think of that contains 500 mg of any vitamin or mineral? Nature only provides nutrients in small and balanced combinations.

Any supplement that comes in mega-doses stimulates the body and creates an imbalance in the system. The body has to work hard to eliminate the excess, and in the process, further depletes its supply of other essential nutrients. A person might ask, "How can that be? When I take certain vitamins in larger doses I feel better." That may be true; the good feeling comes from stimulation, just like when people who drink coffee are stimulated by the caffeine. You feel better because the body has increased metabolism in order to eliminate the supplement, which in that form and quantity, is toxic. Over time, such doses cause more deficiencies and wear the body down. The same stimulative situation applies to some herbal supplements and treatments. The body cannot use, and does not accept, isolated nutrients. It requires specific combinations working together synergistically before they can be recognized as food.

Bottom line—synthetic vitamins are harmful. Tests with rats fed synthetic vitamins found that they died sooner than rats given nothing to eat.[3] The synthetic, incomplete supplements stimulated the animals' systems, increasing their metabolic rates and literally causing them to "burn up" or wear out at a faster rate.

Despite the preceding caveats, supplements can play an important role in paying back deficiency debts to the body created by years of nutrient-deficient food consumption. When selecting vitamin and mineral supplements, make certain they come from whole organic food sources, contain enzymes, and have been made with minimal processing. Such supplements may work with the body slowly, but they also work surely and continuously, without the stress of increased metabolism to remove unnatural, incomplete, and toxic substances.

A diet of natural, raw, organic, ripe, and fresh or undercooked foods provides the body with vitamin and mineral supplies with their complete synergistic components. Good supplements can help make up for non-organic foods that are mineral deficient.

## FOOD SUPPLEMENTS

It is sometimes difficult to differentiate between what is a food and what is a supplement, except perhaps for the quantity consumed at one serving. Several of the foods discussed in chapter 15, such as colostrum, bee pollen, and hemp foods can be used as supplements to a regular diet. Two additional highly concentrated foods that show significant promise as organic food source supplements are marine phytoplankton and stevia leaf.

### Marine Phytoplankton

Phytoplankton are microscopic single-celled plant organisms that are the foundational basis of the food chain for all animals living in the ocean. Many species of whales eat them, develop great strength and endurance, and live to between 80 and 150 years. The largest is the whale shark, which lives to more than 150 years and is sexually active until it dies.[4]

Phytoplankton are responsible for the production of a major portion of the earth's oxygen as well as the regulation of our atmosphere. Through photosynthesis, phytoplankton utilize chlorophyll and light to release oxygen into water and, in the process, convert huge quantities of carbon dioxide into living matter.[5] They also have the ability to convert sunlight, water, and minerals into amino acids, fatty acids, carbohydrates, and vitamins.

Until recently, phytoplankton were thought to be food for water creatures only. But that changed with the research of Tom Harper, an ocean farmer from Vancouver Island in Canada, who grows phytoplankton in a controlled environment as feed for the shellfish he raises. In 2004, Tom was diagnosed with a rare cancer, called mesothelioma, which is most often associated with exposure to asbestos, and from which virtually no one survives. He was told by his doctors that he had only a few months to live. While going about his work of raising marine phytoplankton to feed the shellfish, as an experiment, Tom began consuming half a teaspoon of the concentrated microalgae each day along with a drink of water. Within a few weeks he astounded his doctors with his recovery. A subsequent biopsy examination found no malignancy evident in his body. In addition, the diabetes that Tom had developed had also been corrected. Within six months, he had reduced his daily insulin requirement from 88 units to zero; his blood sugar counts returned to normal.[6] In short, Tom returned to full health.

Dr. Bob Rowe explained that, in his opinion, the nutrition contained in phytoplankton works to repair and regenerate the mitochondria, which are the cell's energy generating components. Healthy mitochondria are keyed to fully utilize sugar and turn it into the energy molecule adenosine triphosphate (ATP), which 90% of cell functions depend upon. Sustained energy is fundamental to the health of all body systems. While Dr. Rowe reports that he is seeing "amazing improvements" in many conditions with his chiropractic patients in a very short time,[7] he also cautions that unique marine algae concentrate "is not a panacea or a treatment for any particular condition. It works by providing essential nutrients needed by the body to stay in an optimal level of health."[8] Some of the health attributes of phytoplankton he has observed are that they are anti-inflammatory, anti-allergic, anti-oxidant, anti-cataract, anti-tumor, and anti-depressant. Phytoplankton appear to be able to repair the liver and the nervous system, improve endocrine function, and correct sleep disorders and weight problems. We are only in the beginning stages of learning about their benefits.[9]

Phytoplankton for human consumption may prove to be a significant breakthrough in building health, reversing disease conditions, and providing a viable and eco-friendly food source for the world. At this early point in its use, phytoplankton appear to provide all the basic nutrients required by the cells of the body in a whole and natural unprocessed food form. Further information on marine phytoplankton can be found at www.umac-core.com.

### Stevia Leaf—A Natural Sweetener

*Stevia rebaudiana,* a natural herb native to Paraguay and Brazil is, in its pure form, 200 to 300 times sweeter than sugar and has no harmful side effects. It is almost calorie-free, does not promote tooth cavities since it cannot be ingested by most common bacteria, contains a nutritious array of vitamins and minerals, and has been noted to have benefits for diabetics and hypoglycemics.[10] Stevia is approved as a food source in South and Central America, Korea, Taiwan, Japan, and China, and as such, is used as a sweetener in many food products.[11] However, in the United States and Canada, probably due in large part to concerns raised by the sugar industry about potential competition, to date, stevia is approved only as a food supplement. It is available at most healthfood stores.

## ANTIBIOTIC ALTERNATIVES

### Colloidal Silver

A colloid consists of minute particles that float within a liquid despite the pull of gravity; they remain suspended. Cloudy liquids such as fruit juice and milk are colloidal examples of water with macromolecules in suspension. A particle of colloidal silver is so small that 750 of them could fit across a single red blood cell. It is this small size and the electrical charge that each colloidal silver particle has that gives it the ability to enter cells and to combine with other trace elements.

Colloidal silver is actually ionic colloidal silver.[12] Using the low voltage method, silver is dispersed into water as very small particles (ions). These ions then cluster to form the colloid. The smaller ionic particles are more readily absorbable, making them much more effective than the larger ones. Although a concentration of 3–5 parts per million (ppm) sounds almost negligible, it has proven to be very potent against pathogens.

Research on colloidal silver shows it to be an effective resource against infections and pathogens, yet very little is known about it by the general public or the medical profession. Prior to 1938 it was in common use by doctors.

According to Alexander G. Schauss, PhD, of Johns Hopkins University, considerable scientific evidence has been published regarding the effectiveness of silver as an antiseptic against "several hundred pathogenic organisms." He also points out that silver is not an antibiotic because, by definition, antibiotics are derived from living organisms.[13]

The Environmental Protection Agency's Poison Control Center considers colloidal silver to be harmless and does not list toxicity levels in its rating for colloidal silver.[14] Colloidal silver can be used topically to combat or prevent infections on conditions such as cuts, wounds, burns, rashes, sunburn, and insect bites. It can also be used to sterilize drinking water,[15] as well as taken orally to combat low-grade infections.[16] The one caution for colloidal silver is that ingesting it in large quantities over a long period of time can result in a permanent blue-grey skin discoloration called "argyria."[17]

Colloidal silver has also been reported to be effective against germ warfare pathogens such as anthrax and bubonic plague.[18] In 1919, Alfred Searle, founder of Searle Pharmaceuticals, indicated that in tests, colloidal silver protected rabbits from ten times the lethal dose of tetanus and diphtheria toxins.[19]

Silver is a trace mineral. It is present in the body in minute amounts and is used by the body to produce healthy cells and maintain the immune system. People previously obtained trace minerals such as silver in adequate amounts from eating plants grown in nutrient-rich soil. But our soils have become depleted of many of their trace minerals. Silver is generally now present in only very small amounts in the soil.

Colloidal silver acts to disable the breathing ability of bacteria, viruses, and fungi, causing them to suffocate and die very soon after contact.[20] It promotes cell repair and tissue and bone healing.[21] Colloidal silver in concentrations of 3-5 ppm is very safe to use and has no recorded side effects.[22] However, silver nitrate or other forms of silver in various concentrations disturb the balance of body salts and are also corrosive and cause pain.[23]

Recommendations for using colloidal silver vary from one manufacturer to another. Some recommend taking one or more teaspoons with meals, while others recommend holding it in the mouth for a while so it can be absorbed. Generally, when you swish a teaspoonful (always use a plastic spoon as the silver will electrically ground to metal spoons) in your mouth, it is rapidly absorbed into the bloodstream and transported quickly to the body's cells. It usually takes three to four days for the silver to sufficiently accumulate in tissues to develop a major bacterial fighting strength. It is eliminated from the body after about three weeks.

Colloidal silver can be purchased from healthfood stores or other supplement companies. For long-term and regular use, a colloidal silver maker can be purchased to produce it for pennies per gallon.[24]

### Grapefruit Seed Extract

Grapefruit seed extract is relatively new compared to the other remedies described in this section which have been known and used for many years. A Yugoslavian physicist, Jacob Harich, discovered liquid grapefruit seed extract around 1985. It is a bitter and acidic mixture made from dried and ground grapefruit seeds that is proving to be a potent alternative to toxic medicines and cleaning chemicals. Its wide variety of applications include its use as a fungicide, antibacterial, antiparasitic, antiviral, preservative in food and medicines, and as a sanitizing and disinfecting agent. It kills germs but does not harm people. It first gained attention from farmers for its ability to protect produce, fish, and poultry from bacteria, fungi, and parasites. Research is showing that grapefruit seed extract is effective on a very broad spectrum.[25]

It is now being reported that some hospitals are using grapefruit seed extract in concentrations of 10 to 15 drops per gallon (3.8 liters) of water to kill streptococcus, staphylococcus, aspergillus, salmonella, and many other pathogens in operating rooms, laundry, and carpets. In addition, it is also being used in inhalers to treat respiratory infections and taken internally for various intestinal problems.[26]

I have found it to be a very useful, convenient, and effective remedy to have in my kit when traveling out of the country, to other parts of the world where one might be exposed to harmful bacteria in food or drinking water that can cause intestinal upsets and diarrhea. Two to five drops in a glass of juice or water, taken as needed until the problem is under control, can be helpful.

### Olive Leaf Extract

Olive leaf extract has been referred to as one of the oldest remedies around.[27] Researchers have determined that it has strong bactericidal, virucidal, and anti-parasitic properties. They claim that it also helps to maintain healthy blood pressure levels, increases blood flow in coronary arteries, relieves arrhythmia, and prevents intestinal muscle spasms. It has been found to act as an antimicrobial agent against at least 140 infectious diseases, among them: anthrax, athlete's foot, and urinary tract infections, Epstein-Barr virus, herpes, hepatitis, viral meningitis, pneumonia, salmonella, smallpox, tuberculosis, vaginal yeast infection, and many more. Olive leaf extract is taken in capsule form.

### Tea Tree Oil

Tea tree oil is made from Australian tea tree leaves. Australian Aborigines have used it for centuries by applying crushed leaves to heal cuts, bruises, and skin infections and by inhaling vapors from crushed leaves to treat colds. Tea tree oil is a very strong antiseptic and anti-inflammatory that easily penetrates the skin to relieve conditions such as eczema, psoriasis, shingles, poison ivy reactions, insect bites, cuts, and minor burns. It is non-toxic for topical applications. It is also valuable when taken internally to neutralize toxins and harmful bacteria in the digestive tract and respiratory system. Only minute amounts are necessary, so you need to educate yourself properly before taking it internally.

As with other remedies mentioned in this section, tea tree oil is available at most healthfood stores.

## THE ROLE OF ANTIOXIDANTS IN HEALTH

Antioxidants play a very important role in maintaining health and slowing the aging process. They are the "soldiers" that keep cellular "terrorists" to a minimum within the body. They are the repair crews that work to correct any damage that has already been done. An antioxidant acts to neutralize oxidation.

The subject of oxidation and free radicals has been briefly mentioned before, but we will explore it in more detail here.

### Oxidation

Oxidation is defined as the process of changing the atoms of an element by combining them with oxygen to form an oxide. When a substance burns or rusts, it is oxidized. Oxygen becomes unstable and, in the process of trying to become stable again, causes a breakdown process in other elements it comes in contact with. The unstable atoms that cause oxidation are called "free radicals." In the human body, this continual destabilization leads to aging and disease. The role of antioxidants is to neutralize and clean up free radicals before they get a chance to do harm in the body.

### Free Radicals

Free radicals are atoms with unpaired electrons, which make them unstable, highly reactive, and capable of causing biological damage. They are strongly oxidizing.

In their reactive state, free radicals are constantly seeking to be balanced. But in attempting to become stable, they rob from stable molecules, thereby causing a chain reaction—similar to rusting—of cellular breakdown in the body. As one atom with an unpaired electron robs an electron from another cell membrane to stabilize itself, the one robbed becomes unstable and damaged, continuing the chain reaction. Free radicals caused by poor diet, smoke, chemicals, and radiation, assault the body and increase cellular damage. In time, the damage extends to all parts of the cell, including the membrane, fats, protein, and DNA. Without antioxidants to counteract this breakdown process, aging results.

### Antioxidant Sources

A healthy diet of raw fruits and vegetables contains naturally-occurring antioxidants. Many supplements, such as vitamins A, C, E, selenium, and coenzyme Q10, are antioxidants. More recently, stronger antioxidants have been discovered and developed. Among these are: pycnogenol, which is a water extract from the bark of the French maritime pine; grape seed extract; tocotrienols; vitamin C ester; alpha lipoic acid; DMAE; and alpha and beta hydroxy acids.

On the other hand, a poor diet, processed foods, cured meats, tobacco smoke, infections, alcohol, stress, air pollution, pesticides, and radiation all promote oxidation in the human body. Even if we are minimizing the effects of the aforementioned free radical developers, given our modern urban, industrialized, and technological lifestyles, we cannot completely avoid them. We therefore need to take active antioxidant steps against them.

## HORMONES OF YOUTH

### Human Growth Hormone

When we reach middle age, our bodies start to exhibit the telltale signs of aging. These include wrinkles, sagging skin, muscle loss, thinning hair, decreased energy, and diminished sex drive. Researchers have now determined that these changes of our bodily state are closely related to decreasing levels of Human Growth Hormone (HGH).

HGH is secreted by the pituitary gland. It is then transported by the bloodstream to the liver where it is converted into growth factors, the most important of which is insulin-like growth factor 1 (IGF-1). This is the factor that is mainly responsible for producing our youthful attributes. But here is the problem: the production of HGH typically decreases in amount from 100% at age twenty to 40% at age forty, and eventually, 5% by age eighty.[28] Our youth factory simply slows down as we age. The good news is that we can now take food-form supplements—HGH precursors— to promote the healthy production of HGH again. In as little as 30 to 60 days, it is possible to begin seeing a reversal of some of the signs of aging listed above.

### Your Own Hormone Production

If you want to increase your own production of HGH, your body needs amino acids and essential fatty acids in natural form. Therefore, make sure that your diet includes good sources of raw protein such as low-heat processed hemp, spirulina, chlorella, algae, and amino acid supplements made from vegetable sources. Essential fatty acids are contained in raw nuts and seeds, fish, fish oils, and cold pressed oils from flax and hemp seeds. These are the building blocks for the liver to make hormones and hormone precursors for the brain and glands of the endocrine system.

### Anti-Aging Supplements

Many companies have jumped on the anti-aging bandwagon after it was discovered that the pituitary gland can actually be fed the necessary precursors that allow it to increase its natural production of HGH. If you decide to look into this mode of supplementation, be sure the product you select is made entirely from natural ingredients. Basically, you need to look for a supplement that will feed the body, not stimulate it.

While we are making new plans to be healthy physically, we also need to be working with our internal creative forces—the thoughts, attitudes, emotions, and beliefs behind what manifests in our physical lives. This begins with cultivating awareness.

~ FOURTH KEY

# BELIEVING

# 17 | AWARENESS

~

*Self-knowledge is the beginning of wisdom.*

J. KRISHNAMURTHI

~

## COMPLETE HEALTH

COMPLETE HEALTH is achieved through awareness. Awareness is fully recognizing who we are now, while in the process of becoming who we want to be. Others call it consciousness, being aware of how we are acting and reacting to events in our lives.

To be aware is to be in a *state of knowing, through an alertness in observing and interpreting what one sees, hears, feels, and thinks.* Awareness requires us to be fully present, to pay active attention. If we are not conscious, we cannot be truly free, because we are operating from pre-set programs in our subconscious mind, beneath conscious awareness. We will not be able to enjoy full physical, mental, emotional, and spiritual health until we have become aware.

Health is not just a matter of the physical body. It is a holistic integration of our physical, mental, emotional, and spiritual bodies. Each of these expressions has an energy body—none is separate; all are connected since everything is energy.

## THE PHYSICAL BODY

Because health shows itself clearly in our physical bodies, we naturally tend to look after the physical aspects of our being in an effort to improve our health. Accordingly, the majority of space in this book is devoted to promoting our awareness of those subjects. But equally important is our understanding of how our minds, emotions, and spirit contribute to and determine the ultimate state of our health. We need awareness of these invisible aspects of our makeup, and how their energies can positively or negatively affect our health and well-being. Ultimately, everything in our lives is formed from spiritual, universal energy.

## THE MENTAL BODY

The mental body is created by the mind. It is the thinking part of us. It is the energy body of our thoughts. The mind is the tool we use to generate thoughts, formulate beliefs, and make judgments. It enables us to become aware, to formulate intentions, make decisions, and exercise free will. The thinking mind is for us to use and direct, but many people are so mesmerized by the constant chatter of the mind, they think they *are* their mind.

### Two Minds
When we make a decision, we say that we have made up our mind. But, we have also heard people say they are of two minds, when trying to make a decision on a certain subject. Very often, that is actually the case because conflicting core beliefs of the subconscious mind are tugging away at the thoughts of the conscious mind. How do these two minds work?

### *Conscious Mind*
The conscious mind is the mind we are aware of. It is what we think with. This is the part of us we use to express personality. It has the ability to think about the past, present, and future. It also gives us the ability to

judge, assess facts, and make choices. The conscious mind is the foundation of our free will.[1] It is active when we are awake, but when we sleep,
the subconscious mind takes over.

### Subconscious Mind

While we are awake, the subconscious mind directs our thinking from
"behind the scenes," even though we are not aware of it. It is the real brains
behind how we think because it has been programmed by our life experiences. Still, the subconscious mind only works in the present. It makes no
judgments; it just responds to the programming of our core beliefs.

Our subconscious mind allows us to operate automatically in activities such as breathing, driving the car, or pulling our hands away from a
hot stove. It can also sort through the vast reservoir of information stored
in our memory bank to help us solve problems, make plans, and find
something we have misplaced. But, until we have changed our core beliefs,
our subconscious mind also causes us to repeatedly do things we consciously vowed not to, such as: repeating losing investments, smoking,
drinking alcohol in excess, or marrying the same kind of person a second
or third time.

The conscious mind's capacity for processing information, compared
to that of the subconscious mind, is minuscule. The conscious mind can
process environmental information stimuli at the rate of about 40 per second; whereas the subconscious mind can process at the rate of 20,000,000
per second.[2] The subconscious mind is like a super computer, an amazing
resource. The key is to make sure it is programmed for positive outcomes
in our lives.

### The Mind Is Always Processing

When we eat processed foods, we cause an imbalance in our bodies.
Without realizing it, we do the same with our thoughts. We process
thoughts about conversations we've had by recalling them and going over
them repeatedly. We spice them by rehearsing words that were said to us,
or with words we wish we had said in response. These silent verbal reviews
are ongoing. Sometimes we vent our anger and vow to seek revenge in our

minds. Eating processed food repeatedly causes dis-ease in our bodies. Processing past thoughts and events repeatedly perpetuates dis-ease in our mental and emotional bodies.

Even though our conscious mind is preoccupied with thoughts that we think we are in control of, it is our super-powerful subconscious mind that is actually directing the show from our embedded beliefs. If it is your conscious mind that enables you to think, and yet the beliefs in your sub-conscious mind direct *how* you think, who do you think you are?

### You Are Not Your Mind

The title of the first chapter of Eckhart Tolle's life-changing book *The Power of Now* is "You Are Not Your Mind." I say life-changing because it was this book that released me from the constant chatter of my thoughts to a life of mental, emotional, and spiritual freedom. It opened the door to a new life of emotional tranquility.

On first glance, the statement "You are not your mind" may sound con-fusing because our thoughts are always with us. However, there is a whole other area to our lives that we may not be aware of. That is because we typi-cally believe, or just accept, that our mind is who we are. We think that what generates our thoughts clearly demonstrates who we are. But, that is only partly true. This may be a new concept, but grasping it can lead to inner peace and an understanding of why your life may be going the way it is.

You are not your thoughts! To understand this statement, realize and accept that, as humans, there are three parts to us: body, mind, and spirit. The body and mind are easy to comprehend because we use them every day. The spirit is not well understood, except in some ethereal or religious context. If you can accept that you were spirit when you came into your body in your mother's womb, and that when you die your spirit leaves your body, then you will follow what I will say next. If you have trouble accept-ing the spirit aspect of human nature, then you may have some difficulty.

Everything in the universe is energy. Energy is never destroyed. It just changes form, and form includes us. Even though we are temporarily occupying a body, we are spirit or energy that will always be. Energy cre-ates matter, be it physical objects or parts of our body; scientists are proving this every day. Our thoughts are energies that create positive or negative outcomes, according to their kind, whether we realize it or not. Thoughts in turn, are created by our mind.

Here is the key to understanding this. You, the real you, are spirit—the central "heart" of you, but not the pumping one! Your mind and your body reflect who you are at the moment. They are your mirrors and your drawing board. They are tools that aid your spirit in expressing who you are in the larger context of who you want to be, but they are not you. As long as your mind commands center stage, it is liable to become your sense of self, what we call the ego.

### The Ego Wants Control

The term "ego" can have many different meanings, but as it is used here, it is essentially an awareness and preoccupation with self. Egoism is a tendency to be self-centered and to consider only oneself and one's own interests—as in pride, selfishness, or conceit. The ego always covers up its limitations by making excuses and casting blame.[3] It can be quick to take offense to something said to us. If we are holding grievances, then our egos are ruling our minds.

The ego is that part of self that is created and perpetuated by constant thoughts associated with our worth or importance as an individual in the family, group, or society in which we live and work. It began when we left the childhood world of innocent spontaneity, and entered the adult world of calculated thought and pretence. We began projecting a self-image to make us appear acceptable to others.

The ego is based on an unconscious identification with the mind, but it is a false self, an imposter.[4] Since the ego feeds on mind chatter, life in the egoic mind is an illusion. When the ego is in control, we respond to life's circumstances like a robot without realizing it. Our real self is the humble, patient, loving, and confident spirit behind the noise, distraction, and confusion in our mind. When we say that we are not our mind, it is more correct to say that we are not our egoic mind. However, before we can see through the mind chatter illusion and naturally operate from spirit, we need to become aware of our emotional body.

## THE EMOTIONAL BODY

Our emotional body comprises the collective energy of our feelings, as well as the memory of our past feelings. Feelings are energy, and stored feelings are stored energy. Emotions are meant to be "e-motion," or energy-in-motion. They are meant to be generated, experienced, and emoted—allowed to move. When we lack awareness, we hold our feelings inside and they become blocked energy. We usually think we are protecting ourselves, but instead, we are blocking ourselves from growing and experiencing the fullness of happiness and joy that life has to offer. Painful feelings and emotions keep us focused on the drama that is in our lives; our spirit self remains hidden, and our spontaneous, authentic child-self is afraid to come out and play.

When our emotions are positive and naturally flowing, our emotional body is relaxed and content. When we are discontented and unaware, the emotional energy becomes blocked and our emotional body takes on a negative charge.

### Our Negative Emotional Charge

Painful experiences collected in childhood and reinforced by other emotional wounds at a later stage build up within us as a negative emotional charge that sits in our subconscious mind, restricting our ability to experience full happiness, success, and joy. It pervades life, coloring our view of everything and preventing the development of true intimacy in our relationships. Our negative emotional charge can manifest in personality traits such as: a pessimistic attitude, being controlling or manipulative, criticizing, being super-sensitive and taking offense, outbursts of anger and even rage, blaming, the feeling of being a victim, lack of self-esteem, and expecting to be short-changed in the abundance and happiness that others seem to enjoy. We can develop a poverty complex or a persecution consciousness, which then perpetuates these circumstances in our lives.

This stored emotional charge, or emotional "pain-body" as Eckhart Tolle calls it,[5] is a negative energy field. It occupies our attention causing us to identify with the pain as part of who we are, but it is only the ego, not the true person we are as loving spirit.

Our subconscious beliefs, reinforced by our conscious experiences, have led us to believe we are our egoic minds. We have lost touch with the original sense of who we are. This causes a great conflict within us because we are not being our authentic selves; we are not living in truth. As a result, we try to run from the mental anguish. We do not want to feel pain, so we resort to methods of sedation; we try to escape. We do not know how to heal the conflict, so we continue to live unconsciously. But, "love, joy, and peace cannot flourish until you have freed yourself from mind dominance."[6]

### Addiction and Disease

As long as we continue to be unconsciously directed by our ego, we have very little control over our feelings and emotions; they happen *to* us. The ego feeds on struggle, and produces a constant flow of self-talk that produces pain in our emotional body. In attempts to escape the emotional pain, we turn to a variety of ways to feel better. Repeated sedations become addictive habits. But the pain always returns. Our innate wisdom is trying to get our attention so we can change our dysfunctional beliefs. A person who is addicted is trapped in a prison of their mind.

Addictions take many forms; some are socially acceptable and some are not. When emotional stress becomes too great, we turn to escapes such as food, sugar, soft drinks, alcohol, nicotine, sex, destructive anger, manipulating and controlling others, gambling, or legal and illegal drugs. When the stress is not alleviated by sedation, which is always temporary, and when it is not addressed by a resolution of the underlying emotional conflict, disease symptoms begin to appear. The addiction problem and the emotional pain continue. In both cases, our collective bodies are mirroring the disease and imbalance in our lives so we can become balanced and grow in freedom as spirit, unencumbered by the ego.

### The Purpose of Emotional Pain

Nothing in life is an accident; everything has a cause and a reason for being. The difficult part for us is realizing this. In terms of emotional pain, this is especially hard since emotional pain is an imbalance of emotions, which impairs our ability to see objectively. But, within this understanding of our inherent imbalance lies the purpose of our pain.

One of my all-time favorite books, which I have owned since I was twenty, is Kahlil Gibran's 1923 masterpiece, *The Prophet*. In a majestic poetical style, the Prophet shares wisdom with others on life's common experiences and challenges. When a woman asks him to speak of pain he says, "Your pain is the breaking of the shell that encloses your understanding." To me, that statement is so profound! When we experience pain as a result of our present moment awareness, rather than trying to block it out, it can lead us to an understanding of the emotional part of us that is crying to be healed. The purpose of emotional pain is to attract our attention so we can change our thinking and beliefs.

## THE SPIRITUAL BODY

The spiritual body is our eternal body. It is the soul energy matrix—the life that we are. The spirit inhabits the physical body at some point while we are in the womb, and leaves when we die. Spirit is the invisible eternal energy that we are. During life, it guides gently to help us create what we want in the physical from our various energies. Our spirit is meant to be in charge of our minds, and in turn, our thoughts. Our spirit wants to create, or recreate, who we really are, which is love and all that it means. When we are in touch with this love source, we create life from spirit, not from the egoic mind.

### Becoming Aware

When we begin to notice our thoughts, we become aware that we are not our thoughts, but rather the observer of them. Here is how Eckhart Tolle expresses that form of awareness:

> You are aware not only of the thought but also of yourself as the witness of the thought. A new dimension has come in. This is the beginning of the end of involuntary and compulsive thinking.[7]

This is when we realize there are two parts to us, our ego self and our spirit self. Until this realization, our thoughts will have been generated and continually recycled under the reactive influence of the ego. But now, as observer of the thoughts, our spirit enters into the picture and begins to exert direction.

**Taking Control**

As we listen to our thoughts, we are in the present moment; we have moved into awareness and control. Our mind chatter is always about the past or the future, but the past is only a memory, and the future is only imaginings. As long as we are rehearsing stressful memories, we cannot move forward into inner peace. This moment we are in right now is the only reality; it is where our power is. Living in the present NOW is where our peace is. We can learn to tell our minds what to focus on.

When we are able to control our minds and direct our thoughts, we naturally begin to feel more confident. We create an empowered present and from that, a future that is in harmony with spirit and life.

Once we are aware of our thoughts, the next step is to become aware of the feelings that are generated by our thoughts. Our feelings create our attitudes and emotions. Becoming aware of our feelings, and where they are manifesting in our bodies, enables us to understand our attitudes and emotions. This is the subject of the next chapter.

# 18 | ATTITUDES AND EMOTIONS

∽

*You can't heal your own pain by spreading it to others.*

Keith Atlea, Ahousaht Chief Councilor

∽

A POSITIVE mental outlook that reflects a balance in the mental, emotional, and spiritual aspects of our lives is essential for a complete program of health. We must take responsibility for our thought lives and deal with negative attitudes, emotions, and experiences that are influencing our behavior and affecting our health, in a corrective and purposeful manner.

## ATTITUDES

Attitudes shape our character and well-being. They are formed from our beliefs and become the steering wheels of our lives. If we have an open heart and a teachable mind, we will be continually learning and improving our character. If we have a closed mind or negative outlook on life, we will tend to lock out opportunities for learning and character improvements, and remain stuck in the past.

## THOUGHTS

In the last chapter, we briefly explored various aspects of our mental make-up. Left on its own, the egoic mind recirculates our thoughts and runs our life from a reactive and judgmental point of view. We do not even realize it is happening. Once we become conscious of the mental chatter, we can begin to act as an observer and see through the illusion that our thoughts are who we really are. But we have to do this on our own. No one can do it for us.

## EMOTIONS

The word "emotion" is derived from the Latin word, "emovere," which means: *to excite, agitate, stir up, or move*. Emotions are strong generalized feelings that have both psychological and physiological manifestations. Strong emotions produce chemicals in our bodies that have definite influences on our health. For example, remember how happy and energetic you felt when you were in love. Conversely, when you are sad or depressed, you have a difficult time dragging yourself out of bed in the morning; you feel tired and lack motivation to get going and tackle the tasks that must be done.

Our thoughts create our emotions and our attitudes influence our thoughts; they are all connected. Being aware of all three is a key part of conscious health. The emotional reaction we have to any experience is directly related to our thoughts about it. Are they happy, hopeful, loving, sad, hateful, fearful, or angry? It is our *perception* of events that determines what we feel. We know the feelings of emotion, but are we aware of them? If we are not aware of our emotions, we are like a ship without a rudder, tossed about by the winds of circumstance in life. Our buttons get pushed and we don't understand why; we just react. We may think someone else is doing it to us, but it is our own attitudes and thoughts about what they say or do that provoke our emotional responses. Our emotional experiences are created by how we talk to ourselves.

338

Instead of masking our painful emotions with outbursts of anger, submission, continual activity, or addictive substances, we need to become aware of our emotions as they are happening by recognizing where they are manifesting in the body, and what the associated pain is saying to us. The body is talking to us, trying to get our attention to help us become whole again. We need to understand its language.

## UNDERSTANDING THE NEGATIVE

Negative attitudes and emotions are not fun. We do not like having them, and we do not like being around those who display them. When we are being negative, or are near a negative person, we feel like putting up our defenses. This emotional reaction has a corresponding pattern in our physical bodies. We operate the same way on a cellular level.

Dr. Bruce Lipton's research has totally revised conventional views on how cells work. Cells don't just operate from the inside-out, taking direction from their genes; they work from the outside-in, taking direction from their emotional and chemical environments. Each cell's membrane, or "mem-brain" as he calls it, perceives what the cell requires to thrive and survive from its environment, and then gives direction to the proteins inside it.[1]

Dr. Lipton shows that each cell has intelligence, and that what applies to one cell also applies to communities of cells. The body is a community of 70 trillion or more cells; it is a vast collection of cellular intelligence. In his book *The Biology of Belief*, Dr. Lipton explains that cells are either growing or protecting themselves. When cells perceive nutrition in their environment, they move toward it for growth. When they sense a threat to their well-being, they go into protection mode and move away.[2]

When we are newly born, we naturally respond to good nutrition and love; we feel energized and supported, and consequently grow. But when the receptors in our bodies perceive toxins or chemicals from emotions that cause fear, we go into protection mode; we retreat and stop growing. Our bodies mobilize for protection using what is known as the HPA axis, or Hypothalamus-Pituitary-Adrenal Axis.[3] They perceive threats via the hypothalamus, which sends a message to the master gland, the pituitary, which then signals the adrenal glands to release the stress hormone adrenaline. Adrenaline initiates a fight or flight response. In the interest of survival, this diverts blood flow from the internal organs and brain to the muscles. We speed up and move to a state of high tension. Digestion and internal nourishment, plus intelligent thinking, take a back seat to brute strength. During this time our immune system is suppressed. We become physically stronger, though intellectually weaker; we are in protection mode.[4]

The critical issue is that positive emotions help us thrive, while negative emotions help us survive.

## LOVE OR FEAR

Our emotions have a purpose. Positive emotions and attitudes such as joy, hope, optimism, contentment, and gratitude are based in love and make us feel good about ourselves; we feel expansive; we develop a positive self-image and grow. Negative emotions such as anger, resentment, guilt, anxiety, and depression have their basis in fear, and in feelings of powerlessness and lack of self-worth. Under the influence of negative emotions, we feel vulnerable and put up our defenses; we stunt our growth. Love encourages us to grow; fear discourages us and causes us to move into protection mode. Love fosters health and energy generation while fear fosters dis-ease and energy depletion.

Negative emotions create disorder in a person's heart rhythms, and disharmony in the autonomic nervous system. On the other hand, positive emotions produce an orderly heart rate variability, balance in the autonomic nervous system, and cardiovascular efficiency.[5]

The chemical by-product of a negative emotional stress response in our bodies is acid. As we have learned, acidic conditions create the environment for disease. We need to be conscious of our negative emotional health habits so we can change them to positive attitudes, which have an alkalizing effect in the body. When we move to positive attitudes, we relieve the body of stress and help it to produce health.

Negative attitudes work against healing, even though they appear to give temporary satisfaction or relief when we express them. Reacting to situations with anger, fear, worry, grief, apathy, or rebellion causes dis-ease in our bodies. This is because the energy of our thoughts, beliefs, and attitudes is connected to our body organs via energy pathways. When we continue to allow a negative view of the world to dominate our thinking, it results in minute changes in energy flow to body organs. Over time, this restricted energy results in cellular change and function which precipitates the development of disease. By the time medical technology can identify its presence, the disease condition is well advanced.

Our mind is where we should begin the process of making changes in our lives. We must be willing to view life and ourselves in new ways to recover from a disease process. This takes courage. A sincere desire for change allows this to happen.

When we take responsibility for our thoughts, and build attitudes of acceptance, gratitude, generosity, forgiveness, humility, and love into our thinking and actions, the negative characteristics of our temperament, such as selfishness, bitterness, guilt, regret, and self-condemnation begin to lose their power and disappear. We have reprogrammed our subconscious mind. We have moved from being self-centered to being other-centered and have learned to live in the present moment.

## BECOMING EMOTIONALLY AWARE

Gary Zukav and Linda Francis wrote the book *The Heart of the Soul: Emotional Awareness*.[6] It is a resource that was very helpful to me in understanding my emotions and becoming aware of my reactions to various situations. By following the explanations in the book, I learned to *feel* where emotions were manifesting in my body, which then allowed me to know whether love or fear was behind my emotion at the time. I was able to observe pleasure or pain in the present moment and stay emotionally aware.

Consciously experiencing our emotions in the present moment, the same as we do with our thoughts, is key to self-empowerment and spiritual development. All power to understand and change happens in the present. Developing emotional awareness is a continuous process of observing and recognizing the changing emotions inside us. At first we might think this to be an onerous task, but once we develop present-moment awareness, it becomes matter of course, a monitoring process of recognizing who we are being. When we do this, our emotions are able to keep moving. They don't become blocked. As we become more proficient in this process, we are able to operate from spirit in our relationships. We develop emotional awareness.

By being aware of our thoughts and emotions as they happen, we can choose the direction we want our lives to take, because our future is created from the present. This is the key to self-empowered emotional freedom.

### Emotional Freedom

We can learn to be in control of our thoughts and emotions by reprogramming our subconscious minds. The most fundamental way of doing this is by identifying the negative thought patterns we want to change and by repeating or holding positive ones in their place often enough and long enough, so they can make their way into our subconscious memory. We *intend* to become a different person, and we do! But it takes time.

There are other techniques we can learn, to bring relief and to change our thought patterns and subsequent life outcomes. They all require personal introspection so we can identify factors in our lives that are not working in our best interest. Some examples are: Neuro-Linguistic Programming (NLP), Emotional Freedom Technique (EFT), and Brain Gym. PSYCH-K™, which Dr. Bruce Lipton endorses, works in a relatively short time to correct dysfunctional subconscious beliefs through left and right brain synchronization. A search of the Internet will provide further information on these programs.

Another program, called "The Healing Codes," has been developed by Drs. Alex Loyd and Ben Johnson. It is based on activating "energy switches" in the body, allowing destructive energy from unhealthy fear-based emotional pictures held in cellular memory to be neutralized. When the perceived threatening factor is removed, the body is able to move into a growth healing mode that is based on love and a healthy self-concept. As this happens, stress is removed from the body "thus allowing the neuro-immune system to take over its job of healing whatever is wrong in the body."[7] This system, although somewhat expensive, claims supporting testimonies for various kinds of healings, including that of Dr. Ben Johnson who was healed of ALS (Lou Gehrig's disease).

Any process for effecting change must involve cultivating an awareness of what is working in our lives and what is not. It must help us deal effectively with our underlying hurts and beliefs by bringing them to the surface so we can recognize them and allow them to pass out of our subconscious pain-body. This process can take some time, so we should be willing to recognize and acknowledge our pain as it comes into our awareness. We need to be focused on the present moment. If we allow our minds to dwell on past experiences, those experiences will keep repeating in our lives. The only reality is the present. The only time we can *do* anything is *now*.

## POSITIVE THOUGHTS AND EMOTIONS ARE HEALING

Unlike their negative counterparts, positive thoughts and emotions have a calming, healing, and regenerative effect on the whole body. Attitudes of happiness, gratitude, thankfulness, love, forgiveness, patience, and so forth, are relaxing, stress-reducing, and supportive to all body functions. Laughter is especially healing.

### Gratitude and Love

Whatever we do, whether it is eating, working, or playing, should be done with gratitude and love. Both attitudes play large roles in our emotional well-being. Thankfulness is a feeling of gratitude and appreciation. And although we are most familiar with feeling love as an emotion, in its pure form, love is a way of being and relating to the world; it is an attitude.[8] Love acknowledges everything to be a contributing part of God's creation.

It embraces the qualities of acceptance, allowing, giving, sharing, and wishing the best for another.

Attitudes of gratitude and love are prerequisites for peace and emotional stability in our lives. They engender humility and modesty in our characters, and help to develop a gentle way of relating to others with an air of unpretentious confidence. Gratitude and love are the keys to harmony, not only in our relationships with people, but in our relationship to the food and beverages we consume. Recall how Dr. Masaru Emoto demonstrated that speaking or thinking words of gratitude and love to water caused beautiful, organized ice crystals to form in the frozen samples. Such harmonious structures nourish our bodies accordingly when we consume them. These words attributed to Jesus urge us to follow this approach: "Always receive with love, for it is love which instructs the food on how to nourish your body."[9]

## GETTING IN TOUCH WITH OUR FEELINGS

If thoughts are the generating forces that create what we want in life, then feelings are our compass. They show us whether we are going in the right direction.

Life, with its pressures and varied emotions, can be confusing. We all enter into decisions, agreements, and relationships that don't work out happily at times. And, many times when we look back on the process that led us there, we can identify a certain degree of comfort or discomfort with those decisions at that time. But chances are, we were not sufficiently aware of what our authentic self was feeling. We need to become conscious of our feelings and emotions as they are happening. We need to be in touch with our hearts.

Research done by the Institute of HeartMath in Boulder Creek, California, has found that the body's physical heart is much more than a pump, it has its own intelligence. Whereas the brain thinks it *knows* about situations by processing information, the heart *understands* at an intuitive feeling level. It influences how the brain functions.[10] Ideally, the heart and brain should work in cooperation with each other. We need to become aware of what the heart is saying as well as what we are thinking.

## OUR FEELINGS SHOW US TRUTH

Our feelings tell us what is true. At our core, at the level of our authentic self, we are in touch with spirit—our real self, our soul. Feelings are the language of the soul.

Each of us wants to know what is right for us in any given situation. The purpose of our feelings is to tell us that very thing. In his book *Questions and Answers on Conversations with God*, Neale Donald Walsch advises us to take the tummy test. Just pay attention to the feeling in your stomach; be aware of whether it is calm, feeling the excitement of anticipation, or if it is queasy or tense with anger. He says the tummy never lies and always knows what is right.[11]

If we don't like what the tummy is feeling, then we know that something is not good for us at this time. The tummy has said that our thoughts on this certain subject are not in our best long-term interests. Maybe we need to change our minds; adopt new thoughts. Emotions always follow thoughts.

## HOW DO WE WANT TO "BE"?

The state of our character can be measured by answering these questions: "Do I love?"— in the true, humble and unselfish sense of the word; "Am I who I say I am?" "Am I being authentic, or do I project a false front to others?" "Is my life deeply satisfying?" "Am I at peace within myself?"

The ultimate objective in life is to achieve a state of inner peace and joy. This is possible if we are prepared to work through our feelings of hopelessness, fear, anger, and resentment, toward acceptance, forgiveness, reason, and loving unconditionally. Ultimately, our aim would be to personify an attitude of compassion toward all others.

## BEING AUTHENTIC

We all have an inner sense of whether we are being real or not. When we are being real, we are authentic and genuine. There is no acting; our true self is coming across. Our authentic self is honest, open, and straightforward; it is free of ego. It makes no pretense of being anything other than who we are; it is transparent. Our authentic self is our child self that is spontaneously natural, because it is always in the present moment. It has no agenda other than being who it is. Being our authentic self opens the door to truth, happiness, fulfillment, and joy in our lives. It helps us learn again who we are as a being of loving intent in all we say and do. It is who we were created to be. If we are not there yet, it is who we came here to become.

## GETTING OUR ACT TOGETHER

Reshaping our characters requires an honest examination and identification of both the positive and negative attitudes that operate in our lives. It means becoming aware that attitudes and emotions influence our health. It means taking responsibility for our attitudes, and making the commitment to change the negative ones. No matter what attitudes our parents, friends, or associates influenced us with, or what our life experiences have been, we are still responsible for our own attitudes. We are the only ones who can change them. Blaming others gets us nowhere except into a rut. Taking personal responsibility for where we are in life is the first step toward improving our attitudes.

Healing on the mental/emotional side comes from being grateful and forgiving, as well as accepting responsibility for the consequences of our own decisions and actions. It is when we run into difficulties that we should be asking ourselves: "What can I learn from this? What am I doing wrong that should be changed?" Challenges and setbacks are opportunities to change our attitudes and beliefs.

Why does our life unfold the way it does? Is there something that drives our life in the same direction it has been going for many years? When we say we want to change, and even make resolutions, why do some of us seem helpless to carry through and achieve different outcomes in our lives? There is an answer, and it all depends on what we believe.

# 19 | THE POWER OF BELIEF

∽

*Whether you think you can or you think you can't,*
*you're right.*

HENRY FORD

∽

## HOW POWERFUL ARE OUR BELIEFS?

OUR BELIEFS are so powerful that they create our health, our happiness, and our lives. The beliefs we hold in our subconscious minds, whether positive or negative, are reflected in our life circumstances.

Every disease is a reflection of a false belief system within us. Our bodies are talking to us. A disease process is evidence that something is amiss in the workings of the mind; that is where the power to effect lasting change resides.[1] The disease distress is the body's cry asking us to change the underlying cause—the beliefs that are not working for our highest good.

Research by Dr. Bruce Lipton, discussed previously, proves that the biology of our cells is controlled by our minds.[2] This is primarily because our thoughts, which stem from our beliefs, cause a different chemical response in our bodies depending on whether we feel safe or threatened, happy or annoyed, positive or negative. By sensing through their receptors, cells react to their environment by either growing or being protective. A healthy environment evokes a growth response, and a toxic environment evokes a protection response.

It is not necessarily what is true, but what we believe to be true, our perception, which is important. That our minds can heal our bodies is now becoming a proven reality in studies on the placebo effect. There have been television documentaries on how people have been healed completely when they truly believed that a reparative surgery had been performed, or that a certain medication had been administered, even though the surgery wasn't performed and the medication was just a sugar pill.

It inevitably disturbs the pharmaceutical manufacturers that in most of their clinical trials, the placebos, the "fake" drugs, prove to be just as effective as the engineered chemical cocktails.[3]

When our minds believe something to be true, this causes our bodies to respond accordingly and make it happen. This is how we create our reality.

## HOW OUR BELIEFS ARE FORMED

As little children, we make agreements in our minds, based on the experiences we have in our homes and cultural environments, about what must be true.[4] When we accept these perceptions, they become our beliefs and we store them in our memory banks. From pre-birth to about age six, we are like computer hard drives, recording all our experiences and perceptions into our subconscious memories. And, just like computers, these beliefs become the programs that direct our lives. It doesn't matter whether they are really true or not; the fact that we perceive them to be true turns them into automatic programs that are the blueprints for our future life experiences. We download our parents' beliefs and behave accordingly.[5] At our core, the beliefs that we are either capable or lacking in ability, worthy or undeserving, safe or at risk, healthy or sickly, for example, become programs that create our reality as adults. Still, the majority of our accepted beliefs are not true.[6] They were formed as a result of our feelings as we interpreted the situations we found ourselves in, or were subjected to. Exactly like cells, or the community of cells, that we are, we adopted behaviors of protection in the interest of survival or of growth as we felt confident and free to explore our world and develop our abilities.

It makes quite a difference whether we were raised in an environment of acceptance or criticism, affirmation or abuse, calmness or anxiety, happiness or anger, security or fear, because these become the filters through which we view the world.

## FROM CHILD TO ADULT

Little children are naturally spontaneous and joyful. They live in the present moment and have no pretense. They don't pretend to be other than their authentic, inquisitive, and responsive selves. They ask innocent and direct questions. They are open and trusting. They hear things literally, and believe what adults tell them is true. Little children operate from spirit. But eventually, they begin to model their beliefs and behaviors according to their experiences and what they perceive to be true.

As negative experiences begin to impact them, children learn to hold back their innocence and spontaneity; they move from authenticity to pretense. Because of discomforting feelings and emotional pain, they start to *think* protectively of the "self." They begin to identify with their minds. The ego, that sense of self-centeredness, begins to form. Their thoughts move out of the reality of the present and into the fantasy of the past and future in which the mind makes up stories in relation to their experiences. As a result, children begin to modify their behavior and *pretend* to be other than their natural spontaneous selves. They learn to bury their pain and hold back part of their complete true self. But this buried pain and pretend-self extract a price. The child self is repressed because of fear and the pretend adult self emerges as a protection. The result is a loss of the authentic self. Children observe the adults in their world and start to emulate them. They begin to operate from the mind.

As adults, if we have not dealt with our dysfunctional beliefs, we continue the pattern of living through our minds, meaning that our dysfunctions keep repeating.

## SENSING SOMETHING GREATER

Down through the ages, across every tribe, nation, and culture, people have sensed, sought, and practiced a mental communication with God, or the Great Spirit—whatever they perceived that force or presence to be. Even so-called nonbelievers turn to a quick prayer in times of extreme crisis. When groups of people share common beliefs about how the spirit world operates, religions are born. They search for meaning, a sense of control, and an understanding of how they fit in the cosmos. Is there a difference between religion and spirit?

## RELIGION VERSUS SPIRITUALITY

Webster's dictionary defines religion as, *belief in a divine or super-human power or powers to be obeyed and worshiped as the creator(s) and ruler(s) of the universe*, and, *expression of this belief in conduct and ritual.*

Spirituality is concerned with *the spirit or the soul, often thought of as the higher part of the mind; showing much refinement of thought and feeling.*

Religion teaches that what happens in our lives is in the control of a power external to us, that our happiness, success, or circumstances are up to the will of this power—whatever it decides—usually according to our behavior and faith.

Religion, for the most part, sees human beings as separate from God. Spirituality sees human beings as one with God, and understands that everything is connected. Religion focuses on an external power, while spirituality focuses on the power within. Spirituality invites us to understand our thoughts and feelings as reflections of the source of creation in our lives.

Oddly enough, the great teachers of the religions have taught that: "the kingdom of God is within you."[7] They have tried to show the way. But, religious groups have missed the point. Followers of all major religions end up worshiping the messenger instead of embracing the message and transforming themselves. Over the centuries, why have we listened and not understood? Why do we still struggle and fight with each other?

## WISDOM OF THE KABBALAH

More than 4000 years ago, the collective wisdom up to that time, called Kabbalah, was recorded in a book entitled *The Book of Formation*. It is said to have been written by Abraham, the founding patriarch of Judaism, Christianity, and Islam. The Kabbalah was later expanded and written into 23 books called the *Zohar* which are said to contain all the instructions for understanding "the game of life."[8] But this information, which was meant to free people from mental bondage, was not appreciated by the religious establishment, which wanted to retain control of the people. So down through the centuries, it did everything in its power to persecute the Kabbalists and destroy their written texts. Fortunately, the establishment was unsuccessful. What has been a secret for millennia is now becoming public knowledge.

### We Live in Two Worlds
We live in two worlds, but we only see one. Kabbalah teaches that our reality is divided into two parts. The physical world perceived by our five senses comprises 1%, while the vast majority of our reality is encompassed by the 99% realm of spirit. The 1% is the source of darkness, and struggle, and chaos in our lives. The 99% is the source of lasting fulfillment, joy, and Light.[9] Light, with the capital L, is the source of our connection with God.

According to the Kabbalah, the common interpretations of religious scripture are misleading because everything was written in code. Scripture is not to be taken literally. What we take at face value is actually symbolic; it has a deeper hidden meaning. Without understanding the symbols, we look in the wrong places for solutions to our problems, and remain unaware of how to access the God-given, miracle making power in our lives.

### Why Can't We See?
What is the reason for the apparent illusion that blocks our understanding and progress in the game of life? There is a force that seems to work against us, and that has been referred to throughout history by many names such as: the Devil, Lucifer, the Dark Side, the Enemy, the Deceiver,

and Satan. The Kabbalah calls this force our Opponent, and the Opponent is none other than our ego![10] It is our false and over-sensitive ego that deceives us and causes us to react to situations that arise in our lives, cutting off our connection to the 99% world of fulfillment, joy, and Light. We react on impulse and get caught in the web of our emotional charge. We don't realize what is actually going on because we are blinded by our reactive emotions. We don't see because we don't understand. When we move from the innocence and clear perception of childhood to the pretense that characterizes adulthood, we get caught in the illusion of our ego; our view of reality becomes obscured. Our ego keeps us stuck in the 1% world unless, or until, we use our free will to resist the urge to react, thereby disconnecting from ego, and moving into the Light.

So, the solution to the problems that develop in our lives is to become proactive, to get out of our mind and stay in the present moment, moving into conscious creation. Down through the centuries, humanity has tried to do this through prayer. But without knowing the "rules of the game," the results have been hit-and-miss at best.

## THE LOST KEY TO THE POWER OF PRAYER

Prayer means different things to different people, but basically it is words spoken to God. Some believe in the power of prayer because of the experience of seeing it work in their own lives. Others, while they may never have personally experienced any tangible results of prayer, nonetheless maintain a private practice of prayer because of their upbringing and the sense of security it seems to bring in times of loneliness. The Bible contains many stories of miracles as a result of prayer. But the big questions are: "If prayer works, how does it work and why? When people pray for others, why does one receive their "miracle healing," and the next one doesn't? If prayer works for one person, why doesn't it work for another? Is there more power in group prayer than in individual prayer?" These are valid questions for which some answers are beginning to emerge.

In most European and Western cultures, the predominant faith is Christianity, and the main scriptures are the Bible. But when we begin to investigate the history of how the Bible was written and assembled, some very interesting facts come to light. Rabbi David M. Hargis, in his study paper entitled *The Constantine Conspiracy* (also mentioned in chapter 5), points out that under the direction of the Roman Emperor Constantine, a large group of bishops, known as the Council of Nicea, met and worked together between the years 318 and 325 AD, to decide church doctrine.[11] This group also decided which ancient texts would be included in what we now know as the Holy Bible.[12]

The Council of Nicea removed important spiritual and life information contained in many original scrolls. It was not until 1946, when the Dead Sea Scrolls were discovered, that this was realized. The Isaiah Scroll was among those documents. It contains information regarding prayer that had been lost until this time. That information is quite astounding: it reveals that the secret to effective prayer appears to be a combination of thought, feeling, and emotion.

In the Bible we are told that, "whatever things you ask in prayer, believing, you will receive."[13] But nowhere in the Bible do we find the wisdom from Isaiah and the ancient Essenes regarding the application of thought, feeling, and emotion as the engines that actually create the manifestation of our prayers.

Could this be the reason that some people seem to have their prayers answered, or why miracles happen for some and not for others? When we understand that everything is electrical, including thoughts, feelings, and emotions, then it seems to logically follow that saying or repeating words in prayer is one thing, but adding the electrically charged power of feeling and emotion to the process of believing or visualizing that it is already accomplished is quite another. Praying with passion appears to be the key to connecting with the universal creative power.

## WORDS ARE ELECTROMAGNETIC AND CREATIVE

In chapter 2 we were introduced to the understanding that everything in the universe is electric. Everything is an expression of energy—even apparently solid matter. All things can communicate at the cellular level because of their electromagnetic nature.

Under the discussion on water and memory in chapter 12, the work of Dr. Masaru Emoto was introduced to show how he photographically proved that different words and sounds result in different crystalline patterns in frozen water. Positive, uplifting words produce beautifully symmetrical ice crystals. Negative, angry, and discouraging words produce totally disorganized and miserable looking ice crystals. Words have creative, or destructive, power.

In the Bible, Genesis 1 is the "creation" chapter. The first verse states: "In the beginning God created the heavens and the earth." Notice that every time God created something, the Bible reads: "God said." God is also referred to in the Bible as, "the Word." Now consider this. Genesis 1:26 reads: "Then God said, "Let us make man in Our image, according to Our likeness." God, the Master Creator, made us to be creators! This is not just a religious statement. The creation key is the words we use as well as our intent and belief. Whether we realize it or not, we are creating our life circumstances by our thoughts, words, and emotions. Further, in Matthew 12:37, Jesus says: "For by your words you will be justified, and by your words you will be condemned."

Even if you choose to be nonreligious or to be a nonbeliever, you need to think carefully, at least about the physical proof of "word effects" as demonstrated in Masaru Emoto's ice crystals. The phenomenon of how words cause physical manifestation changes has since been repeated and verified by other researchers, such as cellular biologist Dr. Bruce Lipton.

Dr. Len Horowitz states that the physics of sound, including those of the spoken word, incorporate electromagnetic phenomena and waves moving through space. Creating miracles through prayer requires both the spoken word as prayer, as well as an attitude of being faithfully and righteously connected to God.[14] The person praying must be in harmony with the universal force of Love. I interpret this to mean having an attitude of loving intent.

### Religion and Science in Agreement

Dr. David Yonggi Cho is a Christian pastor in Korea who built a congregation of 50,000 members. In a discussion he had with one of Korea's leading neurosurgeons, the doctor was telling Dr. Cho that science had recently discovered that the speech center in the brain rules all the nerves in the body. Dr. Cho agreed saying he knew this from the Bible, since it says, "the tongue is the least member of our body, but can bridle the whole body." The medical doctor went on to relate his findings that simply speaking positive or negative words gives one control over the body to be able to manipulate it as one wishes.[15] If one thinks and speaks words to the effect of being tired, weak, sick, or old, then the speech central control gives out those orders to the body; the body responds accordingly and begins to disintegrate. Conversely, thoughts and words of energy, strength, health, and youth are acted upon by the speech control center in the brain bringing about a positive and rejuvenating response via nerves throughout the body.

Words have a tremendous bearing on our health. There have been several books written on the subject of, "What you say is what you get." One such book, by Karen Burton Mains, is *You Are What You Say: Cure for the Troublesome Tongue.*[16] Emerging research is throwing powerful illumination on our own positive and negative creative abilities, and the message is clear: If you want the best of health, happiness, and prosperity, watch your thoughts, because these are the words that create your reality! We all have ability to redirect our thoughts toward the positive.

### AFFIRMATIONS

Louise Hay is a best selling author of 27 books, including *Heal Your Body.* She has discovered that there is a cause for every physical condition in our lives; manifesting symptoms are a result of mental thought patterns. She says she *knows* disease can be reversed simply by reversing mental patterns. *Heal Your Body* contains a quick reference guide of probable mental patterns behind various diseases in the body and provides appropriate healing affirmations that a person is encouraged to repeat many times for a month. This is a good book that has comforted many people, but it may be helpful to take this advice a step further.

Most affirmations are spoken in the present tense regarding something we want in the future. In his book *Law of Attraction,* Michael Losier explains why many affirmations don't bring about the desired results. He says that as you repeat them, the words bring about a subconscious reaction or vibration based on how the words make you feel. For example, if you are overweight and repeat the affirmation, "I have a slender body," you know it's a lie because at the present time you don't have a slender body. There is a conflict and the resulting vibration is negative. This is because your words are not congruent with your present beliefs, feelings, and reality. However, a desire statement such as, "I am excited at the thought of having a slender body," is believable, provokes positive feelings, and can ring true with your subconscious mind. That is, of course, if you are also on a nutrition and exercise program designed to bring about the desired positive result.

Affirmations do not work if they are merely statements of what you want to be true. Affirmations work only when they are statements of something we already know to be true. So, in order for affirmations and desire statements to work, we should be experiencing feelings of excitement, possibility, and hope.[17] Again, as with the secret to prayer, it is emotion that kindles our creative power.

The same creative principle of utilizing emotion also applies to visualizations. You must *feel* what you visualize for it to become activated.[18]

## VISUALIZATIONS

We are living in an exciting time which some call "the end times," and others call the beginning of the "age of enlightenment." I believe it is the end times of "not knowing," and the beginnings of coming into an age of "awareness." It is the end of darkness and the emergence of light. Enlightenment is an experience of awakening to the true nature of the universe, and learning to function in harmony with it. The intent of this book is to help shed light on this process with regard to health.

Also helping to make this new understanding accessible are a number of extremely gifted young people, often referred to as Indigo or Crystal children. One such gifted person is a young man named Adam. He has the innate ability to see energy patterns and emanations around living beings, even at the cellular level, and to help rearrange these energies for health.

Adam says that we all have the ability to harmonize our energy and heal ourselves. The main tool he teaches for doing this is visualization. Briefly, it is a process of mentally visualizing an area of bodily dysfunction becoming well again and *seeing* the healing happen in the mental pictures we create. More information on Adam can be found at www.dreamhealer.com.

Visualization works with the creative capacity of our conscious and subconscious minds. An accomplished hypnotist told me that the subconscious mind sees in pictures. What it hears, it converts to a visual image, believes it, and reproduces it in the person's life. Whether the hypnotist is working to entertain, or to help people heal their lives, he taps into this automatic creative process within all of us.

## CHANGE YOUR BELIEFS, CHANGE YOUR LIFE

The series of *Conversations with God* books, by Neale Donald Walsch, distill down to two questions we need to ask to determine why we are here: "Who am I?" and, "Who do I want to be?"

As human *beings*, we are body, mind, and spirit. The body is the temporary physical home of spirit. The mind is our thought generator, our tool of creation. Spirit is the energy of who we are; it is the eternal part of our being.

God, or Creator, or Universal Power, or All That Is, or whatever term we may wish to use, created the universe and everything in it. The universe continues to create itself and expand. As discussed earlier, we are also creators. We create our own reality. We are responsible for everything in our lives.

Our spirits want to create, or recreate, who we really are inside. But here is the critical point: we can only create based on what we think or believe at our very core. We can only engage the process using the data programs that are running inside us, similar to a computer. Our bodies are manifestations or reflections of our beliefs as well as those that are held at the cellular level. Do you operate from a base of anger, resentment, and fear, or from a base of forgiveness, gratitude, and love?

Love is the creative force of the universe. As part of this creative energy, our souls are also pure love. As the loving essence of who we are, our souls or spirits always want the best for us. Behind the scenes of our conscious awareness is the eternal master, spirit. The mind is the servant, but, like an unruly child, it wants to be in control through the ego. The subconscious mind can only operate in logic through our core beliefs—what we think of ourselves deep down. If our core beliefs are of insecurity, scarcity, illness, or aging, it will, and can only, act to create these in our lives. On the other hand, if our core beliefs are centered on security, abundance, and wholeness, then our subconscious mind obediently works to create these in our lives.

Our bodies function from stored subconscious memories, but our spirits always urge us to become the very best vision we can hold of ourselves. Soul/spirit is the real creative power, but like God and as part of God, it will never interfere with our decisions or right of free choice. It continues to gently suggest. The fact that you are reading this book is a result of your spirit leading you to this information and knowledge for your consideration. Knowledge is power, and the power to change and become a greater version of who you are at this moment always begins with thought.

Our bodies are energy systems that can be directed by our thoughts. The key to a healthy body, in addition to the food we eat, is to program our subconscious mind with positive, healthy thoughts. We need to watch our self-talk as well as visualize the health we want to have. We need to control the energy messages we send to our subconscious mind.

You may be saying, "Alright, but how do I do that?" The following story provides the solution.

## CHANGE AND HEALING

Lila Dahl lives in Victoria, B.C., Canada. She is the author of a small but powerful book entitled *Change Your Mind Change Your Life.* After Lila had cancer for the second time and was very ill, her doctors told her she only had two months to live. What happened next was an amazing testimony to the power of spirit and creativity within all of us. She returned home, made a decision in thought form: "No one is going to tell me when I will die," and shouted out loud, "I am going to live." This opened up a whole new life for her. In her words, "I realized that I had to disconnect from my unhealthy thought patterns."

Lila's book leads us through a detailed process of identifying the unhealthy, rooted decisions, or core beliefs, we hold at a subconscious level about ourselves and life. She shows us how to disconnect from those beliefs, and finally, how to record and anchor healthy decisions and beliefs in their place. What results is a new creation of our own ongoing reality. Our inner data programs are renewed one at a time so our outer experience can change.

## SCIENTIFIC RESEARCH CONFIRMATION

Dr. Bruce Lipton asserts that we are not victims of our genes; we have an enormous potential to determine the outcome of our health. It is up to us to change or control our environment, something we do through the energy created by our thoughts and beliefs. It is now understood that cells can rewrite existing gene programs that had been created mostly from our perceptions and beliefs during fetal development and early childhood. Dr. Lipton explains that during this period, we are mostly in the hypnotic states of theta and delta consciousness. This is our main period of subconscious programming, similar to the programming of the hard drive of a computer.[19] This is the stored source of the negative emotional charge many of us have and carry into our adult lives. So, whether we are fearful, pessimistic, confident, happy, or optimistic, our cells take their orders from our thoughts and begin acting accordingly by moving our health toward dis-ease or harmony.

Our outer world is a reflection of the subconscious beliefs that are creating our realities. Conscious health is becoming aware that this is happening and directing the process with intention.

## INTENTION—GIVING DIRECTION TO OUR LIVES

Whatever we accomplish in life—no matter how large or small—comes through a process of creation. It begins with intention. We think of a goal, we consciously *intend* to reach it, and we set in motion mental and physical actions to achieve it.

Dr. Wayne Dyer, building on understanding from Carlos Castaneda's book *The Active Side of Infinity*, explains that intent is a force, an energy field in the universe that we tap into and that "sets up the path to attainment."[20] Intention is more than just deciding to do something; it is a universal power that sets the stage for creation in our lives. Still, where the ego is in control, the power of intention is deactivated.[21]

Everything already exists as energy in the form of spirit. The process of creation is one of connecting to spirit to bring our desires into manifestation. We are always creating our life circumstances but most of us are not aware of it; we do it *unconsciously* through the ego. However, we also have free will to *consciously* connect to the universal energy with intention and spirit, thereby creating the lives of health, happiness, and harmony we all desire.

In the next chapter we will discuss a fundamental understanding of how this creation process works while suggesting some practical ways of clearing and organizing our minds to connect to this energy field of consciousness. We can create new lives if we wish to.

# 20 | CREATING OUR OWN LIVES

~

*Everyone thinks of changing the world,*
*but no one thinks of changing himself.*
LEO TOLSTOY

~

## EVERYTHING IS CONNECTED

All people and events in our lives are connected because they are part
of one energy system in the universe. This is inherent in the meaning of
the word universe, which is: *all created things turned into one system.*
Nothing is separate; everything is part of the one system, including us.
The difficulty for us is that we see each other as individual physical bodies, and therefore we think we are separate. However, this is an illusion,
because everything is energy in different forms. We, as energy beings, are
part of universal energy. So, if we are part of this great oneness, how can
we synchronize our energy to be in harmony *with* the universal energy?
How do we fit in? Why do some people seem to have more problems than
others?

## WHY ARE WE HERE?

Have you ever wondered about your purpose for being here? Why are you
in the body you have, in the family you were born into, with the job or

relationships you find yourself in? Great questions! Probably the most important ones you could ask. The answer is simple to state, but more complex to understand and put into practice. Our purpose is nothing more and nothing less than to discover who we were created to be, and to learn to express that. It is to move from unconsciously creating our lives to consciously creating them; we have to see through the illusion that our thoughts are who we are. This requires that we get past the distractions of our noisy minds and controlling egos.

## DISCONNECTING FROM EGO

In chapter 17, we learned that the ego is based on an unconscious identification with the mind—that it feeds on mind-chatter. The ego is also perpetuated by pain. It indulges in criticism, gossip, and comparison with others. Underlying its mental behavior are feelings of insecurity, low self-worth, and not being loved enough to satisfy its desires. By allowing the ego to control our lives, it blocks the very things we want most, which are continual feelings of happiness, joy, peace, well-being, and fulfillment. The ego is reactive, always in thought and emotion based on remembrances of the past or fears of the future. Like a magician, it keeps us focused on the illusion. It keeps us in the dark, unable to see the light of true reality.

To disconnect from the ego's control, we have to be willing to get off the rollercoaster; we have to give up the thoughts that constantly feed our pain-bodies with impulsive, reactive desires. We must be willing to give up our grievances and practice true forgiveness. We have to learn to be in the present moment. Actually, just learning about what the ego is and how it operates puts the odds on our side; we are already on the road to success because our consciousness is being raised. Becoming aware is always the first step. This means learning the rules for the game of life. It means moving into en-*light*-enment, dispelling the darkness of non-understanding. We are learning to create our lives consciously, on purpose.

## MOVING FROM REACTIVE TO PROACTIVE RESPONSE

The secrets to overcoming the ego are *present moment awareness* and *resistance*. We become aware of our thoughts as they are happening, and we resist the urge to play the ego's game of reacting impulsively. We relate with people in the focus of the present moment, uninfluenced by emotional sensitivities of the past or fears of the future. When we are in the present, we are able to be totally authentic.

The proactive power to create our lives is in each present moment. We stop taking things personally and resist the impulse to react. We drop the urge to express anger, and as we do, we gradually lose our fear. We observe, and allow things to happen with the realization that everything happens for a reason. We step out of the combative role, into a proactive one. Instead of working against the energy, we work with it. When we consciously practice this, we achieve a spiritual transformation and begin to create our lives in the 99% world of positive emotional vibrations. When we are controlled by our egos, we live and react in the 1% world.

Whenever we feel frustrated, angry, upset, and are reacting to a situation, our ego is operating; the counterfeit part of us is crowding out our real, authentic self. At that moment, we can choose not to react. We can move away from the negativity of criticizing and blaming other people and events for our problems, because this is what prevents us from breaking free and achieving peace of mind. We can choose to drop the reactive response and become proactive. We can move from attitudes of defensiveness, into love, acceptance, and harmony in our minds and actions. We can move from being self-centered to being other-centered; from wanting to receive to desiring to share.

## FORGIVENESS—THE KEY TO FREEDOM

Complete forgiveness of everyone who has hurt or wronged you, and more importantly, forgiving yourself, is the key to freedom and peace of mind.

This will not happen without true forgiveness. When we free another in our minds, we also free ourselves. When one understands, it is easy to forgive others because you realize they are only living their own movie from their thoughts, acting out their own fears and hurts. They are being controlled by their egos; they are reacting. Only when we forgive will the cords that bind and hold us be cut. We are then free to move on in peace to become the person we would like to be. This is how Jesus was able to express compassion for those who crucified him: "Father, forgive them for they know not what they do."[1]

Being bound to a person through unforgiveness reminds me of a practice from ancient Greece. Evidently, when a person was convicted of murdering someone, the corpse of that person was tied to the murderer and s/he was forced to drag it around with them. That's sort of how it works when we won't forgive someone who we think has wronged us. They continue to plague our mind and drag us down. True forgiveness cuts that connection and sets us free.

At first, forgiveness is a conscious act, but as we habitually practice it, even when we feel annoyed at someone, it becomes an attitude and a way of being which develops inner peace within us. We give up judging others.

## THE FEELING OF FREEDOM

The feeling of being free to be who I truly am, being authentic and living in the present moment is the greatest joy I have ever experienced. I have an inner peace that I have not known in my life before. I am finally in control of myself with no blame, malice, or thought against anyone else.

When we are free to be who we are, with honest and loving intent, we are no longer bound by fear. Behind anger there is always fear. People who are angry try to control and influence others through force. Force is not power. Love and truth are power. A good example is how Mahatma Gandhi, through the power of passive resistance and standing on truth and human dignity, broke the oppression of the British Empire and its subjugation of the people of India to win independence in 1948. Gandhi used power; the British tried to use force. True power always wins in the end.

## ACCESSING OUR SUBCONSCIOUS POWER

The powerhouse of our lives is our subconscious mind. Knowing how to connect to it is key to creating the life we want. When we are able to control the thoughts in our conscious minds, we can use them to give our subconscious minds different instructions. We do this by opening the subconscious mind to suggestion. This is the same process that a hypnotist uses. He relaxes his client's mind and implants a suggestion. Their subconscious mind believes it and reproduces the condition or habit in their life circumstance. At the suggestible moment, the belief that they are hot, cold, unable to walk, can bark like a dog, or whatever, will be literally acted on by their subconscious mind and reproduced in their experience. We can access our subconscious power by purposefully setting up this state of suggestibility for ourselves.

The interface between the conscious and subconscious mind is greatest when we are in stage two consciousness, the alpha state. It is a time of stillness, when the portal to the subconscious mind is open. This is the feeling we have just before we fall asleep, or when we first wake up. It is a state we can reach in meditation, the purposeful stilling of the mind and entering the present moment. It is when the conscious mind can talk to the subconscious mind, when it can gently and confidently make suggestions to be acted on by the subconscious mind. As these are repeated frequently enough, the subconscious mind accepts them as directions to be reproduced in life. Whatever we desire in the way of health, prosperity, success, or relationships, for example, must be programmed into our subconscious minds. That is how our thoughts become our reality; it is how we create our own lives. An excellent book for more detail on this process is *The Power of Your Subconscious Mind* by Dr. Joseph Murphy.

## MY PERSONAL BELIEFS

In this section, I share my own beliefs about why we, as individual spirit beings, came to be here on earth in the persons we are, and in the families we find ourselves in. You, the reader, are urged to form your own conclusions about what is true and real for you. Remember that most of our beliefs about what is true have been conditioned—they came from someone else. This section is meant to be a stimulus to encourage you to think for yourself, "outside the conditioned box," and to realize the wonderful person you are, and were created to be. At the spirit level you are Love, the prime force of creation in the universe.

We are in a continual process of evolving to become more like God, or Prime Creator, who is pure love. In this context, love is not a feeling; it is a way of being. A belief I share with others is that we are not physical beings having a spiritual experience, but rather spirit beings having a physical experience. We have come here to learn and grow. As spirits, we always were and always will be like God, because we are part of God. God is not in physical form, but experiences physically on earth through us. We are created in God's image. That means that, every second, with every thought and every word, we are creating our own realities. We have been given free choice to decide what that reality, our lives, will be. In other words, God says, "Don't cry about it, if you don't like your present reality, change it." God created us to be able to change our thoughts, beliefs and words, and therefore, to create new lives. That's how it works. We have choices. We are not victims of our circumstances unless we decide or believe that we are.

I have come to believe that, as spirit beings before we came to earth, we chose to be born into the families we are part of; we knew the possible challenges beforehand. We chose our specific family because it afforded us the perfect context in which to grow spiritually and achieve the spiritual goals we set for ourselves for this lifetime. When viewed this way, we are not victims, but rather the very initiators of our own trials and joys. We are responsible because we chose to be here in the first place. The unfortunate downside to this is my realization that we humans are also stubborn, myopic, and have a tendency to feel sorry for ourselves. As we develop our lives, we often neither "see the light," nor change and grow without the stimulus of pain. The question for each of us is, "Have I had enough pain yet?" At age 62, I finally began to see the light and said, "That's enough." I opened my eyes and "saw." I understood. I finally stopped being controlled by my ego and moved into spirit. If you haven't already done this, at what age will you say, "Enough already. I'm moving on to claim my freedom to be who I am inside. I am taking my power and my peace back."

It is always your choice and only your choice. God gave us free will to be or not be whoever we decide at each moment. He allows us to create our own movies. Nobody else can make the choices for us. And nobody else is ultimately to blame for our circumstances either, because that is to still be stuck in victim mode. That is why Jesus said to his followers— if they believed and practiced the truths he was telling them—"You will know the truth, and the truth will set you free."[2] However, throughout the Bible, Jesus always expected the other person to take the first step. When the desired change, such as a healing had happened for a person, he would say, "Your faith has made you whole."[3] The truth is that from our thoughts and deep beliefs (faith), we create the present reality we find ourselves in.

### The Process of Creation in Simple Terms

The creative process from our thoughts to manifestation can be explained quite simply. Actually, everything is one and simultaneous with no divisions, but it may help to compartmentalize the process as shown in figure 20.1.

We have two parts to our minds: conscious and subconscious. Conscious thoughts are thoughts we can control once we are aware of them. The subconscious mind is like a dutiful, unquestioning servant. It takes whatever the conscious mind thinks about and stores it for literal duplication, without question. It is like a photocopier, reproducing exactly

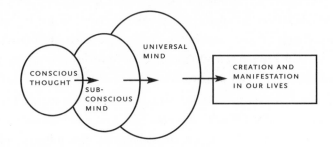

**Figure 20.1   Creation and manifestation process**

the thoughts fed into it. There is also the God-Mind, or Universal Mind. This is where all knowledge in the universe is and where the creation process takes place for manifestation into our lives. Here is the secret: Our conscious minds can not access the Universal Mind (or Universal Power) directly, but the subconscious mind can. So whatever we store in our subconscious minds via our conscious thoughts, positive or negative, gets transferred to the Universal Mind for creation in our lives.

Just like the computer programming aphorism—"Garbage in; Garbage out"—as long as we feed our subconscious minds thoughts of negativity such as fear, poverty, unworthiness, and disease, this is what gets translated into our reality. But when we reprogram our subconscious with positive thoughts of love, abundance, worthiness, and health, then these will eventually manifest in our lives. That is what Lila Dahl's experience was all about. By using this exact process, she beat the so-called incurable cancer that the doctors had sent her home to die from. She re-created her life.

### Relationships

There is no greater teacher or mirror for us to see who we are being than our relationships with others. Relationships, especially intimate ones, are the primary vehicle for our transformation and growth. That is their main purpose.

Everything we say in a relationship, intimate or otherwise, is all about ourselves![4] It has nothing to do with what the other person says or does. That is their own movie. What we think, say, feel, and how we react, is our movie, how we are creating our own lives. The key to creating a positive life is being aware of our actions and reactions as they are happening.

The greatest gift we can give to ourselves and our loved ones is to stand in confident love, not anger, for who we are, and become the wonderful, secure, happy, magnificent human being that spirit inside us knows we are. We were created to develop ourselves fully through intimacy in relationship; it is an essential part of balanced health.[5]

Every physical thing in the universe is manifested energy. Because it is energy, every physical thing vibrates. Different things vibrate at different frequencies. Different thoughts and beliefs vibrate at different frequencies also. Fear operates at low frequencies. Pure love vibrates at the highest frequency. I mention this scientific truth to highlight that the loving intent and truth we hold in our beliefs, or who we are in our process of evolving, will determine the frequency our individual beings vibrate at. As we grow in love and live more of our truth, we raise our vibratory frequency.

The law of energy physics is that things of similar frequency vibrate together; like attracts like. In other words, we attract people of similar frequency to us, and similarly, we are attracted to them. We do this for the purpose of reflecting our state of growth to ourselves. If we don't like what we are seeing around us in our relationships, we can change who *we* are being. As we change our attitudes and behaviors, we change our frequency, and consequently, different people will be attracted to us.

As we begin to change, a person at the lower vibratory frequency in a relationship wants desperately to hold us at their level. Another way of saying it might be, "misery likes company." They cannot stand to see or feel us grow. They instinctively know we are growing away from them but are afraid to look inside themselves and make changes. So they try to control us. When we allow this, we lose the freedom to be who we are; we are no longer being authentic.

Remember that people we are in relationship with are there for a reason, for example, as Gabor Maté points out:

> Couples choose each other with an unerring instinct for finding the very person who will exactly match their own level of unconscious anxieties and mirror their own dysfunctions, and who will trigger for them all their unresolved emotional pain.[6]

To me, this means that when we feel pain, it is a signal to look inward to identify the pain and to move through it by correcting the false assumptions or beliefs that caused it in the first place. When we start to grow while the other person is still caught in their dysfunctions, it can be very difficult, but no one should stay in the presence of manipulation and abuse. Through it all I try to keep in mind the respect and integrity I have for myself. That has to be paramount. We must always love and respect ourselves in order to be able to love and respect others.

### Everything Happens for a Reason

It is my belief that everything happens for a reason. Nothing is accidental or coincidental, because everything in the universe is connected. Everything that happens in our lives is what we have attracted so that we can see and feel where we are in the act of creating our lives. Even black clouds have silver linings, if we will just look for them. When we finally break out of the grip of the ego, we can look back on the difficult times and see the purpose behind them in our evolvement to become who we are now. Again, events and experiences are mirrors, messengers, or challenges for us to overcome so we can move into a closer harmony with our souls. There is a masterful purpose behind everything. Ultimately, all creation is from Spirit. The only true and complete healing of any kind is a return to perfect wholeness via Spirit.

## PLANNING YOUR LIFE'S DIRECTION

The remainder of this chapter is intended to offer some practical ideas that one may think through and record on paper as an organizational framework of their personal life priorities and direction. This is an important step in sending clear messages to the subconscious mind. Unless we are clear about what we want in our lives, how can we expect happiness and success to manifest? This is a very worthwhile exercise.

### Life Purpose

To have a feeling of direction in your life, you need to be connected to your passion. Your life purpose can be distilled from your thoughts, dreams, and expectations.

To get in touch with your purpose, ask yourself the following questions and write your answers down:

1   What do I enjoy doing the most?
    - What do I enjoy doing so much I lose track of time?
    - What would I do without pay just so I could do it?
2   What am I good at?

- What are my natural talents?
- What do I have to contribute?
- What do I feel good about doing?

3  What do I want to accomplish in life?

4  What am I willing to do to accomplish it?

- Am I willing to go outside of my comfort zone?

5  If failure were not a possibility, what would I be doing with my life?

Become the best you can be, and live it—BE IT!

You will know your purpose because: It will be simple. You will feel it. It will inspire you.

Your purpose will be your passion—what you feel excited about!

## Values

We need to base our thinking, decisions, and actions on a clear set of values that we adhere to in our relationships and life activities. These are what form the basis of our character. Values can vary somewhat from person to person, but the following are basic examples: honesty; integrity; loyalty; commitment; respect; trust.

Remember: "Right is still right, even if nobody else is doing it. Wrong is still wrong, even if everybody else is doing it."

## Priorities

To give us direction and a sense of peace in carrying out our daily activities, we need to have our priorities clearly determined as the basis for making decisions. The priorities that work well for some people, in order of importance from highest to lowest are: Spiritual life; spouse; children; job or vocation; life interest or life purpose activities. When our activities or pursuit of money and status are our top priorities, it inevitably causes imbalance and leads to unhappiness in our lives.

When our values are firm and our priorities are well defined, we can display strong character, act with integrity, and give direction to our activities and relationships while working toward true success in life. From these bases, we can pursue purposeful goal setting and planning.

## Written Goals

In 1953, a study on the effectiveness of goals was done with students at Yale University in Connecticut. Only 3% of the graduating class reported that they had specific written goals. When these same class members were surveyed twenty years later, it was discovered that the 3% group with written goals had financial income exceeding the total of the remaining 97%.[7]

A goal is a dream with a deadline. If it is not written down, it is just a wish. We need to have desire and vision. We need to follow our spirit to where we want to be, and know what we want to achieve. We need to know where we want to go. There is a saying that, "If you don't know where you're going, any road will take you there." If our goals are just indefinite dreams, then we have no clear expectations for them to become reality. When our goals are defined, our thoughts, energies, and creative talents focus on their achievement. Whatever we are fascinated by, whatever we define as an objective and focus our attention on, we tend to bring into our lives.

Work on your inner qualities first, and be committed to personal growth. The things that help us to grow are:

- The people we meet and associate with.
- The books we read; tapes, lectures, and sermons we listen to; the seminars we attend.
- How well we get to know, understand, and accept ourselves.

Personal growth takes effort and commitment. Growth and change only happen when we venture out of our comfort zones. The answers to your life are *within you.* Are you growing and learning? Meditate, and dwell on your questions, and the answers will come to you.

Goals are many and varied, but they must be real. Goals can be short-term, medium-term, and long-term. They can be internal and external. To formulate and define your goals, start brainstorming without qualification, and write each one down. Next, divide your list into categories such as: spiritual, social, health, material, career, recreational, financial, and relationship, identifying what value each one fulfills. Next, look at your listing within categories to see if you have balance in your life. Do the majority fall into one, or into a few categories? What is the motivation behind each goal? What are you trying to accomplish?

In order to be effective in leading us toward a sense of lasting fulfillment, our goals and visions must be:

- Based on our values.
- Positive, active, and creative. (Passive, spectator activities such as watching TV can pass the time enjoyably, but they are not truly recreational. They do not "re-create" and help us grow.)
- Something we start on right now and work toward.
- Time limited, with a clear date objective and aim for their accomplishment.
- Written down and referred to, so they become objectives of our subconscious mind.
- Specific, so we can know how they directly relate to what we want in our lives.
- Formulated in a plan with a series of action steps leading to their accomplishment.
- Something we really desire. (If we don't truly desire something, it will not happen. Desire is the starting point, the fuel of achievement in life.)

Finally, goals focus our activities so we can achieve objectives. But remember, your life focus should also be enjoyable. Goals are there to give direction. Use them as a guide, without allowing them to be so set that you become a slave to them. Slavery in any form is a curse, and counterproductive to the pursuit of happiness and health. www.talklisten.com/exchange/2001/october/ is a website with helpful information on goal setting.

**Planning**
A plan is a map to get us where we want to go. It is our plotted route toward the achievement of our goals and success. Most people don't *plan* to succeed, nor do they plan to fail either. They just fail to plan. Make your planning choice organized, with a purpose in mind.

Making a plan is a process of taking a goal we want to achieve and breaking it down into its simplest action steps. A good method of planning is to start with the end result or goal we want to achieve and then work backwards to where we are now. Having identified the path backwards, we can then map out step by step, with time objectives for each step, the plan that we think will best lead to the achievement we want.

Good planning takes into consideration the priority of activities in terms of our values and needs. This is an important identification process to go through so that we are making an efficient and profitable use of our time. In other words, it is good time management. The saying "more haste, less speed" is often true. If we just bolt ahead without much thought to get the job done, we often either complete the task or project at a poorer standard than we are capable of, or we subsequently have to redo parts of it. Similarly, if we have several tasks to complete, and we just start working on them more or less at random, we are probably not making the best use of our time.

When we are able to sort our activities into priorities, we can reduce our stress level, increase efficiency and the quality of our output, as well as accomplish more of what is really important in our lives.

### Moving Toward Your Purpose

Once you have a clear vision of your purpose, have defined your values, priorities, and goals, and have formulated a step-by-step plan, you can begin to put the plan into action. Having a clear outline in our conscious minds and going over it periodically prepares our subconscious to begin creating the future we envision. Our lives can move forward. We have motivation to improve. We are in a better position to make the attitude changes that are needed, which will assist us in achieving our goals. We can adopt attitudes that will help us, such as being relaxed, assertive, patient, confident, determined, calm, and caring.

You must be able to focus your attention to create and achieve your purpose. Focus on, and stay committed to a particular project, career, or relationship. It is a universal law that we attract to ourselves what we focus on. Focus on progress, achievement, abundance, and success. Spending time judging, resisting, complaining, criticizing, fearing, or worrying is counter-productive and does not contribute to achieving a positive purpose, nor to a healthy physical body. A statement by Vladimir Kuskoff summarizes this truth: "Where the majority of your thoughts lie, there lies your destiny."[8]

A new and improved life—physically, mentally, emotionally, and spir-itually—is there for your making. Start with a vision that gives you a pic-ture of what you want. Create a plan of how you will move toward it. Work each step of your plan with determination and commitment. Enjoy the challenges, successes, and progress along the way. As you do these things for yourself, you are consciously making a new reality, creating your own enthusiasm for life.

Now that we have covered the first four keys toward *Conscious Health*, let's move into action—putting this knowledge into operation. In the next few chapters we will discuss the practical aspects of changing over to a health-ier lifestyle. If we have knowledge but don't put it into practice, nothing changes. It is like a light switch that we never turn on. Knowledge allows us to form beliefs, but beliefs must be implemented before we can profit from them.

# IMPLEMENTING

# 21 | CHANGING OVER

~

*A journey of a thousand miles
begins with a single step*
CONFUCIUS

~

## MAKING THE TRANSITION TO A HEALTHIER DIET

WHEN YOU have made the decision to change to healthier lifestyle practices, over time you can expect to see improvements in your health. To help you realize the progress you are making and to give yourself encouragement, as you begin your changeover program, it is recommended that you write down on paper all the troubling symptoms you have. Make a baseline, a starting point for yourself. Date this list, then review and record your progress every two or three months. This is very helpful because most people forget about some of the symptoms that are no longer bothering them. They just concentrate on the ones that concern them at the time, not realizing that their list of complaints is getting shorter.

### Cooked Foods Are Addictive

No less than alcohol, drugs, or nicotine, cooked foods are addictive. Overcoming any addiction takes understanding and personal discipline. Over time, with perseverance, the addiction to cooked food can be overcome. Our taste buds can be re-awakened to detect the superior taste of prime raw fruits and vegetables, making cooked foods less appealing. As cells throughout the body start to get healthier from the intake of true nutrition, the body's innate intelligence begins to function more efficiently, increasing the body's desire for living foods.

### Calories in Raw Food

Calories essentially have nothing to do with nutrition because a calorie is only a measure of heat energy. Raw foods contain calories as well as all the other live factors necessary for their utilization.[1] Cooked foods contain calories, but few or no live factors required for their utilization. A diet of mostly cooked food eventually causes the body's channels of elimination to become inefficient. As this happens, food calories that are not eliminated have to be stored in the body as fat. If, on the other hand, the body has become adjusted to a mostly raw food diet, all organs begin to function more efficiently; complete nutrition is obtained from the food eaten while any excess calories are easily eliminated via bowel movements. As a clear indication of how much less heat a healthy body requires to function properly, raw foodists typically have body temperature readings that are 1.8 degrees Fahrenheit (1 degree Celsius) lower than cooked food eaters.[2]

### How to Change Over

This is very important. Depending on how toxic your present diet is and how quickly you make the change over to healthy eating practices, the reaction symptoms your body manifests as it eliminates toxins can vary from mild to quite severe. For example, as poisons are eliminated, they are dumped into the blood and circulated through the brain. As a result, nerve endings are irritated and react, causing the pain of a headache. In cases of serious illness, there may be little choice because the need for a rapid detoxification of the body and replenishment of nutrients is the overriding concern. In other cases, it may be preferred to eliminate wrong foods by gradually replacing them with better choices. This will mean that detoxification reactions will be slower, but the health benefits will also be more gradual in making their appearance. It is a matter of personal choice and determination.

The ultimate objective is to eliminate toxic foods. They cost the body energy and nutrients to process them into and out of the body. The toxins they introduce remain in storage, contributing to disease. The first foods to go should be caffeine, nicotine, sugar, table salt, dairy products, alcohol, and red meat (to a large extent). Desserts, with their typical high sugar content and because they are usually eaten after meals, are very hard on digestion. This practice should be eliminated. These foods are all strong acid-producers.

The key to changing over to a healthier diet is not to focus so much on taking wrong foods out of the diet right away, but rather to start adding more of the right, raw foods into it.

Changing to healthier foods should not be seen as a "take-away diet," but rather as an "add-to diet." We should move to fruit or fresh fruit juice for breakfast and a large salad containing a variety of raw vegetables with lunch and dinner. As we add more raw fruits and vegetables to our meals we will naturally begin to eat less of the other foods. As time goes on, and as the body begins to respond to the supply of fresh wholesome nutrients, we will find that the old foods start to lose some of their appeal. What we used to eat every meal or every day, we begin to eat every other day, then twice a week, then once a week, and so on.

To occasionally "fall off the wagon" is no reason to feel badly. The thing to do is not to *gorge* on the wrong foods. For instance, eat a piece of pizza but not three or four. When we eat out and really have no choice, we should eat more of the salads, with smaller portions of the other foods. We can supplement with digestive enzymes to help digest the food. The next day, we simply get right back to the healthy routine.

The best addition we can make to our diets is freshly-made fruit and vegetable juices. They are to be consumed slowly and by themselves. Take them as a meal or between meals. Freshly-made juices are better than any store-bought vitamin and mineral supplements, and will produce detoxification and health-rebuilding results faster than anything else. They are whole living foods that are easy for the body to digest.

Make a transition plan for yourself or your family that each week, you will move a little closer to an ideal diet. Decide that one or two years from now, you will be eating according to, or close to, the suggestions outlined in the *Healthy Lifestyle Checklist* (see later in this chapter). Above all, don't make it hard on yourself or others. It takes time to change habits and tastes. Just move forward with purpose, and as you add more of the right foods, the amount and frequency of wrong foods will decrease over time.

Making the transition to a better diet and a healthier lifestyle and seeing the positive health changes in your body is an exciting and rewarding process. It is worth all the effort and patience taken through the healing phases. You will be rewarded in the long run with more energy, less illness and pains, a stronger and healthier body, and renewed enjoyment of life. That's what this book is all about. Reread portions that mean the most to you once in a while, so that the information becomes part of your handy knowledge base.

### Simple and Effective

The most simple and effective change that everyone can make is to drink one or two glasses of water with the juice from one-half or a whole lemon upon first rising in the morning. For lunch make and consume a green smoothie (see Appendix 7). These two practices alone can produce health benefits in a surprisingly short period of time.

## RESTORING ACID-ALKALINE BALANCE

By checking the pH levels of our saliva and urine, we are able to monitor how well our bodies are coping under the conditions of our lifestyles; we are also able to determine the health of the alkaline mineral reserve in the body. Remember, checking your pH is a health index evaluation process, not a disease identifying process.[3] To check your pH, you will need a supply of good quality, fresh (not old) pH papers having a range of 5.0–8.0. Check health food stores and drug stores. Some networking companies also sell them.

The discussion and comments provided here are brief and a summary at best. Readers are urged to obtain a copy of Dr. M. T. Morter's booklet *pH, Your Potential for Health,* or other books on pH testing for more detail. It should be stressed that a person should not try to draw firm conclusions based on one day's readings. An average of pH numbers over several days is a more reliable indicator.

Generally speaking, the more the initial urine pH reading, after awakening, is below 6.8, the weaker the body's alkaline mineral reserve and the more acidic the fluids inside and outside the cells. Such a reading also means cellular oxygen is at deficient levels, thereby providing a welcome medium for harmful organisms, and setting the stage for degenerative disease.

### Testing

Using pH reagent strips, check saliva before getting out of bed. Move your tongue a bit and swallow two or three times to get the saliva flowing. Touch the pH strip on your tongue to wet it, then remove it and take the reading. Next, get up and go to the washroom to check the pH of your urine. You can quickly place the pH strip into the urine stream and remove it. Or, you can urinate into a receptacle and then quickly dip the strip in and out again. Record both saliva and urine readings.

The ideal first reading for both saliva and urine is approximately 7.0. During the day, both the saliva and urine readings will vary, depending on what we eat and drink. Because the body excretes excess acids from protein in the food we eat, urine pH during the day will usually be lower. Ideal saliva pH readings should be: 6.8 on awakening; 7.0 after rising but before eating; and 8.5 after breakfast.[4]

When initial morning saliva pH numbers are below 6.8, one should be looking at his or her level of emotional stress and any ways to make improvements. Underlying emotional patterns over the months and years can have an exhausting effect on the body. This inevitably depresses the immune system and overall health. Even vegetarians, whose food is mostly alkaline, can have low saliva pH readings due to negative attitudes or emotional stress. Dr. Morter states that saliva pH should always rise immediately after a person has eaten. If it does not, this indicates that alkaline reserve minerals in the body are lacking and need to be replenished.[5]

Initial morning urine pH numbers are easier to interpret. When body pH is in healthy balance, the urine has very little odor, and has a pH in the range of 6.8 to 7.2. When the pH is lower than 6.8, you have a clear indication that you need to increase your alkaline mineral reserves. To do this, eliminate as many of the acid-producing foods and beverages as possible and increase your intake of alkaline foods and drinks.

*Note: In cases of serious illness, as discussed in chapter 10, the initial morning urine test results can be misleading. When the body is fighting serious conditions, such as cancer, it is so acidic that the kidneys begin to produce ammonia as a temporary damage control measure. This would give a fairly normal pH reading, but it would be false.*

### Checking Your Mineral Reserve

Testing your urine pH gives the most accurate indication of the mineral reserves in the body. Consume only alkaline fruits, vegetables, and beverages for two days. On the third morning, test your urine pH as described above. The lower the reading is under 6.8 will indicate the extent of body acidity, and the extent of alkaline reserve depletion. Acidosis begins to occur when the initial morning urine pH is lower than 6.8. Extreme acidosis occurs when the initial morning urine pH is 5.5 or lower. This indicates that there is no alkaline reserve, and that an alkalizing diet of raw fruits and vegetables may be required for several months to rebuild the body's store of alkaline minerals.[6]

### When Body pH Is Very Acidic

When initial morning urine pH tests are consistently acidic, below 6.1, this is an indication that the body is seriously deficient in alkaline minerals, especially organic sodium and potassium. These must be replenished for true health to occur. A stricter adherence to a diet of alkaline foods and beverages plus alkaline supplements if needed, and an avoidance of acid-producing foods is necessary to bring the body into a healthy acid-alkaline balance. The number one addition to the diet should be green smoothies (See Appendix 7). However, these dietary changes should be made gradually to allow the body time to adjust to new foods.

This degree of an acid condition indicates another, seemingly contradictory, problem. Although the body is overburdened with too much acid, the stomach is not producing enough acid to properly convert food in digestion. The reason for this is that the stomach's parietal cells, which produce acid for digestion, are so toxic they cannot work efficiently. Supplementation with betaine hydrochloride plus digestive enzymes may be required as a temporary measure. The more acidic the system of the individual is, the more will acid supplementation be required to relieve their symptoms of digestive discomfort.[7] These symptoms are often indigestion and heartburn, for which the standard remedy is antacids. Unfortunately, this is exactly the opposite of what is required because it does not address the cause, which is a weak presence of stomach acid.[8]

My preference in these situations, as a temporary measure, is to use unpasteurized apple cider vinegar, which is rich in organic alkaline minerals. One teaspoonful to one ounce (5–30 ml) can be taken in a little water before meals. This provides a remedial medium in the stomach and intestines that promotes digestion and assimilation of minerals. Unpasteurized apple cider vinegar is a live food which is acidic in the stomach, but which leaves an alkaline ash in the body after digestion. It is the #1 food source recommended by Dr. Gabriel Cousens for maintaining the body's vital acid-alkaline balance.[9]

Unprocessed sea salt is very helpful as a source of organic sodium and other minerals. One-half to one teaspoon of sea salt in a glass of water, right after getting up in the morning, or as necessary, can be taken. For serious acidic body conditions, a more alkalizing salt may be required. (One example can be found at www.excelexgold.com/water_alive.) Unprocessed sea salt is natural salt. Do not use table salt, NaCl, which is toxic and cannot be utilized by the body; it only contributes to a worsening of health problems.

## Baths Are Helpful

During the period when one is attempting to correct an acid pH condition, it is also very helpful to use regular soaks in the bathtub. Three or more baths per week for 30 to 40 minutes each can be taken in very warm water to which two or three handfuls of crystallized sea salt has been added. Afterward, towel dry but do not shower off. The advantages of baths are twofold: one, toxins are drawn out of the body; and two, alkaline minerals from the sea salt are absorbed into the body to bolster its alkaline reserves. Water for the bath should be filtered to remove chlorine since it is quite harmful to the body.

## Be Patient and Persistent

A body that is very acidic is lacking in alkaline minerals, and has probably been that way for many years. It can take several months of alkalizing to fully correct a pH imbalance. Be patient but persistent during this process. Note that when one switches from unhealthy eating to healthy eating, and has started using alkaline foods and alkaline supplements, urine pH numbers can actually go down, becoming more acidic at first. Don't be alarmed because this is quite normal. As alkaline minerals are being supplied, the body will begin eliminating acid minerals from the areas it was previously forced to store them in. It will work to correct the most unhealthy acid terrain conditions immediately. In time, as an abundance of alkaline minerals continues to be supplied, steady progress will be noted as pH numbers move upward toward acid-alkaline balance.

Once acid-alkaline balance has been reached and has become stabilized, we can occasionally be less strict about the diet. By monitoring our urine pH, we can make diet and supplement corrections as needed to keep cellular terrain in optimum oxygenation condition.

## ULTIMATE OBJECTIVE

The ultimate objective for those who are really serious about being healthy is to eliminate all cooked and processed foods from their diets. Remember that, even though some of the Pottenger cats were fed one-third of their food raw, they degenerated over three generations until they died out.

Work toward reducing cooked food from your diet in stages. The very minimum for removing disease conditions and regaining health, without the use of many enzyme and other supplements, is 75% raw and 25% cooked. A better ratio would be 90% raw and 10% cooked. The ultimate objective is 100% raw, unprocessed foods and beverages. Also, remember to keep the ratio of alkaline to acidic foods at 80% or more alkaline and 20% or less acid foods.

## POSSIBLE FOOD SENSITIVITIES OR ALLERGIES

In the beginning, when a change is made from consuming wrong foods to introducing more raw fruits and vegetables into the diet, many people experience difficulties with digestion. There can be a lack of hydrochloric acid and digestive enzymes plus existing inflammation in the intestines because their digestive systems have been weakened from years of abuse. Symptoms can be similar to irritable bowel syndrome. The digestive system is sensitive and unaccustomed to breaking down raw, fibrous food, and it enters the intestines incompletely digested, which can cause irritation of the mucus membrane linings. The system needs time and assistance to adjust.

Although proper foods are now being consumed, one is not able to fully digest them to receive their benefits. Further, incomplete digestion produces toxic byproducts that draw energy from the body and hinder the healing process. If discomforts of excess gas (stomach and bowel), bloating, and tenderness in the lower abdominal area are evident, it is often an indication of insufficient stomach acid. By avoiding offending foods for a period of time, taking appropriate supplements to correct excess acid conditions, using digestive enzymes with meals, and improving intestinal flora, the digestive system is able to heal and strengthen to the point where these foods can be gradually introduced into the diet again. Many people are experiencing fairly rapid improvement with just adding green smoothies to their diets.

## PRODUCING BALANCED HORMONES

Good health results from healthy lifestyle practices. When properly nourished, the body naturally produces hormones in balance. However, when diet has been deficient for many years, where there is excess stress in a person's life, where there has been surgical intervention such as a hysterectomy, or as we move into middle age, hormones can move out of balance, with estrogen levels increasing out of proportion with the other hormones.

The three main hormones (in both males and females) that must be in healthy ratios to each other are estrogen, progesterone, and testosterone. Although estrogen dominance can emerge at an early age, a typical pattern for both sexes is the emergence of estrogen dominance as women move into menopause, and men move into the menopausal equivalent called andropause. This can occur from approximately age forty-five on, becoming more noticeable after age 55 to 60 in most people as progesterone and testosterone levels decrease.

Estrogen dominance can arise as a result of many factors, including the intake of estrogen-like chemicals via our foods and environment, hormone replacement therapy, drugs such as birth control pills, improper diets, and prolonged stress. Associated health problems that can develop are: weight gain (mostly around the waist), decreased libido, anxiety, depression, lack of mental clarity, and lack of energy. Women can experience difficult menstrual periods, painful breasts, and cyclical mood swings. Men can begin to notice the development of female-like breasts, loss of muscle mass and strength, and prostate problems indicated by a frequent need to urinate, difficulty in starting the urine stream, and a feeling of being unable to completely empty the bladder. If left unaddressed, this condition can lead to prostate cancer in men.

Natural progesterone can be of assistance in bringing hormone ratios back into line. It is a key factor in the creation of other hormones, as it performs many functions in both female and male human bodies.[10] Progesterone opposes estrogen dominance and allows testosterone levels to rise. Progesterone supplementation is best accomplished by using skin creams that contain natural progesterone, since it is readily absorbed and assimilated by the body this way. Oral supplementation is reported to be much less effective because progesterone is fat-soluble and can therefore be disposed of by the liver.

There is a simple hormone balance check that can be done by sending a saliva sample to a laboratory for analysis. I strongly recommend that anyone who may suspect they have a hormonal imbalance problem seek further assistance on hormone balancing and saliva testing. One possible information source is www.helpforhormones.com.

## LISTENING TO YOUR BODY

The section on *Symptoms versus Causes* in chapter 6 talked about how your body communicates with you. Our main problem is that we have not been taught to listen, understand, and respond in a supportive way to the signals the body gives when its needs are not being met. The body always wants to return to a state of health.

As the body begins to detoxify and heal, the signals it sends become easier to read. It is as if the fog has started to lift. When you have indigestion, gas, or a bloated feeling after eating, you know there is a cause you can help to correct without using a drugstore remedy that only works to eliminate the symptom temporarily. Diarrhea and constipation are not mystery ailments; they are reactions of your body requiring your cooperation to correct. A headache is not caused by a deficiency of analgesic pain relievers, but is from a stressed body due to emotional pressures, or toxins in the blood that the body is trying to eliminate.

You need to listen to your body and respond in a supportive way. Illness symptoms have causes. They are our friends. They are cries for us to cooperate with the healing process so the underlying causes can be corrected. As uncomfortable reactions manifest, think about what you did or ate recently that provoked the reaction. From these experiences, learn to avoid doing those things that are irritating to your body. Keep your eye on the goal of good health and increased vitality. Our mission is to build a healthy body and a strong immune system for the long term, not just to look for a quick-fix remedy for the symptom. Each step of the way, try to help your body become more efficient and stronger. Don't contribute to wearing it down if you can possibly avoid it.

## A WORD OF CAUTION

A person who is taking medication on the advice and direction of their physician should continue doing so. Any change in diet or medical treatment should be made in consultation with your personal holistic physician. Realize that drugs are for emergencies and should be taken only as long as the emergency persists. Your goal should be to strengthen your body with natural nutrition and rejuvenating lifestyle practices.

## FOOD PREPARATION TIPS TO MAXIMIZE NUTRITION AND DIGESTION

- Grains should be sprouted.
- Breads made from sprouted grains are best.
- Raw nuts and seeds should be soaked overnight to deactivate the enzyme inhibitors that are in them to prevent premature sprouting. Soaking nuts and seeds makes them more digestible and increases their enzyme content by up to twenty times.
- Excellent milk substitutes can be freshly made in a blender using living water plus a few raw almonds, sunflower seeds, sesame seeds, coconut powder, or a combination of a couple of these according to your taste. Blended hemp seeds and water alone makes an excellent milk substitute.
- Sweet corn is most digestible when eaten raw or at least very lightly cooked.
- Consume raw fresh fruit and vegetable juices regularly.
- Consume organically grown food when possible.

- Scrub fruits and vegetables to remove sprays, toxins and dirt, after soaking for 10 or 15 minutes in water that has had a tablespoon or more of unpasteurized apple cider vinegar added to it.
- Lightly steam vegetables; they should still be a bit crispy after steaming.
- Lightly stir-fry vegetables with water, unsalted butter, or olive oil.
- Use a minimum of hot spices.

## JUICING

Consuming fresh raw fruit and vegetable juices regularly can be one of the fastest ways of returning to vibrant health. Fresh juice has many benefits due to its alkaline nature, and an abundance of enzymes and other live ingredients. The majority of juices consumed should be vegetable. Keep in mind that fruit juices are loaded with the simple sugar fructose, and that without the fiber from the whole fruit, they quickly raise the level of sugar in the bloodstream.

Why should we consider adding fresh juices to our diet? There are several reasons. Due to our typical diets, virtually everyone has a digestive system that is stressed and underfunctioning, an intestinal tract with a diminished store of flora, congested underfunctioning organs of assimilation, and an overload of toxins entering the system on a regular basis. We eat the wrong foods, which do not supply the nutritional needs of our bodies. Commercially-produced fruits, and especially vegetables, are now deficient in vitamins and minerals due to the overfarming of soils and the use of chemical fertilizers. These may satisfy our acquired tastes and hunger, but unfortunately, their mineral and vitamin content does not satisfy the body's cellular requirements for nutrition.

### Advantages of Fresh Raw Fruit and Vegetable Juices
The advantages of consuming fresh raw fruit and vegetable juices over eating the actual fruits and vegetables are that they:

- are an alkaline meal with concentrated nutrients.
- are foods with the living enzymes intact—if consumed soon after juicing.
- require little digestion (about 10% of that required by solid food), and are easily assimilated by the body.
- conserve energy for the body to divert to healing.
- are balanced nutrition.
- aid greatly in the detoxification of the body, making it less acidic.
- are one of the keys to fast track healing. One month on a straight juice diet can produce the same results as six months on a healthy diet of solid food, with emphasis on raw fruits and vegetables.

### Disadvantages of Fresh Raw Fruit and Vegetable Juices

- Fiber is separated from the juice and discarded, thereby depriving the colon of its benefits. This situation can be mitigated somewhat by adding fresh-ground flax seeds to the juice.
- Root, such as carrots and beets, are less nutritious than their green tops.

### Guidelines for Making and Consuming Fresh Juices

- Use only good quality produce.
- Fruit and vegetable juices should not be mixed. Exceptions are apples which will mix compatibly with vegetable juices, and celery and lettuce which will mix with fruits. Tomato juice and carrot juice do not make a good combination.
- 80–90% of the fresh vegetable juice should be from your geographic area when available.
- Juices should not be heated or allowed to stand for long, as this kills the live enzymes within them.
- Seasonings should not normally be added, with the exception of a few grains of naturally dried sea salt, if desired.
- Consume juice as soon as possible after juicing because it begins to lose nutrients through oxidation after it is prepared.

- Juices should be consumed slowly to allow them time to mix properly with saliva and digestive juices.
- It is best to not drink juice with meals. A glass of juice is a meal in itself. Combining juice with solid food can overload digestive capacity.
- A healthy regimen of juicing would include a full glass of fruit juice and another of vegetable juice each day. For correcting more serious health problems, more can be consumed in lieu of solid food. For serious illnesses, a total juice diet for one week to one month or longer is sometimes recommended, but this should be done in consultation with a health practitioner. Fruit juice should be limited to no more than two glasses daily. Vegetable juice should comprise the majority of juice consumed.
- An excellent combination for nutrition and for deacidifying the body is 80% carrot, plus celery, parsley, beet, and fresh ginger.
- A similar combination is carrot, celery, parsley, plus spinach for its iron content.
- Apple is compatible with vegetable juices and may be added to sweeten any combination.

For more detailed information and instruction on juicing and its benefits, there are many juice books available.[11]

> **Note:** *People who have an insulin problem should avoid juicing fruits and root vegetables because of their high sugar content.*

### An Encouraging Juicing Story

As mentioned in chapter 4, a man I know made a wonderful comeback in his health when he started to drink a combination of freshly made vegetable juices. This gentleman (who we will call Bruce) and I had met as friends several times to discuss various foods and supplements that might help him in his battle with cancer. He was searching for a solution and was making his own decisions regarding treatment. He had decided to use natural methods and had resisted the standard medical treatments except for the drug Lupron, a testosterone blocker to reduce his prostate PSA count. He had had one session of radiation because of his worsening condition in the later stages. For about a year and a half he ate as naturally as possible and drank juices that he made. But as he related, the juicing was random, and did not follow any particular combination or formula. For six months during this time, he also spent thousands of dollars and consumed copious quantities of live-source supplements, but something was missing because his condition continued to worsen.

When I met with him he looked like a "dead man walking"; he told me later that he had begun to plan his own funeral. He was discouraged, thin, and getting very low on energy. During the next week his anemia became severe and his complexion turned white. Blood tests at that time showed very low iron, and a red blood cell count of 89 compared to the normal of about 140. His doctor suggested that he take iron pills but he wanted to research natural sources of iron first.

Bruce began reading *Fresh Vegetable and Fruit Juices* by Dr. Norman Walker. He decided to try one of Dr. Walker's vegetable juice formulas for the treatment of anemia. This consisted of a combination of carrot, celery, parsley, and spinach in certain proportions. Each morning he made the juice and drank 1.5–2 liters of it. Within a week his blood condition had stabilized and by the end of the second week his blood counts were rising. Bruce also started juicing a whole lemon, minus seeds, in a blender with up to a liter of water and a little maple syrup and drinking it as his first food each morning.

Whether Bruce will ultimately be successful in maintaining his gains and returning to full health, remains to be seen. He has financial difficulties and a considerable amount of stress in his life. In my opinion, the main reason for his turnaround as described above was due to the live nutrients and the flood of alkaline minerals in the fresh juices, which began to reduce the acid condition in his body. I am convinced that a healthy acid-alkaline balance is fundamental to eliminating disease conditions.

## All Juices Are Not Equal

A word of caution is appropriate regarding citrus juices. Juices made from mostly orange and grapefruit, if substantial amounts are consumed regularly, can cause problems for the body. This is not the case when eating whole, ripe fruit in moderation. Most citrus fruits are harvested before they are ripe, making their juices much more acidic.

There are further problems with commercially made juices. First, all canned and bottled juices are heated, which kills their enzymes. Second, acid is added to juice concentrates to make them last longer. When a glass of juice comes from a concentrate, it takes about eighteen glasses of water to neutralize the acid it contains.[12] Third, most present-day commercially-harvested fruit is loaded with toxic chemicals such as preservatives, artificial colorings, pesticide sprays, and wax. Some of these are bound to be consumed because the whole fruit, skin and all, is squeezed by powerful presses in the extraction process.

## All Juicers Are Not Equal

Juicing machines that remove most or all of the fiber from fruit and vegetables also remove food value along with the pulp. The more moisture there is in the pulp, the more nutrients there are in the discarded fiber.

A Norwalk-type juicer presses juice with a hydraulic press from ground fruit and vegetable pulp to extract all the minerals. It has been reported that even animals will not eat the remaining pulp because it has no nutrition left in it.

Some centrifugal juicers do a fairly good job of extracting maximum juice from fruit and vegetables; others do not. The drier the pulp expelled, the more efficient the juicer.

Fruits and vegetables that have been finely blended in a Vita-Mix® blender retain all their nutrients as well as the fiber. The Vita-Mix® operates at a very high speed, grinding food to a fine, smooth texture. Obtaining juice this way is the healthiest because one gets to consume the whole food, as nature intended. Digestion is aided because the food has already been broken down. Remember that this kind of juice is a whole food, and needs to be mixed with saliva and consumed slowly.

## ORGANIC FOOD

Eating foods that have been grown organically is much healthier for the body because the soils they are grown in contain more trace minerals. Organic farming is based on a system that replenishes and maintains soil fertility. Using organic matter, compost, or animal manure enhances soil quality. Chemical fertilizers are not used. Studies have shown that organic produce contains significantly higher levels of minerals and fewer heavy metals than conventionally grown crops.[13]

## READ THOSE LABELS!

We need to become aware of the ingredients that are in the products we consume, put on our body, or clean with. To do this, we must read labels!

If you are not already in this habit, you may be in for a surprise. For instance, most brands of toothpaste contain three ingredients that pose health risks if too much is ingested. They are: sorbitol, a liquid that keeps toothpaste from drying out and acts as a laxative that can cause diarrhea in children; sodium lauryl sulfate, used in garage floor cleaners and engine degreasers, is potentially carcinogenic and a very strong irritant; and fluoride, a poison if too much is swallowed. Some toothpaste labels contain a warning to seek professional help, or call a poison control center immediately, if someone has accidentally swallowed more than the amounts normally used for brushing teeth. Some toothpaste products contain TSP, tri sodium phosphate, a strong all-purpose cleaning chemical that carries the general precaution: "Whenever handling TSP, be sure to wear rubber gloves or other protective material."

Many antiperspirants contain aluminum, which is a toxic heavy metal associated with Alzheimer's and other diseases.[14,15] While the function of underarm deodorants is to close skin pores so that one doesn't perspire in these areas, some of the deodorant's chemicals are absorbed into the body where they become stored as toxic waste. If you do choose to use an antiperspirant, read the labels to ensure that they are all natural ingredients.

Additives such as chemical flavor enhancers, dyes, and preservatives in food products can cause or contribute to problems ranging from allergies to cancer. All synthetic additives are strong acid producers.

The bottom line on processed food products, cleaning agents, or personal hygiene items that come in contact with our bodies, is: if it isn't natural, the body cannot use it for health. Further, it may be outright harmful.

Wherever you go to purchase products at the grocery store, drug store, or health food store, the guideline for reading labels and selecting products is, as soon as you have found an ingredient that is a chemical or a word that you can't pronounce, put it back! Your health depends on it, and your body will thank you for it.

## HEALTHY LIFESTYLE CHECKLIST

### What to Consume

- Natural whole foods—local, organically-grown when possible.
- Food that has not been genetically altered.
- Living, structured water.
- Green smoothies.
- Freshly prepared fruit and vegetable juices.
- Alkaline ash forming foods—raw fruits, vegetables, nuts and seeds. (Except for peanuts and peanut butter which are difficult to digest, contain the least calcium, and are the most allergenic of the nuts.)
- Whole grains. Sprouted grains are easiest to digest.
- Acid-forming foods in moderation. (See appendices 1 to 4)
- Foods in compatible digestive combinations.
- Digestive enzymes, when eating cooked, processed, or irradiated foods.

- Digestive enzymes on an empty stomach to achieve therapeutic health gains.
- 2 or 3 ounces (60 to 90 ml) of aloe vera juice per quart (or liter) of water, to feed the intestinal tract and regenerate the villi, thus improving absorption of nutrients.
- Organic, whole-food concentrate, low-dosage vitamin and mineral supplements that contain live enzymes.
- A supplement of cold-pressed flax oil for the first while, then hemp oil to ensure an adequate supply of essential fatty acids.
- A limited amount of cooked protein. However, each meal should contain some quality protein source that will combine properly with other foods. Hemp protein is excellent.
- A good probiotic product to ensure a healthy population of friendly bacteria in the colon.
- Antibiotics and drugs in situations of serious health crises only. When you do, immediately follow up with probiotics.

### What To Do Regularly

Detoxification and the replenishment of enzymes and nutrients for the body are ongoing and central components of a good health program. Our lifestyles, the foods we eat, and our use of supplements should always have these two purposes behind them.

- Drink one or two glasses of pure warm water with fresh lemon juice upon first rising in the morning to flush and cleanse the digestive tract; then allow 15 minutes before eating anything. (Some people like to use unpasteurized apple cider vinegar, with or without honey.)
- Supplement meals with good plant-source digestive enzymes.
- Drink green smoothies.
- Use unrefined sea salt as a seasoning; add a small pinch to drinking water.
- Use oils that are high in Omega-3 and Omega-6 essential fatty acids. Hemp oil has the best natural balance. Oil blends and fish oils from cod and halibut are also good.

- Don't eat full meals in the morning, wait until you are hungry. A lighter meal such as juice or fruit helps the body cleanse from the day before.
- Eat the heaviest meal for dinner to allow enough time for its complete digestion. Ideally lunch should be predominantly carbohydrate, which is easier than protein to digest and is a quicker source of energy.
- Don't eat food in the evening after the dinner meal.
- Drink fluids half an hour before, or two hours after meals.
- Drink fluids that are neither too hot nor too cold, to reduce stress on the stomach.
- Combine foods properly.
- Don't overeat at a meal (20% less is a good objective); eat more often, if necessary. Six small meals are easier to digest than three large ones.
- Chew each mouthful thoroughly before swallowing. Remember that digestion begins in the mouth.
- Eat mostly raw fruits and vegetables, nuts, grains, and seeds. Ideally, twice as many vegetables as fruits.
- Include a quality protein in each meal (raw vegetable, or nut is best).
- Periodically fast for a day or so on pure water, fresh juices, or watermelon. This gives the organs of digestion, assimilation, and elimination a chance to rest and rebuild.
- Consume fresh raw fruit and vegetable juices.
- Eat only foods that you could enjoy as a one-item meal.
- Read food product labels, including those from health food stores, to check for the presence of additives. Avoid those with non-food names.
- Fry and cook sparingly. Only use water or broth. Do not cook with fats or oils at high heat. Whatever can be cooked in an oven, should be; the temperatures on stovetop elements are too high.
- Steam vegetables, but leave them a bit crispy.
- Eat a variety of foods, so your body can acquire the many minerals it needs for health. Use the edible skins of vegetables and fruit.
- Take care of your skin—brush with a vegetable fiber brush or loofa. Do not use, or use sparingly, soaps (except oil-based), lotions, or sprays. Do not use deodorants that contain aluminum.

- Install a carbon filter unit on your shower to remove chlorine from the water, so it won't be absorbed by your skin.
- Take care of your teeth—brush regularly. Avoid fluoride, amalgams (fillings) that contain mercury, and root canals. A good resource on self-care (without the dentist) for healthy teeth can be found on the Internet at www.mizar5.com.
- Wear loose-fitting clothing made from natural fibers. Avoid synthetics —nylons, acetates, et cetera, as these interfere with the body's electrical balance.
- When possible, expose your skin to sunshine for brief periods each day. Vitamin D, manufactured by the action of sun on the skin, is needed for health. Avoid tanning lotions because they clog pores; instead, you can use hemp oil. It thoroughly penetrates the skin and contains a natural SPF of 15.
- Get involved in exercise such as walking, swimming, skipping, using an electrically tuned mini-trampoline, aerobics, strength training, stretching, and so forth.
- Have times for breathing deeply, including diaphragm breathing, to increase oxygen absorption and reduce stress.
- Get adequate sleep and rest, including naps if required. These are the periods when your body heals and generates new energy.
- Relax and take time to do things you enjoy.
- Adopt positive attitudes of gratitude, appreciation, forgiveness.
- Define your purpose in life. Set goals, and make plans to achieve them.
- Build relationships with others. Express appreciation, love, and forgiveness. Be honest about your feelings. Listen in order to really hear and understand the other person. Practice a relaxed patience. Accept responsibility for learning from your experiences. Avoid criticizing, blaming, or finding fault. If you want a friend, be a friend, without conditions.
- Look for solutions instead of focusing only on problems. Look for communication agreements instead of disagreements. Do things for others without being asked. Remember the golden rule.

**Foods to Avoid**

- Beverages: Alcohol, coffee, tea (non-caffeine herbal teas are okay), milk and all dairy beverages, soft drinks, cocoa, instant coffees and coffee substitutes, diet drinks. Beverages with added sugars, preservatives, salt, and colorings. Commercially frozen and pasteurized fruit juices. Tap water that has not been run for some time to flush out copper and plastic residues which have been absorbed while standing in pipes. Fluoridated, chlorinated or otherwise contaminated water. Soda water and carbonated beverages.

- Caffeine, nicotine, sugar, table salt, red meats (to a large extent), strong spices, chocolate (made with sugar), trans fats and hydrogenated oils, fried foods, dairy products (except unsalted butter in moderation), refined grains and flours and their products, nonorganic-source or high potency or synthetic vitamin and mineral supplements, 'enriched' foods and foods with chemical additives.

- Genetically altered foods.

- Cereals, grains, and seeds that are processed, boxed, puffed, flaked. Roasted commercial cereals. Cereals with sugar. White rice. Roasted and/or salted or rancid seeds. None of the above with preservatives or additives, including added vitamins and minerals.

- Eggs: Instant egg preparations, eggs from commercially farmed chickens that have been fed antibiotics or commercial feed. Hard-boiled or hard cooked eggs. (Eggs are very nutritious provided they are from free-range chickens, are undercooked, soft-boiled, soft-poached or lightly scrambled.)

- Cheeses: Most should be avoided—especially colored, processed, creamed and fancy cheese spreads. White cheese made from unpasteurized milk is okay.

- Sugars and sweets: White, brown, refined, all processed sugars, glucose, fructose, et cetera. Candy, chocolate, desserts, gums, artificial sweeteners. (Unpasteurized honey and maple syrup are okay in moderation.)

- Wheat and wheat products (except the original varieties of spelt and kamut).

- Breads and pastries: Bread made from any commercial flour, white flour, or flour that is more than 48 hours old. Macaroni, spaghetti, pasta. Breads that are high in salt. Over-cooked toast. Rolls. Pastries, crackers, biscuits, cookies, cakes, pies, pancakes, waffles, pizza. Potato and corn chips, pretzels, fried snacks, and doughnuts.
- Fats from animal sources: None, except unsalted butter. All foods fried in fats. Lard, shortenings. All fat meats.
- Butter: Salted butters, stale, rancid. Any that has been stored unfrozen for months.
- Oils: All oils that have not been cold-pressed or that have been extracted with chemical processes. Commercial mayonnaise and salad dressings. Stale, rancid oils. All margarines and hydrogenated oils.
- Nuts: Roasted and salted, stale. Nuts that have been out of the shell a long time. Any nut that is off-color and possibly moldy.
- Fish: Contaminated, smoked, salted. All shellfish, catfish, or scavenger fish.
- Meats: All scavenger animals and birds. Pork in any form— bacon, ham, et cetera. (Pork contains many parasites. Tests have shown that pork parasites remain alive after the meat has been cooked to a char.[16]) All canned, processed sandwich preparations. Sausages, bologna, salami. Smoked, salted, colored meat, or meat that has been treated with nitrates or nitrites. Meat that is well done or overcooked.
- Seasoning: Pepper, table salt, or any preparation containing salt. Monosodium glutamate (MSG), hydrolyzed vegetable protein (MSG), aspartame.
- Vegetables: Overcooked or cooked until mushy-soft, or when color, taste, and consistency have undergone marked changes. Canned, frozen (except corn, beans, peas), stale, sulfured, or high sodium versions.
- Potatoes: French-fried, chips, grilled, and roasted without skins. No soft, mushy, reheated, stale, or instant.
- Salads: None with iceberg lettuce. No sulfured, pesticide, or chemically sprayed produce. Commercial coleslaw, because of preservatives.
- Soups: Canned, creamed, dehydrated with chemical additives, instant, or powdered.

- Fruit: Canned, frozen, sprayed, sugared, preserved. Sliced and left exposed to the air. Picked and shipped green or unripe. Sulfured or artificially colored, or treated with preservatives.
- Juices (fruit and vegetable): Canned or frozen concentrates. Sugared or artificially sweetened. No synthetic, instant, powdered juices.

## NUTRITIONAL HOME RUNS TO HEALTH

In a baseball game, there is nothing that wins the game faster than home-runs. It's the same in winning the health game. Reversing degenerative disease conditions and regaining good health can be achieved more quickly by doing those things that have a very influential impact on the body's ability to heal.

It's really quite simple. Stop doing the wrong things and start doing the right things. A great example of a nutritional homerun is juicing. Presented below is a brief list of the main nutritional routines to adopt, in order to expedite and retain health gains.

- Eliminate all harmful foods from the diet.
- Fast regularly on fresh fruit and vegetable juices and watermelon.
- Drink energized water, or water that is slightly alkaline.
- Drink fresh raw juices regularly.
- Eat sprouted seeds and grains regularly.
- Eat only when hungry.
- Eat 20% less at each meal for more efficient digestion and fewer calories.
- Eat 80% alkaline, 20% acid ash foods.
- Eat 75% raw and 25% cooked food. (More raw is better.)
- Combine foods properly.
- Supplement with digestive enzymes, bowel bacteria, and quality oils.
- Supplement with plant source, whole-food preparations.
- Use essential oils.
- Detoxify the colon regularly by taking a gentle cleansing product that utilizes herbal or oxygen formulations.

- Cleanse the liver.
- Adopt positive thoughts and attitudes.

## WORKING WITH YOUR BODY

Working with your body, means:

- Introducing the *Nutritional Homeruns to Health* into your lifestyle.
- Practicing the principles found in the *Healthy Lifestyles Checklist*.
- Recognizing the symptoms your body is giving you to signal that it needs your cooperation for it to correct the underlying causes of your health challenges.

## WHAT DOES HEALTH LOOK LIKE?

Some of the characteristics of a totally healthy person, devoid of all toxins, would be the following:[17]

- Neither overweight nor underweight.
- Solid muscular build.
- No weakness or fatigue.
- Bright eyes, whites not yellow or blood shot.
- No presence of disease or illness.
- Quick healing of injuries.
- Clear, soft, and smooth skin.
- Sweet breath.
- No body odor.
- Craving for natural foods.
- Loss of desire for toxic foods and substances.
- The consumption of toxic foods and substances produces immediate cleansing reaction: vomiting, diarrhea, fever, cold symptoms, sluggishness, et cetera.

- Regular bowel movements (1 to 3 per day).
- Fruity odor or no odor of stools.
- Well formed, floating stools.
- Urine that is not too strong in odor or too dark in color.
- Saliva and urine pH of 6.8 to 7.0 (initial morning samples).
- No tiredness, only drowsiness at bedtime.
- Rests and sleeps well.
- Wakes up refreshed and energetic.
- Enthusiastic about life.
- Ability to handle stress.
- Sense of fulfillment and accomplishment.
- Love, forgiveness, and acceptance of self and others.
- Clarity and sharpness of thought.
- Good memory recall.

## NATURE'S GREAT HEALERS

- Faith—belief in yourself and in the innate intelligence of nature within your body.
- Hope—the strongest healing force. Hope of recovery, hope of loving and being loved, hope of succeeding.
- Joy. Humor. Laughter. These are very powerful.
- The power of our minds. Decision. Determination. Discipline.
- Positive attitudes.
- Positive lifestyles—free of excesses and abuses.
- Sleep. Rest. Relaxation.
- Diet and nutrition.
- Clean blood. Blood circulation. Exercise.
- Self control. Moderation.
- Cleanliness.
- Your body's innate wisdom. Let it take care of itself. Provide it with what it needs.

Remember that no drug, or artificial, synthetic, refined, processed, chemically treated food, pill, supplement or substance exists that has the ability to create new cells or to heal the body.

The really good news you need to hold on to is, "There is always hope for health." No matter what the disease condition, as long as the body has life and a little energy, it knows how to get well. Your body is capable of healing, but it needs your full cooperation.

The next chapter shows you why there's always hope.

# 22 | THERE'S ALWAYS HOPE

∼

*While there's life, there's hope!*
ANCIENT ROMAN SAYING

∼

THE QUOTE displayed above is such a wonderful saying! If you have learned anything from reading this book, it should be that the human body is wondrously created. It has innate intelligence. It doesn't make mistakes, we do. It always strives to survive and become healthier, but it needs our help. It needs good materials to work with as well as the proper mental attitude from us. It needs you to apply the 5 Keys so it can create life and reverse the degenerative slide toward disease, premature aging, and early death.

## IT'S NEVER TOO LATE

There are many cases of people who have recovered from so-called "death sentence" diseases. I will relate a couple here. The following is taken from an interview I had with Michael O'Brien, who is a former medical doctor. Michael cured himself after his wife had been told that he would not live through the weekend. As a result of this experience, he left the medical field and became a researcher and teacher on natural health and a formulator and manufacturer of health-restoring supplements. The following two stories are in Michael's own words:[1]

### Michael O'Brien—Colon Cancer, Liver Cirrhosis

I had colon cancer, and also had cirrhosis of the liver. The doctors said that I would never get over that, but I got over both of them.

The problem that people have is that, when they have been sick and become well again, they think they know the answers. When they think they know the answers, they think they can cheat again with their food. The part people don't understand is that, when they get into a crisis with their health again, they think they can always change to a healthier diet tomorrow. But tomorrow never comes, and before long you are in a crisis and depending on people who don't know what you know to get you back to health again.

The colon cancer I had was so serious that the doctors told my wife to have any necessary papers signed immediately, because I wouldn't live through the weekend. They gave me less than two days to live. I decided to take massive quantities of enzymes, even though they were not in the strengths that we have today, and I recovered. All I did was ask God to show me how to get well. I was not interested in getting healed. One of the problems we have is that people who get healed haven't corrected the problem. They go on doing the same things. Two thousand years ago, when he healed people, the man called Jesus said, "Now go your way and sin no more, lest your second condition be worse than the first." So I came to understand what caused my cancer, and I stopped doing those things to my body. I also understood what the body needed to recover. This is what gave me the ability to handle Dr. Bernard Jensen's case.

### Dr. Bernard Jensen—Prostate Cancer, Bone Cancer, and Paralysis

Michael was called in to see if he could help Dr. Bernard Jensen, who had been a long-time friend, but had been given only eight days to live:

I learned a great deal from Dr. Jensen and other early natural healing practitioners. He was very famous for cleansing and detoxifying the bowel, and was a tremendous influence in my life.

When he was eighty-five, Dr. Jensen had prostate cancer that had metastasized into the bone. His wife called me and asked if I could help. His family and employees had visited him for the last time, and his doctors had given up hope. As far as everyone was concerned, Dr. Jensen was dead.

When I first came to see Dr. Jensen he was down to 76 pounds. He was skin and bone and just wanted to die. So I asked him, "Do you want to live? And if so, why?" The first thing we had to do was kindle his desire to fight for his life. I reminded him about all the old friends we had worked with over the years, the ones who were the 'great-greats' and who are all gone now. I said, "In the world we are living in today, one of the great-greats has to face the crisis, and overcome it so that the world will know we can win, and not submit to the other factors that take everybody out. Somebody has to do this, and you are the only one of the great-greats who is left. If you don't do it, no one will." That gave him the inspiration to say, "Yes, maybe I ought to take this on, and show the world that you can do this with natural means."

From Dr. Edward Howell's studies we learned that when you are out of enzymes, you are out of life. So, we loaded Dr. Jensen with digestive enzymes. Every drink he had was loaded with enzymes, between 200 and 500 each day, in powder form. We also gave him large amounts of active bowel bacteria. These two supplements returned the workers back into his body, which had been completely exhausted over his years of traveling and eating cooked foods. We also gave Dr. Jensen food for his liver and body in the form of TOCO™ which is a product that I formulated.[2] With the workers and complete proteins returning to his body, Dr. Jensen started to rebuild and gain energy. In fact, just eight weeks and one day later, I was walking with Dr. Jensen on the hills of his farm in California. He was fully recovered.

A sequel to this story is that, approximately six weeks later Dr. Jensen was paralyzed from a car accident. Doctors told him that he would be in a wheelchair and never walk again for the rest of his life. Again, we loaded him with enzymes and complete food for the body, in the form of the tocotrienol/amino acid complex. He came out of that one too! He got rid of his wheelchair.

You see, the human body is so wonderfully created and has such natural, built-in mechanisms for recovery from injury, illness, and disease. When we understand this, and give it the materials it needs to clean and feed itself, some very surprising things can happen.

## CUTTING TO THE CHASE

The human body has an innate intelligence. It knows how to be healthy, and it knows how to correct disease conditions. It never makes mistakes and always strives to return to homeostasis, or perfect balance. But it can only do this if we remove the major health-detractors from our lifestyle. These stresses take many forms, including emotional, nutritional, physical, and environmental factors. Anything that causes undue stress on the body reduces its ability to produce health.

To a great extent, this means that health and the reversal of rapid aging come down to how much we want it.

## WHAT THE BODY *MUST HAVE*
## TO RECOVER FROM MAJOR DISEASE

- The replacement and replenishment of its "workers"—enzymes and bowel flora. This must be done in significant quantities over a short period because a person's "time," in the case of a terminal illness, has almost run out.
- Replenishment with concentrated foods to feed and rebuild the body—fresh juices, whole complexes of vitamins, minerals, amino acids, and antioxidants.
- Replenishment of alkaline reserves.
- Detoxification of the bowel, liver, and all tissues of the body.
- Improved digestion and absorption of nutrients.

- Rest, especially during times of illness and healing reversal reactions.
- Clearing negative emotions and energy blockages.

## RESTORING YOUR HEALTH

Read, reread, and thoroughly incorporate the knowledge from chapter 11, *What Your Body Needs for Health,* into your lifestyle. Remember that harmful microform bacteria cannot live in the presence of oxygen; when cellular oxygen is high, diseases cannot manifest. Keep your alkaline mineral reserves high. Use concentrated green vegetable drinks every day. Avoid acid-producing foods and all sugars, as well as foods that convert to sugar. Drink six to eight glasses of good water each day.

The human body can and will renew itself if it has the materials and the proper environment within which to work.

Nourish and detoxify your body. That's about as simply as it can be put. Nourishment means eating live food, and honoring your body with positive attitudes and beliefs. Detoxification requires continuous attention to the removal of toxins and wastes so the body can work more efficiently, while becoming less acidic.

It is my opinion that real progress in restoring one's health in the face of long-standing disease symptoms and nutritional deficiencies requires the use of appropriate supplements. This is because most of our modern day foods lack the complete range of nutrients required by the body. When selecting supplements, check to ensure that they have been formulated by taking into account the electrical integrity of the component combinations, and that they have been prepared at low heat. Remember that each combination of foods or herbs produces a different group of electrical matrices, and that the body can only use natural electrical matrices from whole foods for health.

Try not to become discouraged when you embark on your health program. It took a long time to get to the health condition and age you are now. Your existing conditions cannot simply be corrected in a week, or a month, or even a year in most cases. You will go through some times of feeling that things are "tough" as your body reverses its path and starts to correct past disease and injury conditions. Your progress will depend on your determination and your ability to consistently supply your body with the necessary whole foods, detoxification, enzyme and food supplements required, so it can then do the job of healing and returning to a state of health, energy, and youthful appearance.

Remember also, from chapter 13, that your body heals from the inside first, and then on to the outside. What you are going to experience in the way of noticeable progress in the beginning will be increased energy as your organs and glands become healthier. Wrinkles and sagging skin will be worked on later. Although most of us want to look younger right away, smoothing out wrinkles is not as critical to our health as restoring the efficient functioning of our internal organs. Skin quality will be improved as a matter of course when the body is ready. The body knows what the priorities for health are—which things to work on first. Just cooperate with it by giving it what it needs, instead of trying to dictate what it has to work on. Let it do its job and it will serve you as the loyal and wise servant that it is.

## What Will This Cost?

### Discipline

Old, harmful habits and cravings must go—gradually or quickly—but they must go. You will have to change the way you think about health, food, drugs, and supplements. Your whole approach to eating must be to convert over to mostly raw, fruit and vegetable foods.

### Money

Where time is not critical, the most inexpensive alternative is to move quickly towards a mostly raw, whole-food, fruit, vegetable, fresh juices, and green smoothies diet, from organic sources. All the ingredients for moving back to health are contained in these foods.

In cases of very serious illness, it can, but does not necessarily have to, cost several thousand dollars for specific supplements in a period of 60 to 120 days. Critical conditions require serious action. Thereafter, the costs reduce considerably, but a maintenance program should be continued in order to further build health. If you think all this is a lot of money, consider the cost of alternatives, like being an invalid, or going to a remote country for an uncertain cancer treatment.

In some cases, people who are serious about eliminating lesser disease conditions and regaining a more youthful vitality and health spend several hundred dollars each month to cleanse and rebuild their bodies more quickly. Eventually, monthly costs can reduce to a lower amount for maintaining an ongoing health-rebuilding and maintenance program.

There are no hard and fast rules. To regain health, you have to do what you can, at your own rate, and spend what you can afford on supplements that will help your body. But remember that based on your new way of eating and living, you will be spending less than you spent on the food you used to buy and the previous habits. You may therefore not be spending that much more, but rather only transferring the focus of your expenditures. In the long run, spending money and effort on your own health is the best investment you can make.

### If You Cannot Afford Expensive Supplements

If you can't afford supplements, don't despair. There is still a lot you can do. You may not have the money to buy the expensive supplements that can work to speed your recovery, but you can work on the basics fairly inexpensively. You can incorporate all the rules and recommendations for healthy eating, sleeping, exercising, and thinking. Here are some specific suggestions:

- Do regular colon cleansing.
- Use a fresh lemon drink first thing in the morning.
- Drink green smoothies every day.
- Use unpasteurized apple cider vinegar and natural sea salt to re-alkalize your body.
- Make and drink as much fresh juice as possible, mostly vegetable. Good used juicers can often be found in the classified ads.
- Use marine phytoplankton food concentrate.
- Buy cold-processed protein powder, such as hemp, rice, or tocotrienols.

417

- Other useful food-form supplements could be: molasses, sunflower and pumpkin seeds, flax seeds, and raw almonds.
- Periodically, buy and use a probiotic such as acidophilus with bifidus.
- Work to remove and replace negative emotional causes of physical malfunctions.

For chronic conditions that won't respond to anything you've tried, you must aggressively work on detoxifying acids from your body. This is an indication that your pH levels are still significantly out of balance.

### You Can't Be a Cheater

What if you have been on your new program for a few months, and still, not much is changing? Your health problems are still persisting as usual. What could be wrong?

*If* you have really changed your diet to include much more raw food, and *if* you have been detoxifying your body and working on educating yourself about the things that contribute to renewed health, and your physical problems don't seem to be healing, there can only be one logical conclusion—you are cheating! In fact, your first in the morning urine pH will tell you the story. You are still eating foods that are poisonous to your body—sugar, salt, coffee, ice cream, or those baking and cooked food specials you really enjoy. That is, you are eating enough of them to counteract the healing effects of the good food you are eating, as well as the live supplements you are taking. Your body has to divert its healing efforts to deal with toxins that are still coming in.

Your body doesn't make mistakes. It is very intelligent, but it is not a miracle worker. If you give it good materials to work with, it will work to produce good results. If you give it mediocre materials to work with, it will be capable of producing only mediocre results.

It always comes down to our choices and our decisions. If we are unable to give up those things we like to eat, which we know are not good for us, then we will have to live with the discomfort that comes with degenerative conditions as they develop.

Be forewarned. When working to improve your health, everything you do has a consequence, sometimes long-term and sometimes short-term. If you cheat, you only cheat yourself.

## OVERCOMING SERIOUS CONDITIONS

If you want to overcome a serious condition such as cancer, you must be dedicated.

First, you must understand fully how your body works and what it must have in the way of food and supplements. You have to know, and you have to believe. Without belief, very little is possible.

Second, you must detoxify, detoxify, and detoxify, in order to reduce the acid condition of your body. You *must* bring the acid-alkaline ratios into balance. Only in this way will cellular oxygenation be maximized. Remember that harmful microform bacteria and cancer cells cannot live in the presence of oxygen.

Third, nutritional imbalances that have built up in your body over the years are considerably large, and cannot be corrected by simply switching to more raw food. Your body must have the workers and building materials it needs in concentrated supplement form—lots of them.

Detoxification must begin in a major way. This is where a lot of people have difficulty. Because they are used to taking pharmaceutical drugs, they seem to equate food supplements to drugs. They are not! Food supplements of enzymes, probiotics, antioxidants, and complete amino acid protein powders are concentrated working elements of food. They are building blocks of life. Don't be overwhelmed by the sight of several bottles or canisters of these supplements on your counter, or feel uncomfortable about taking 10, 20, or more, digestive enzyme capsules at a time, on an empty stomach. In very serious cases, when time is short, your body needs its workers back, NOW. It may need them by the 100s for a period of time. Remember that this is your *food*, only in concentrated form. This is "medicine" that your body needs and knows how to use.

You have switched from eating bulk food to eating concentrated food during the recovery phase. Dr. Bernard Jensen's story related earlier in this chapter clearly illustrates this. Also, do not overlook the healing power of marine phytoplankton, discussed in chapter 16.

### Every Case Is Different
Remember that:

- Each body is different, has its own unique problems, challenges, and deficiencies.
- Each person's mental and emotional attitudes are different.
- Results depend on your understanding of how the body works to heal itself, and the extent to which you cooperate with it by supplying the factors it needs to do its job and allowing it to do that job without interference.
- The only guarantees are that the natural health principles contained in this book have proven to be true; the stories of healing are true.

## NEVER GIVE UP

### There Is Always Hope
You've heard of the saying, "Where there's a will, there's a way." It's true. Your body always has the knowledge and roadmap to health. But, it needs inspiration. It needs you to have the will, so it can accomplish what it has set out to do.

From this book, you have been presented with some of the best health knowledge available. You have been shown the keys to great health that have proven effective over and over again.

If you are suffering from a serious illness, my suggestion is to read, and reread this book. Read especially, the parts that seem most pertinent to you, until the information becomes part of you. This will help form your new outlook and become part of your new thoughts and beliefs. Remember that your mind is your "creation machine." It creates thoughts;

thoughts become your underlying, core beliefs, and eventually become your physical reality.

### The Truth about the Human Body

Remember these truths about the human body:

- As long as there is life, the body wants to be healthy.
- The body knows how to be healthy.
- The body will return to health if it is given the proper "tools" to work with.

### 120 Days to Freedom

Michael O'Brien is of the firm opinion, based on his extensive experience of helping many people overcome critical illnesses, that any disease condition can be overcome in 120 days, *if*, as in the Dr. Jensen story, the person does all the right things. As Michael says, "Clean and feed your body." Detoxify it of its acid waste stores, balance pH, replenish its supplies of enzymes and bowel flora, and feed it complete amino acid proteins for rebuilding. These three food forms must be consumed in sufficient quantity, along with lots of good water. All non-healthy foods must be strictly avoided. We must also address our attitudes and beliefs. When this is done he says, "Healing will happen. I've never seen it fail."

## NO INCURABLE DISEASE

Here is a quote from Dr. Christopher based on his experience:

> There are no incurable diseases, only incurable people who do not, or will not, work with Mother Nature.[3]

Michael O'Brien teaches that there are five reasons why people do not get well:

1  They believe it is their time to die!

2　They like being sick; it affords them lots of attention!

3　They believe their problem cannot be fixed!

4　They are unable to follow instructions!

5　They haven't learned to love or forgive! (Learn not to hate or fear. Let go of negative emotions.)

I would only make one addition to this list:

6　They are not willing to give up their addictions to the unhealthy beverages, cooked meals, sweets, and other acid-producing foods they like.

All of the above are choices, whether based on attitude or will. Health is a choice. But so is disease! If we truly want to get healthy, we have to use the approach that really works. This is what Dr. Joel Robbins advises:

> We can whine, cry, psychoanalyze, blame, run, relive the past, hide the past, or resign ourselves to a particular wrong frame of mind or attitude. We can also attempt to cover up or over, drown our sorrows through sensationalism, sensuality, drink, drugs, food, or any other form of escape that we want to, in an attempt to get relief from the struggles of life, *but none, none of these approaches will truly solve the problem, nor permanently resolve it.*
>
> Don't be overwhelmed by all that needs to be done. The fact, literally, that you are still breathing, indicates that God feels that there is *hope.* Take it the same way God does: one day at a time. It is an exciting, challenging process. *You can do it!* 4

For those who are healthy, or who have regained their health, there is still another option, and that is to stay youthful well into old age. The next chapter discusses factors that will help to rejuvenate the body and slow its rate of aging.

# 23 | SLOWING THE AGING PROCESS

~

*The only thing that overcomes hard luck is hard work.*

HARRY GOLDEN

~

## AGING GRACEFULLY

SOME PEOPLE age gracefully; they are active and appear to be much younger than their chronological age. Others age more quickly, and may even "die before their time." Aging is inevitable for all of us, but the rate at which we age is variable. It is dependent on how well we cooperate with our bodies. We *can* age more slowly and maintain many of our youthful qualities well into our advanced years. As we renew our health, we can also regain some of the youthful vitality we have lost.

This chapter is for those who want to feel vibrant and more youthful in their senior years. It focuses on reversing disease conditions that cause rapid aging, and on maintaining a more youthful body. It is for the dedicated health-seeker, not the dreamer or the wisher. If you really want a more youthful body, you must be the kind of person who has the desire, faith, vision, self-discipline, determination, perseverance, and financial willingness to rejuvenate your body. This entails a readiness to forego some of your current pleasures in favor of a better prize a few years down the road. You also have to be prepared to "tough it out" through the cleansing and healing crises that may occur.

Who wouldn't like to feel and look younger? Just a dream? For most people—yes. But for those who are willing to do what is required, it can happen!

## SLOWING THE AGING CLOCK

Rapid aging and disease happen because body tissues become overburdened with acid wastes. As a result, vital organs and endocrine glands become less efficient; the generation of oxygen and energy in the cells is reduced; free radicals have an increasing capacity to take a toll on the body.

Reversing disease damage, and slowing the rate of aging already underway in the body, requires a detoxification of both body and mind, the restoration of a strong acid medium in the stomach, healthy bile flow, correction of hormone imbalances, achievement of pH balance, minimization of free radical damage, and the maximization of energy production in the mitochondria within cells. This is easier said than done; it takes time, but it can be achieved. It must become a lifestyle program.

## RAW IS THE WAY

When it comes to age reversal, nothing beats a totally raw diet—but it must contain sufficient greens. Green smoothies appear to be the best way to ensure this. It must be noted however, that after years of eating mostly cooked food, it may take the body's digestive system a little time to adjust to a raw food diet. The following story, told by Michael O'Brien, illustrates the rejuvenating effects of a totally raw food diet beautifully.[1]

### The Japanese Army Officer

Perhaps the best story I could tell illustrates how the human body is capable of responding when it is fed as nature intended it to be. It is able to reverse its condition to one of youthful vigor and achieve a state of sensitive oneness with its environment. You might remember the true story about the Japanese army officer, who fought the war in the jungles on one of the Philippine islands for thirty years after World War II, not knowing that it was over.

This man was on the Boston show which is like *Good Morning America*. It was amazing to look at him. For thirty years, he hadn't brushed his teeth and he had the most beautiful teeth I had ever seen. This was a man who was putting live, active foods into his body. They took him back to Japan and ran him through medical tests because they hadn't seen a man who had lived for thirty years without seeing a doctor. They put him on a treadmill but couldn't wear him out. He had the ability to return to the homeostasis of a twelve to fifteen year-old boy. It was exciting to see him because he was fifty-nine when he appeared on the show, but looked younger than the age of twenty-nine when he had left Japan to fight in the war. He had recaptured his youth by living on raw, enzyme-active foods, because he had been afraid to start a fire in case the enemy found him. He was on a wholesome diet for so long that he became hypersensitive to his environment. He knew when people were coming, and could hide. He knew exactly where they were. His innate intelligence became predominant in his life.

## IT TAKES DEDICATION

Restoring some of the youth you have lost, or retaining it, takes dedication, perseverance, and hard work! The older you are when you start, the longer it will take, and the more difficult it could be. But it can be done. When physical difficulties and disease symptoms begin to leave, it is a very gratifying feeling. As health returns, benefits such as energy, strength, stamina, clear thinking, better sleep, sexual capability and desire, plus a general feeling of optimism about life, start to increase.

Health can be yours. You can feel and look younger. You now have the knowledge; the rest is up to you. Go for it! You deserve it! A couple of years from now you'll be glad you did. I am, and am still working at it. It feels so good to have energy and enthusiasm, and to be free from the degenerating physical conditions that one has suffered with for many years. After all, consider the alternative of just continuing to slide and ending up in a medical institution or care home where your freedom is gone, where others make the decisions about what goes into your body, and what you are allowed to do.

Just make a decision and stick with your program. Good health is there for you. Go out and get it!

## THE NECESSITIES

Every *body* is different, and has different challenges. The body needs everything going for it to reverse the aging process. In point form, the following are the necessities:

### Detoxify, Detoxify, Detoxify!
To rejuvenate your body you must remove all acidic waste products, especially the old ones.

- Consume sufficient fiber. Green smoothies, psyllium hulls, and fresh-ground flax seeds are excellent sources.
- Use a good colon cleansing supplement product regularly. Periodic colon hydrotherapy is very effective.
- Consume mostly alkaline foods and drinks that contribute to making your body less acidic.
- Use fresh juices and alkalizing supplements.
- Grow and eat your own sprouts (mostly alfalfa).
- Complete enough liver/gallbladder cleanses to remove all stones from your liver.
- Install and use a shower filter to remove chlorine. Finish off showers with a couple of minutes of cooler water.
- Make minimal use of soaps and use only pH-balanced products.

**Help Your Body to Balance Hormones**

Hormone balance is natural in a clean, healthy body. When the colon and the liver are clean, there are no acid wastes in the body. When the body is being fed a natural, predominantly raw food diet containing enzymes, probiotics, essential fatty acids (oils), and essential amino acids, and sufficient green foods, it produces its own hormones. There are no problems such as diabetes, thyroid disease, PMS, menstrual difficulties, hot flashes, prostate, hormone-based emotional problems, or sexual dysfunction problems. So, the objective in restoring health is to return the body to this state and let it produce its own hormones. As we move into our elder years, we can give our bodies some assistance with natural HGH precursors.

To achieve this balanced objective, the body *must* be fed the raw materials it requires for the liver to initiate the hormone production process. The necessary raw proteins are contained in foods such as raw greens, hemp, spirulina, chlorella, and other cold-processed protein supplement foods. Supplementing meals with digestive enzymes further helps the digestion and nutrient conversion process.

You are encouraged to do further reading or consult with alternative health practitioners who are able to provide detailed instruction on how to balance hormones.

**Feeding Your Body**

Provide your body with:

- Food that is full of life and nutrition—raw, organic, mostly alkaline.
- Water that is pure—8 to 10 glasses per day; that is, water that has been filtered to remove toxins, and energized to facilitate hydration and energy production.
- Fresh, clean air.
- Moderate, but regular exposure of skin to sunshine.
- Supplements, if necessary, that supply enzymes, alkaline minerals, complete amino acids, and colon cleansing herbs.
- Antioxidants.

- Growth hormone precursors.
- Ionic minerals—a few drops in each glass of "purified" water, if you must use this kind of water.
- Juice of a half, or whole, lemon in a full glass of water, immediately upon rising in the morning.
- Green smoothies.
- One or two glasses of fresh juice—carrot, celery, spinach, beet, ginger, parsley, apple (or some other appropriate combination), every day.
- Consume quality proteins and oils that your liver can use. Hemp foods are good examples.

**Caring for Your Body**

Make the following part of your lifestyle:

- Regular, moderate exercise, such as brisk walking, swimming, and rebounding. Daily use of a Chi Machine is beneficial.
- Some kind of weight bearing exercise three times per week.
- As health and vitality returns, increase exercise to raise pulse rate and bring on perspiration. This improves cardiovascular function and releases toxins through the skin and breath. It also works to generate more energy.
- Get the full rest your body needs. Try to keep regular sleeping hours. Review *Rest* in chapter 11.
- Protect yourself from harmful EMFs and geopathic radiations.

**Address Underlying Emotions and Beliefs**

- Learn to identify and reverse the effects of negative emotions, limiting beliefs, and the energy blockages caused by them. (Review chapters 17–20.)

**Other Lifestyle Practices**

- Work to get your mental, emotional, and spiritual life in balance. Attitudes of forgiveness and loving intent are very powerful. Vibrant health cannot happen without them.
- Reduce stress in your life.

## WINNING THE PRIZE

The prize to win is a healthy and youthful body with abundant energy and a life with more joy and fulfillment. Your degree of success in getting there will depend on the extent to which you can internalize and put into operation the basic health principles in this book. It all depends on the priorities you choose for your life. You are the only one who has the full power to control your destiny. Take your power back. Take responsibility for your own health.

To achieve anything worthwhile in our life we must want it. We need to be focused on our objective and know how to accomplish it. Being healthy comes from being conscious of how the body operates and what it requires to produce health. We must keep the main points in mind and make them a consistent part of our lifestyle; we must be health conscious. Let's take a quick review.

# 24 | BEING HEALTH-CONSCIOUS

∾

*It is never too late to be what you might have been.*
GEORGE ELLIOT

∾

CONSCIOUS HEALTH means choosing health. It means choosing health with understanding, awareness, intention, and vision. Conscious health is the active and deliberate creation of a vital body, mind, and spirit, with full knowledge, understanding, and belief. We create our lives, and we have the power to re-create them. When we are fully conscious, we can take responsibility for our own health. We can make the necessary choices and decisions. We can determine our health destiny.

The preceding words are the same as those at the beginning of the *Introduction* to this book. The only difference is that we now have a deeper understanding of their meaning.

Having read this far, let us now pause to review and reinforce what it means to be health-conscious and consciously healthy.

We have learned that there are three separate aspects to the body's health. If we want optimum health, we must remain aware of all three. Weakness in any one of the areas leads to malfunction, disease, suffering, and a shortened life. Let's review what we have learned about health.

## THREE ASPECTS TO THE BODY'S HEALTH

1   Electrical Energy—life and vitality are all about electrical energy.
2   Chemistry—optimum health happens only with pH balance.
3   Belief—our reality is created by our thoughts.

We can think of health as a bank account. In each area highlighted above, we are either making deposits to, or withdrawals from, our account balance. As long as the account is being replenished, the body will continue to serve us. When withdrawals exceed deposits, disease begins to appear; in time, the balance goes to zero and the account is closed—we die.

### Electrical Energy

The body is an energy system that operates on, generates, and stores, electricity. For comparison, nerve pathways are our transmission lines, and every cell is a miniature generator and storage battery. Energy to replenish body reserves comes from the food we eat. Only raw, living food contains restorative energy that can be made available for transfer to the body. Any food whose enzymes have been destroyed by cooking has lost its electrical energy. When it is consumed, it becomes a drain on the body's electrical potential because the body must draw on stored energy to process the dead food.

We must be conscious of our diet and choose to eat adequate quantities of electrically active food. Living food leads to health and vitality. Dead food has no electrical energy; consuming disproportionate quantities of it leads to lower energy reserves, disease, and an early death.

All food, including supplements, must contain live enzymes to be electrically alive and health-building.

### Chemistry

The human body was designed to operate in a slightly alkaline state. In optimum health, blood has a pH of 7.4; cells operate best at a pH near 7.0. Body pH is determined by the predominance of alkaline or acid minerals the body must process and store. Raw fruits and vegetables are the main sources of natural alkaline minerals for the body. Most other foods contain minerals that produce strong acids in the body, which then must be neutralized and eliminated. This neutralization process depletes the body's stores of alkaline minerals.

A healthy diet should contain approximately 80% alkaline and 20% acid foods and beverages. Having knowledge of which foods supply the mineral requirements for pH balance, and consciously choosing to consume them, empowers us to work with our bodies toward health. By regularly checking the pH of our first in the morning urine, we can monitor the body's need for additional alkaline minerals.

## Belief

Ultimately, everything in our lives is determined by our conscious and subconscious beliefs. Thoughts are energy, which in turn, creates our reality. Our thoughts and emotions produce either harmony or disharmony within our bodies. Positive thoughts have an alkalizing and regenerative effect; negative thoughts have an acidifying and degenerative effect. Becoming aware of what we think and feel is the first step in creating a life of health and happiness. All our beliefs are determined, reinforced, or changed by our thoughts. What we repeat in our self-talk eventually manifests as health or disease in our bodies, and as happiness or sadness, fulfillment or disappointment in our lives.

Life is an experience we create; this happens whether we are aware of it or not. Our purpose for being here is to become aware, to consciously create the life we want; our power to do that increases as we become more conscious.

When we begin to understand that our ego is a false self, we open the door to self-awareness. The ego works to keep us self-centered and reactive. It works to retain control of our mind and keep us unaware of the true self, which is spirit.

The first step to overcoming the ego's control is resisting the urge to be reactive, and letting go of our tendency to take offense. Realizing that those people we feel have hurt us in some way were only acting out of their own blindness and lack of awareness, allows us to forgive them. Forgiveness is the key to emotional freedom. Gratitude is the path to peace of mind. Unconditional love is the force that creates harmony with all.

## THE PROCESS OF BEING HEALTHY

Whether we are ill at the present time and want to be healthy, or are healthy and want to remain that way, we have an inner desire to know the answers. We want to become aware of what is involved so we can be independent of others for our own healthcare. Throughout this book, we have learned that we live in an organized universe and that everything happens for a reason. If we understand the *cause*, we can take action to influence the *effect*; we can be personally responsible, and can proactively create our own life.

## THE 5 KEYS TO HEALTH FREEDOM

There is no greater privilege in the world than freedom—being independent and able to pursue our interests and desires in a healthy body that serves us well. Life is an exciting adventure, but without awareness it seems to be a series of inevitable ups and downs, good and bad times, and unpredictability. As we cycle between our states of comfort and discomfort, it is easy to think that God or some force outside our control is doing it to us, that life is more or less a game of chance. Nothing could be further from the truth. The truth is that we were designed to be creators of our own lives. But, in order to do so, we have to learn to become conscious directors. We create our lives consciously or subconsciously from our knowledge, beliefs, and actions. We need to become conscious directors of our own lives and fully aware of what is involved in doing this. Achieving optimal health requires that we incorporate the 5 Keys to health in our lives.

**Key # 1: Learning**

Awareness happens as we gain knowledge about what the body requires for health, why it develops disease symptoms, and how we can cooperate with it to produce health.

- The body is designed to always work for health, but it depends on us to supply its needs.
- Disease happens as a logical consequence of nutritional deficiencies, toxic build-up in the organs, and faulty beliefs.
- Cooking and processing destroys the life-giving properties of food.
- Conventional healthcare views the body only as a chemical entity, and ignores the energy factors of life proved by quantum physics since 1925. Drugs can be helpful in crisis situations, but they are unnatural stimulants, and ultimately incapable of creating and sustaining life.
- Disease symptoms are the body's cries for help to correct imbalances and toxic buildup.
- The absolute fundamental requirement for health is an acid-alkaline balance so cellular oxygen is always at an optimum.

**Key #2: Cleansing**

Efficiency of body system processes is assisted as we detoxify on a regular basis. Toxins that have been stored in organs and tissues must be moved out of the body.

**Key #3: Feeding**

Construction of healthy tissue and generation of energy reserves and immunity happen as the body's requirements for building materials are met.

- The water we consume must be free of pollutants and, ideally have hexagonally-structured molecules.
- Real food for the body is organic, fresh, and living. It should supply all the necessary enzymes, amino acids, essential fatty acids, minerals, vitamins, and probiotics we need.

435

- Supplements, if needed, should be natural complexes made from live, whole organic food sources, with their enzymes and electrical properties intact. The best supplements are those that are prepared with minimal processing.

### Simple, Effective Health Program

- Start the day with a full glass of water with the juice of ½ freshly squeezed lemon.
- Eat only raw fruit until noon.
- Drink a green smoothie (Appendix 7) every day.

### Key #4: Believing

The door to self-empowerment is opened by becoming aware of our thoughts and emotions as they are happening in the present moment. All aspects of our lives, including our health, are created from our subconscious beliefs. When we become conscious and aware of our thoughts, we can take control and create our lives purposefully.

- Work with the concepts, tools, and resources suggested in chapters 17 to 20 for becoming aware of your thoughts, emotions, and beliefs.
- Take time at the end of each day to review the events of the day as well as the associated thoughts and emotions you had and felt at these times. Notice whether your behaviors were reactive or calmly active.
- Try to identify whether the emotional beliefs underlying your thoughts and behaviors come from a basis of love or fear, peace or anger, acceptance or resistance.
- As time goes by and you progress in your reflective awareness of the beliefs that govern your actions, move to being aware of them as they are happening—in the present moment.
- Work to move from the reactions of ego to the gentleness and confidence of spirit.
- Believe that you are love, and become it.

**Key #5: Implementing**

Positive change in our lives and health happen when we implement our knowledge; we must take consistent and persistent action.

- Become knowledgeable about how the body operates and what it needs to be healthy. Read and reread this book, and refer to it as a reference, until you can explain the concepts to others. Continue to learn, but don't stray off the fundamental understanding that the body is electrical in nature, that everything put into it to build health must contain live energy. Food, beverages, and drugs that are not electrically compatible to the body undermine and destroy health.
- Make the intention that you are going to be healthy. Everything starts with thought, belief, and decision. Create a vision of your body in health.
- Replenish your body's reserves of workers, building materials, and alkaline minerals in sufficient quantities to do the job.
- Decide on your nutritional supplement program, and stick with it until you get results.
- Stay focused. Don't be like the thirsty dying man in the desert who keeps changing directions on the advice of each new person he meets when he is trying to find the oasis.

## ACHIEVING RESULTS

When working to eliminate disease conditions and regain health, keep in mind that each individual is different. Just because someone experienced great results in a certain amount of time does not necessarily mean everyone will. Some conditions can be reversed quickly, while some can take a year or more before there is a breakthrough to positive results. The timing for things to begin happening depends on the following:

- Genetic make-up—health of ancestors.
- Diet as a child.

- Diet since childhood.
- Lifestyle habits of eating, drinking, smoking, drugs, exercise, rest, and attitudes.
- Stress in the person's life.
- Exposure to environmental toxins, EMFs, and geopathic stress.
- Belief system.

As well, a commitment to:

- Healthy attitudes.
- Wholesome diet.
- Regular exercise.
- Health-building supplements that cleanse the body and replenish its workers.
- Continual understanding of symptoms and causes.

Whenever we have a physical problem, or symptoms of a malfunction, or disease within the body, we should be asking:

- What is causing this?
- Why is my body acting this way?
- What is it telling me?
- What is it trying to correct?
- What experience(s) in my past could be contributing to my present condition?
- How can I cooperate with my body to assist it in its detoxifying and corrective healing efforts?
- Is what I am eating, taking as a supplement or drug, helping or hindering my body in its efforts to cleanse itself and replenish its enzyme and bowel flora workers and body-building nutrients?
- Is what I am doing acting only to suppress my symptoms to make them go away?
- Am I working for short-term relief or for long-term health?

The extent to which we understand and apply the principles of natural health to our own lifestyles will determine our results, and also the timing of those results. Every human body naturally wants to travel back up the road to health. The lifestyles we have had, the physical and emotional challenges we have, and our openness to reexamining our thinking about health will determine how long that road back will be.

## HEALTH IS A GIFT AND A CHOICE

Health is a natural expression of the innate intelligence of the wonderful human body we were given. What we do with this gift is our choice. We can ignore it, squander it, abuse it, or we can honor and nurture it. Everything begins and ends with our thoughts and intentions.

What we do about our health, how we direct our efforts, and how we spend our money are always our choices. Most people think very little of spending thousands of dollars on a newer car, a vacation trip, or putting money into an uncertain stock market, but squirm at the thought of investing in their own health and well-being.

Spending the effort and money required to regain our health so we can remain healthy well into advanced years brings invaluable rewards.

## WITH HEALTH, EVERYTHING IS POSSIBLE

With health, everything is possible. Without health, nothing matters. If we have lost our health and have regained it, life becomes enjoyable and exciting again. New possibilities can open up. We don't have to deteriorate with age, as we see many people doing all around us.

Health is a choice, when we know the 5 keys to *Conscious Health*. We can choose whether the lifestyle decisions we make will contribute to a health process in our bodies, or to a disease process. It's up to us!

Even after doctors say there is nothing more they can do for you, you now know there are many things *you* can do. With this knowledge, the power to be healthy is within you. The best doctor there is, is your own body intelligence. Take back your power to make your own decisions to be healthy, and begin putting it into action—today! The final decisions are always yours, and so are the rewards.

I wish you the very best of health, happiness, joy, and fulfillment.

Life is here for our creation and re-creation.

Life is all about choices.

Create yours—consciously!

# APPENDIX 1

## ACID-FORMING AND
## ALKALINE-FORMING FOODS

MANY FOODS of one type, as they pass through our bodies, are acted upon by the body chemistry so that they produce an acid or alkaline residue (ash) that is the opposite of their original chemical composition. That is, foods that are acidic, will alkalize, and vice versa.

The following foods and non-foods are listed in order, from most alkaline to most acidic; or, in other words, from most healthy to most harmful for the body.[1,2]

### ALKALINE-FORMING
- Raw fruits and their fresh juices
- Dried fruits
- Raw vegetables and their fresh juices
- Herbal teas
- Frozen fruits and vegetables
- Lightly steamed fruits and vegetables
- Raw nuts (almonds, pecans, et cetera)
- Raw seeds (sesame, pumpkin, squash, sunflower, et cetera)
- Sprouted grains

### ACID-FORMING
- Some raw fruits and vegetables (cranberries, plums, prunes, squash)
- Whole grains—cooked
- Overcooked fruits and vegetables
- Dairy products (cheese, milk);
- Eggs
- Sugar and refined grains
- Spices (dried mustard, nutmeg)
- White meats (fish, fowl)
- Fried foods

- Coffee and tea
- Red meats (beef, lamb, pork)
- Refined salt
- Soft drinks
- Alcohol
- Drugs and medications
- Tobacco

> **Note:** *A healthy diet should consist of at least 70–80% alkaline foods and 20–30% acid foods. The average North American diet is the reverse of this ideal.*

ALKALINE FOODS

**DEGREE OF ALKALINITY** (*Diet should be 80% alkaline foods*)
Lists of food & non-foods are ordered with the highest degree of alkalinity at
the top of each list, through moderate to lowest alkalinity at the bottom.

| Raw Fruits | Raw vegetables | Beans |
|---|---|---|
| *High alkalinity* | *High alkalinity* | *High alkalinity* |
| Melons | Asparagus | Green |
| Lemons | Carrots | Lima |
| Grapefruit, | Celery | |
| Limes, | Parsley | *Mild alkalinity* |
| Mango, | Sea weed—kelp, algae | Other beans |
| Papaya | | Peas |
| Bananas | *Mild alkalinity* | String bean |
| | Beets | |
| *Mild alkalinity* | Cabbage | |
| Oranges | Cauliflower | |
| Cherries | Corn | **Herbs/Spices** |
| Tart apples | Kale | |
| Cucumbers | Leeks | *High alkalinity* |
| Tomatoes | Mushrooms | Chives |
| Zucchini, | Onions | Garlic |
| Bell peppers | Peppers | Vegetable salt |
| | Radishes | Cayenne |
| | Potatoes with peel | Apple cider vinegar |
| | | (unpasteurized) |
| | | |
| | | *Mild alkalinity* |
| | | Most herbs and spices |
| | | Sea salt |

## Grains

*High alkalinity*
Arrowroot flour
Essene (manna) bread
*All grains are alkaline when sprouted.*

*Mild alkalinity*
Amaranth
Millet
Quinoa

## Protein

*High alkalinity*
Bee pollen
Royal jelly

*Mild alkalinity*
Vegetable proteins
Milk from almonds
and hempseeds
Natural cottage cheese
Yogurt

## Nuts

*Moderate alkalinity*
Almonds
Fresh coconut

## Oils

*Mild alkalinity*
*Most cold pressed, fresh, untreated oils are neutral to slightly alkaline forming*

## Seeds

*High alkalinity*
Most sprouted seeds

## Sugars

*High alkalinity*
Unpasteurized honey
Stevia

## Beverages

*High alkalinity*
Fresh fruit juices
Vegetable juices

*Mild alkalinity*
Herbal teas:
   Strawberry
   Raspberry
Herbal teas:
   Alfalfa
   Clover
   Ginger
   Comfrey
   Ginseng
   Mint
   Sage

## Other

*High alkalinity*
Digestive enzymes
green vegetable drinks
chlorophyll

**DEGREE OF ACIDITY** (*Diet should be 20% acid foods*)

Lists of food and non-foods are ordered with the lowest degree of acitity at the top of each list, through medium to highest acidity at the bottom.

| Raw fruits | Grains and Cereals | Dairy, Meat, Fish, Fowl |
|---|---|---|
| *Low acidity* | *Low acidity* | *Low acidity* |
| Blueberries | Barley | Unpasteurized dairy |
| Cranberries | Rye | Eggs |
| Plums | Spelt | |
| Prunes | Corn meal | *Medium to high acidity* |
| | Buckwheat | Meat |
| *Medium to high acidity* | Unrefined cereals, crackers | Fish |
| Green or overirpe fuit | Popcorn: plain or butter (unsalted) | Fowl |
| | | Processed dairy |
| | | Ice cream |

*Medium to high acidity*
Rice, wheat (especially
  white), oats
  pancakes
  waffles
  muffins
Refined breads
  pastas
  pastries
  cereals
  crackers

| Nuts |
|---|
| *Low acidity* |
| All other raw nuts |
| |
| *Medium to high acidity* |
| All roasted and salted nuts |

## Oils

*Medium to high acidity*
Hydrogenated oils

*Avoid all heated and
hydrogenated oils.*

## Seeds

*Low acidity*
Unsprouted seeds
    (*most*)

*Medium to high acidity*
Roasted and salted
    seeds (*all*)

## Sugars

*Low acidity*
Maple sugar
Pasteurized honey
Molasses
fructose
turbinado

*Medium to high acidity*
White, processed sugar
artificial sweeteners

## Beverages

*Medium to high acidity*
Coffee and substitutes
Black tea
Liquor, beer, wine (*all*)
Soft drinks
Carbonated drinks

## Other

*Medium to high acidity*
Most fast food
    products
Table salt
White vinegar
Drugs, tobacco (*all*)

# APPENDIX 4
## ALKALIZING BROTH

ONE OF the least expensive, yet very effective ways of improving your health and raising your pH to less acidic is to drink mineral-rich vegetable broth. This can easily be made at home by using alkaline vegetables and a good vegetable salt. The broth will be rich in potassium, calcium, magnesium, and sodium. Four or five cups of broth can be consumed for each day that one is on a detoxification and rejuvenating program, or while one is concentrating on raising the urine pH back to a normal level of 6.8 to 7.0.

### Directions
Select and use a few organic vegetables from the mild and high alkalinity lists in Appendix 2, or as follows:

Thick potato peelings (discard rest of potato)
Carrot tops
Beet tops
Parsley
Celery leaves and some stalk
Other green vegetables, such as kelp, kale, et cetera

Chop vegetables and place in a stainless steel pot with purified water. Bring to boil and simmer for 20 or 25 minutes. Let it cool a bit, then strain out the vegetable pieces, keeping the broth. As you are straining, squeeze the liquid out of the vegetable mass with a large spoon or potato masher to harvest all the mineral broth. Season the broth to taste with a vegetable salt such as Vegex®, or Vege-Sal®. Refrigerate. Warm up portions as you consume them.

THE PURPOSE of an enema is to efficiently and effectively clear the colon of toxic wastes when the body is unable to do this adequately on its own.

Enemas are recommended while one is fasting, undergoing an acute cleanse (healing crisis), during periods of detoxification for any serious or degenerative disease (can ease headaches at such times), or when there is a chronic constipation problem. Chemical laxatives are not the answer and should not be used.

Enemas are safe when used according to common sense instructions. The body does not become dependent on them when a person has stopped eating the toxic foods that caused the constipation problem in the first place and has begun to eat foods that rebuild the body and restore health. In time, the colon will heal itself, remove impacted fecal matter (the assistance of gentle herbs helps), slough off the mucus coat, and return to normal bowel function on its own. Taking enemas in the meantime helps the body rid itself of toxins so it can heal faster. It also exercises and tones the colon muscles so they can begin working on their own again.

---

*Note:* *If the dietary habits that caused the colon problems are not stopped, there will not be any healing of the condition, and no matter what method is used to clear the colon—laxatives or even enemas—these will appear to be habit forming. One must work to correct the cause of the problem.*

---

**Instructions**

1   Use a standard enema bag that can be purchased in most pharmacies. It should be able to hold 1 to 2 quarts (or liters) of water. The nozzle should be a regular nozzle, approximately 4–6 inches (10–15 centimeters) long.

2   Fill the enema bag with about a quart (or liter) for teenagers and adults. (Children would require one half or less this amount.) Use water that has been filtered to remove chlorine, fluoride, et cetera. The water should be of a temperature that is comfortable to the wrist—slightly warmer water (do not use hot) can bring on more contractions, while cooler water has a toning effect on the colon walls.

3   Hang the enema bag on a towel rack (or that approximate height), using a coat hanger if a hook is not provided with the bag.

4   Lubricate the nozzle and rectum with K-Y gel, a vegetable oil, or an ordinary ointment. (Do not use a petroleum product.)

5   Kneel on the floor near the toilet, in the 'head-to-floor' position so that the rectum is higher than the shoulders. This position allows the water to run more easily into the colon. If for some reason it is not possible to assume this position, an alternate is to lie on the right side or on the back.

6   Insert the nozzle gently. If it will not go in all the way, it should do so once the flow of water is begun. It will be necessary to hold the nozzle in place throughout the enema session, as the body will tend to push it out.

7   Once the nozzle is in place, begin the flow of water from the enema bag into the colon. Regulate the flow of water into the colon so that it enters at a slow rate. Pinching or bending the hose does this. Some enema bags come with a flow regulator device.

8   As the water is flowing in, should any discomfort or an urge to expel the water be felt, stop the flow of water, take a few deep breaths and then resume the water flow as the urge passes.

9   Empty about 5 or 6 ounces (150–180 milliliters) of water from the enema bag into the colon. Should this be hindered because the urge to expel the water is too great, remove the enema nozzle, sit on the toilet, and expel what water is in the colon into the toilet. It should now be possible to resume the 'head-to-floor' position and empty another 5 or 6 ounces (150–180 milliliters) of the water in the enema bag into the colon. If not, allow in what can be comfortably held in the colon.

10  Once the water is in the colon, remove the nozzle from the rectum and lie on the floor resisting the urge to evacuate. Lie first on the left side, and then roll onto the back, then to the right side, then onto the stomach. Each position should be held for approximately 30 seconds. While lying on the back, the stomach/colon area can be gently massaged to promote better clearing of fecal matter.

11  Now sit on the toilet and expel the water. It may take several minutes for the water and contents to work their way out of the colon. One needs to be patient while waiting for the successive urges to evacuate.

12  Should a good evacuation not be experienced, or if insufficient water was introduced into the colon, the enema bag can be immediately refilled and the entire process repeated. This may be done several times if necessary.

### Problems

Should the colon not be able to expel any or all of the water, introduce some water at a little warmer temperature into the colon, or slowly take another enema until some cramping and urge to evacuate begins. Likewise, should the colon be overactive—not allowing any or very little water to enter—use cooler water. If only a small amount of water is able to enter into the colon, no more should be forced. Simply work with what will enter; it will be of benefit providing it is stimulating a bowel movement.

In times of severe illness, enemas may not be sufficient. Colonics are much more effective and can be life-saving.

> **Note:** *This type of enema allows for a gentle release of toxins and built-up fecal matter from the lower end of the colon without stressing the body. It does not upset the overall electrical balance of the colon or eliminate bowel flora.*

THE FOLLOWING recipes are presented as samples only. For more complete listings and ideas, refer to recipe books mentioned in the *Resources and Recommended Reading* section. Several of the books listed have quite large sections devoted to menus and recipes.

### GREEN SMOOTHIE

Green smoothies are probably the most nutritious meal one can eat—especially when made with organic ingredients. They are quick to prepare and tasty. A good blender can be used, but a VitaMix™ blender is more powerful and efficient. The basic green smoothie instructions are—for one person—blend a handful of greens, such as spinach, kale, romaine lettuce, or parsley, with two glasses of water. Then add two ripe bananas or apples or any sweet fruit, and blend the mix until it is creamy. You can vary the recipe each day, according to your taste, enhancing it with mint, dill, lemon juice, or whatever you find appealing.

> **Note:** *To freeze bananas, peel and place separated on a cookie sheet. Freeze overnight. Then place in plastic bags for later use.*

### Other Smoothies or Fruit Shakes

Almost any combination of fruit may be combined and whizzed in a blender, combined with water, juice, hemp seeds, and almond or cashew milk to make a delicious and nutritious meal in a drink. Some examples are:

### RAW POWER DRINK

Blend the following ingredients in a blender until smooth:

> The water and meat of 1 young coconut (almond milk may be used if young coconut is not available.)
> 1 avocado
> 2 cups fresh berries or fruit (frozen is okay)
> 1 tablespoons unpasteurized honey
> 2 or more tablespoons raw protein powder

### MORNING PEP DRINK MEAL

Soak overnight in the refrigerator:

> ¼ cup shelled, raw, unsalted, organic sunflower seeds
> 2 cups good water

In the morning, blend the seeds and water for 3 minutes, at high speed. Add:

> 1 tablespoon brewers yeast
> 1 tablespoon blackstrap molasses
> 1 tablespoon acidophilus powder (or another probiotic product)

This is a full meal. Sip and chew to mix well with saliva for proper digestion. For a more concentrated drink, double the quantity of sunflower seeds.

## SPROUTED SEEDS AND GRAINS

Soak for 7 or 8 hours:

    1 cup organic rye grains
    1 cup organic barley grains
    1 cup organic sunflower seeds
    ¼ cup organic sesame seeds

Rinse under cold water and drain well. Spread the drained grain and seeds on glass, non-ceramic plates, or sprouting dishes. Let sprout for 15 to 16 hours. During the time they are sprouting, rinse them under cool water at least 2 times or they will acquire a musty smell and taste. At the end of 16 hours, rinse well under cool water and strain. This mixture will last at least 3 days in the refrigerator.

To eat, mash a ripe, raw banana in a bowl and add 1 or 2 tablespoons of natural strawberry jam. Add 1 cup, or desired amount, of sprouted seeds and grains. Mix well.

## RAW CRACKERS

Raw crackers are made with the use of a food processor or a strong blender, such as the VitaMix™, plus a food dehydrator that has a variable temperature control, such as an Excalibur™ (the choice of most raw food eaters). Cracker ingredients are dried at a temperature under 110°F (43°C), which retains the live enzymes. These crackers are nutritious, an excellent source of fiber, and a healthy replacement for cooked crackers and breads. An excellent resource for how to make raw crackers is *Igor's Live Flat Bread*, available at www.rawfamily.com. But with a little practice and experimentation, you can easily make recipes of their your own. A sample recipe I have created is printed here—but I seem to change it every time I make a new batch of crackers! Vary the ingredients according to your taste preferences and amounts desired. Organic ingredients are best.

## SAVORY CRACKERS

> 2 cups freshly-ground (to a coarse size) flax seeds (a dry VitaMix™ container or coffee grinder may be used)
>
> 2 cups water
>
> 4 bell peppers
>
> 3 or 4 ripe tomatoes
>
> ½ to 1 bunch of greens (spinach, kale, broccoli, or …)
>
> 1 bunch parsley
>
> 3 or 4 cloves of garlic and/or fresh ginger
>
> 3 carrots
>
> 1 small to medium zucchini
>
> 1/4 cup cold-pressed oil
>
> 1–1½ teaspoon sea salt
>
> Sprig of fresh rosemary or dill
>
> ⅛ to ¼ teaspoon cayenne pepper
>
> 1 or 2 cups sunflower seeds, soaked in water overnight to begin sprouting. In the morning, rinse for use.
>
> Sesame or hemp seeds

In a food processor or VitaMix™, puree peppers, tomatoes, greens, parsley, and garlic or ginger until smooth. Add oil, sea salt, rosemary or dill, and cayenne pepper. Blend again to mix thoroughly. Pour into a large mixing bowl. Grate carrots and zucchini and mix with other ingredients. Mix in the sunflower seeds plus other seeds, if you decide to use them. When this process is complete, in a separate bowl add the water to the ground flax seeds and stir well. Add to other ingredients immediately and mix thoroughly as the mixture will begin to thicken quickly. Let stand for ten minutes. If the mixture is too thick, water may be added; if too thin, more ground flax can be added.

Next, scoop 2 or 3 medium ladles of the dough mixture onto non-stick teflex dehydrator sheets and spread evenly with a spatula to about a ¼ inch (.6 cm) thickness. (Excess mixture can be frozen and rethawed later to dehydrate another batch of crackers.) Dehydrate about 6 hours, then flip over and remove the teflex sheets. (If the cracker mix still sticks to the sheets, dehydrate a while longer.) At this point, the still-moist crackers may be cut into small squares, then returned to the dehydrator for an additional 5 or 6 hours, or until thoroughly dry. If kept in a dry place, these crackers will remain fresh for up to two months.

## COOKED CEREAL GRAINS

Mix several grains such as oat groats, buckwheat, rye, barley, brown rice, bulgur wheat, kamut, millet, cornmeal, flax, and sesame seeds in water. Bring to a boil. Put on the lid, and turn the stove off. Let stand overnight. In the morning, add water as necessary and heat. Add the following to taste, as preferred—sea salt, paprika, nutmeg, coconut, crushed nuts, raisins, date pieces, vegetable gelatin. You can also substitute fruit juices for water, and add raisins, pineapple bits, nuts, et cetera.

## VEGETABLE CHOP SUEY

1 cup carrots, chopped
1 cup celery, chopped
½ cup green pepper, chopped
¼–½ cup red sweet pepper, chopped
½ cup onion, chopped (optional)
1 cup broccoli pieces
¼ lb. fresh mushrooms, whole or chopped
2 cups chicken stock
2 tablespoons tamari soy sauce or Braggs Liquid Aminos
2 tablespoons arrowroot powder or rice starch, tapioca starch, et cetera
1 cup or more fresh bean sprouts

*Add as desired,*
½ teaspoon chopped fresh ginger
1 teaspoon chopped garlic
2 tablespoons black bean sauce

In a Chinese wok or heavy-bottom pot, stir-fry the vegetables (starting with the more solid ones first) in a liquid, such as water or chicken stock, until just tender but still crispy. Add chicken stock and tamari sauce and simmer, stirring constantly. (Seasoning, such as garlic or ginger, can be added to the stock beforehand to impart its flavors to the liquid.) Dissolve arrowroot powder in cold water, and add gradually, stirring until the mixture is cooked and the chop suey has thickened. Add raw bean sprouts just before serving. May be served with steamed brown rice.

## CHICKEN CHOP SUEY

Same as above, but add 2 cups of cooked chicken cut in 1 inch pieces at the same time as chicken stock is added. Since a protein has been added, it is best for proper food combination purposes, to eat this meal without a carbohydrate such as rice or bread.

## NUT MILK

Good milk substitutes can be made in a blender using raw almonds, cashews, and sunflower or sesame seeds. Take one cup of water, preferably living water, and add about ¼ cup of raw nuts or seeds. Blend at high speed for 2 or 3 minutes, until thick white milk is formed. It is best used as it is, but may also be poured through a sieve, gauze, or nut milk bag to remove the pulp.

## HEMP SEED MILK

Hemp seeds, being high in protein and essential fatty acids, make an excellent milk substitute. Make it using the same recipe as Nut Milk. Vary the amounts of water and hemp seeds according to your preference.

## SIMPLE HEMP PROTEIN SMOOTHIE

In a blender, mix fruit juice, water, a piece or two of fruit and blend. Then add one or two tablespoons of hemp protein (rice protein is okay too). Blend again. Modify ingredients according to your taste. (Just make sure the protein powder you use has not been heat-processed.)

## HEMP PROTEIN SMOOTHIE

In a blender, combine the following (or your own combination) according to your taste. Blend, adding liquid as needed.

   1 cup or more of water or fresh juice
   1 or 2 tablespoons hemp seeds

1 tablespoon hemp oil
Apple and/or banana, strawberries, et cetera
1 (or several) tablespoons hemp protein powder
1 teaspoon greenfood concentrate powder

*Optional—add one or more of the following:*
Flavoring, such as cinnamon or oil of orange
½ teaspoon powdered enzymes
Rice protein powder
Carob powder

This is very concentrated food. Drink it slowly, and mix it thoroughly with saliva in the mouth. This nutritious combination contains everything to live on and build health in your body.

### FRUIT ICE CREAM

Use frozen bananas, strawberries, raspberries, or blueberries alone or in combination, and run through a Champion™ juicer, with the solid screen cover in place, or process in a Vita-Mix™ blender. Tastes great, and is nutritious because it still contains natural enzymes and has no sugar or other additives.

### NATURAL STRAWBERRY JAM

2 cups fresh or frozen strawberries (can also use raspberries)
4 or 5 rings of dried pineapple
Unsweetened pineapple or orange juice

Soak and rinse dried pineapple in water to remove any sulfur. Cut dried pineapple into small pieces. Combine all ingredients, and let set until dried pineapple is soft. Blend in blender until smooth. Juice may not need to be added if the strawberries have enough liquid. This is natural raw fruit. It is a good idea to put it in small containers, and freeze any amount in excess of what you will use in a few days.

THE FOLLOWING meal alternatives are presented as samples only. For more complete listings and ideas, refer to recipe books mentioned in the *Resources and Recommended Reading* section. Several of the books listed have quite large sections devoted to menus and recipes. Note that some of the cooked food suggestions and ingredients apply more to a transitional diet when one is changing over to healthier choices.

My personal diet has simplified over the years until now I typically eat only fruit until noon. Then I consume smoothies, especially green varieties, along with dehydrated crackers. I snack on raw veggies or fruit with a few nuts and seeds, or dehydrated crackers. On occasion, I eat something different for variety, but I try to make it a healthy choice. I seldom eat after 6 or 7 pm.

### NUTRITIONAL AND DIGESTION GUIDELINES

- The more relaxed you are, the better your digestion works.
- The more you chew your food, the better it digests.
- Eat only when hungry.
- Do not overeat.
- Combine foods properly.
- As fruits pass out of season, they should be used less.
- Use a balanced variety of foods, not the same ones.
- Work toward a ratio of 75% fresh, raw foods, including juiced, in the diet. Foods minimally cooked at low temperatures can be included.
- Soak nuts and seeds before eating them (to activate enzymes).
- Consume nuts and seeds with a citrus juice for more complete digestion.
- The basic core of all meals is vegetables and salads.
- Skins of fruits and vegetables contain valuable minerals.
- Supplement with digestive enzymes, as needed by your body.
- Foods, if cooked, should be steamed, stir-fried with water, slow cooked or broiled—not boiled, fried in oil, microwaved, or cooked in a pressure cooker.

**BREAKFAST ALTERNATIVES**

Upon rising, drink one or two glasses of warm water containing the juice of half a lemon. This is an excellent body cleanser and alkalizer. An alternative to lemon could be a teaspoon of pure, unpasteurized apple cider vinegar. Wait 15 or 20 minutes before eating anything else.

- Freshly made fruit juice (minimize the use of citrus fruits).
- Watermelon or one-half cantaloupe or honeydew melon, grapes.
- Fresh fruit of your choice.
- Sliced bananas and a nut or seed milk, such as almond, cashew or sunflower.
- One or two soft-boiled eggs.
- Lightly toasted whole grain bread (preferably not wheat) and butter.
- Cooked cereal grains, served with a nut or seed milk made in the blender, plus a little honey or maple syrup as desired.
- Sprouted seeds and grains with mashed banana and natural strawberry jam. Optional—add blackstrap molasses, lecithin, ground flax seed and/or a balanced oil blend. Chew slowly and thoroughly.
- Morning pep drink meal (see appendix 7).

**LUNCH ALTERNATIVES**

- Green smoothie.
- Raw crackers with hummus or avocado.
- Large fruit salad from a mixture of bananas, pineapple, grapes, coconut, apples, mangoes, pears, et cetera.
- Large glass of freshly made vegetable juice from a combination of carrots (80–90%), celery, spinach, beet (small piece), ginger, parsley, plus others as desired. (Sip slowly; this is a meal in itself.)
- Large, mixed vegetable salad. Whole grain muffin with butter. Herbal tea.
- Homemade blender soup: One or more cups of mixed vegetables and greens, tomato, natural spices, natural sea salt, cup of boiling water, ½ teaspoon (2.7 milliters) unpasteurized apple cider vinegar (to release calcium). Blend at high speed for 30 seconds. (Can use vegetable, poultry, or fish stock.) Crisp rye or flat bread. Herbal tea.
- Homemade soup. Add miso paste, kelp, dulse, as desired.
- Closed or open-faced sandwich of Essene bread or whole rye, with butter lettuce, mashed avocado, sprouts, green or red peppers, Mrs. Dash® spice seasoning as desired.

- Small mixed vegetable salad. Lentil soup. Whole grain crackers or flatbread.
- Fresh vegetables and white cheese made from unpasteurized milk.
- Assorted vegetable sticks with sesame tahini. Sourdough rye bread, lightly buttered.
- Salad and sardines (packed in their own oil or olive oil).

## DINNER ALTERNATIVES

- Green smoothie—with or without raw crackers.
- Homemade tomato juice. Large salad with cold-pressed oil dressing, unpasteurized apple cider vinegar or lemon juice can be added. Baked potato with a little butter. Green beans and/or broccoli lightly steamed.
- Lightly stir-fried (use water) vegetables and cashews or almonds, with tamari sauce or Braggs Liquid Aminos® (from a healthfood store) for flavoring. Baked squash.
- Mixed salad. Broiled or steamed fish (salmon, trout, halibut) and lightly steamed vegetables (not potato or rice). Sliced tomatoes.
- Spinach and tomato salad, with oil and lemon dressing. Roasted chicken or turkey, with arrowroot sauce as gravy. Steamed broccoli, carrots and celery.
- Vegetable sticks. Lentil soup, with rye bread, or flatbread.
- Lentil loaf, with steamed brown rice and a large salad.
- Chicken chop suey, and fresh bean sprouts.
- Vegetable chop suey, and steamed rice.

## SNACKS

- Raw crackers and hummus.
- Freshly-made vegetable juice.
- Fresh fruit, or dried fruit (unsulfured).
- Fresh coconut cut in small chunks, with dates.
- Nut, seed, or hemp seed milk.
- Banana smoothie.
- Fruit ice cream, made in Champion juicer or strong blender.
- Oatmeal-date cookies.
- Raw nuts (chew very well).
- White unpasteurized milk cheese.
- Rye-crisp crackers with avocado.
- Herbal tea.
- Vegetable soup.

## APPENDIX 8
### PURCHASING SUPPLEMENTS

WHEN SELECTING and buying supplements, remember that:

- Nature's vitamins heal; synthetic vitamins stimulate the body but do not heal.
- Natural complexes come from live, whole organic food sources, with their enzymes and electrical properties intact. They have been manufactured with minimal processing.
- No supplement should be taken in concentrations greater than those found in food.
- The body cannot use, and does not accept, isolated or synthetic nutrients.

Use these guidelines when assessing the suitability of a supplement product you are considering for purchase and use.

# ENDNOTES

## INTRODUCTION

1   Lipton, Bruce, PhD. *The Biology of Belief.* 2005.


## CHAPTER 1

1   Robbins, Joel, DC, ND, MD. *College of Natural Health Extension Course.* 1995. Lecture note.


## CHAPTER 2

1   Elliot, David A. *The Electric Universe.* 1996. p. 9.
2   Ibid. p. 13.
3   Becker, Robert O, MD and Selden, Gary. *The Body Electric: Electromagnetism and the Foundation of Life. 1998.*
4   Hiestand, Denie and Shelley. *Electrical Nutrition.* 2001. pp. 35, 36.
5   Irons, V. E., Dr. *The Destruction of Your Own Protective Mechanism.*
6   Jensen, Bernard, DC. *Breathe Again Naturally.* 1983. pp. 48, 50.
7   Robbins, Joel, DC, ND, MD. *Health Through Nutrition.* 1992. p. 36.
8   Arlin, Stephen; Dini, Fouad; Wolfe, David. *Nature's First Law: The Raw Food Diet.* 2000. p. 89.


## CHAPTER 3

1   Robbins, Joel, DC, ND, MD. *College of Natural Health Extension Course.* 1995. Sec. 4, p. 23.


## CHAPTER 4

1   Robbins, Joel, DC, ND, MD. *Health Through Nutrition.* 1992. p. 16.
2   Lipton, Bruce, PhD. *Biology of Belief.* Video. 2001.
3   Lanctôt, Guylaine, MD. *The Medical Mafia.* 1995. p. 157.
4   Robbins, Joel, DC, ND, MD. *College of Natural Health Extension Course.* 1995. Lecture note.
5   Meinig, George E., DDS, FACD. *Root Canal Cover-Up.* 1993. pp. 6, 28, 183–187.

6   Roy, Leo, MD, ND. *Mastery Over Cancer*. 1997.

7   Roy, Leo, MD, ND. *A Microsketch of Cancer*. 1997.

8   Gdanski, Ron. *Cancer Cause, Cure and Cover-up*. 2000. p. 56.

9   Warburg, Otto, Dr. "The Prime Cause and Prevention of Cancer," Lecture delivered to Nobel Laureates. June 30, 1966. Lindau, Germany.

10  Read in Chapter 16, how the man who first harvested phytoplankton concentrate for human consumption recovered from cancer and diabetes.

11  Ryan, Robert, BSc. "Cancer Research—A Super Fraud?". http://www.rense.com/general9/cre.htm.

## CHAPTER 5

1   Petereson, Wes. "Raw Food—One of Your Keys to Outstanding Health." http://www.mercola.com/2002/may/22/cooked_food.htm.

2   Ibid.

3   Pottenger, Francis M. Jr. *Pottenger's Cats: A Study in Nutrition*. 1995. pp. 9–18.

4   Meinig, George E. DDS, FACD. *Root Canal Cover-Up*. 1993. p. 8.

5   Pottenger. Op. cit. pp. 12–13.

6   Arlin, Stephen; Dini, Fouad; Wolfe, David. *Nature's First Law: The Raw Food Diet*. 2000. p. 67.

7   Moss, Ralph. "The War on Cancer." *Townsend Letter for Doctors and Patients*. Nov. 2002.

8   Morrison-Kelly,Carol, MD, FACC; Kelley, William, D. "Cancer Ignorance. Part II." http://www.drkelley.com/what_is_cancer.htm.

9   World Health Organization. "New Health Life Expectancy Rankings." *World Health Organization Report*. June 4, 2000.

10  *Strategic Investment*. Newsletter. Nov. 2000.

11  Robbins, Joel, DC, ND, MD. *College of Natural Health Extension Course*. 1995. Sec. 1, p. 4.

12  Arnst, Catherine. "Is Your Reproductive System in Danger?" *Business Week*. Sept 14, 1998. http://archives.foodsafetynetwork.ca/agnet/1998/9-1998/ag-9-7-98-1.txt.

13  Sims, Katherine. "New Insight on Age and Fertility Rate." *Physicians Practice*. Sept/Oct 2002. http://www.shands.org/professional/ppd/ppd_article.asp?ID=44.

14  Robbins, Joel, DC, ND, MD. *Health Through Nutrition*. 1992. p 29.

15  Cohen, Robert. Speech at Kansas City Symposium. Nov. 14, 2000. http://www.animalconnectiontx.org/issues/KC.htm.

16  Irons. V. E. *Vit-Ra-Tox: The Gold Book*. 1996. p 11.

17  Keon, Joseph, PhD. "The Arguments for Eating Organic Foods." http://www.positive-health.com/permit/Articles/Organic%20and%20Vegetarian/keon47.htm.

18  Robbins, Joel, DC, ND, MD. *Health Through Nutrition*. 1992. p 12.

19  http://www.cam.net.uk/home/Nimmann/healing/microwaves.htm.

20  http://www.proactivenews.com/html/microwave.html.

21  Olsen, Joan. "Tracking Seed to Shelf." *Farm Industry News*. Nov. 1, 2000.

22  http://www.news.cornell.edu/releases/May99/Butterflies.bpf.html.

23  http://www.racoon.com/dcforum/DCForumID7/269.html.

24  Meinig, George E., DDS, FACD. *Root Canal Cover-Up*. 1993. p 8.

25  Braden, Gregg. *The God Code*. 2004. p 49.

26  Braden, Gregg. "Mystery of the Essenes Lost Science of a Forgotten People." *Sacred Spaces/Ancient Wisdom*. Fall/Winter 2000. 5.2. http://www.greggbraden.com/news letter.php3.

**CHAPTER 6**

1  http://www.med-ed-online.org/volume6.htm.

2  http://www.med.unc.edu/nutr/nim/FAQ.htm#anchorteachnutrition.

3  http://www.newstarget.com/z002706.html.

4  Lipton, Bruce, PhD. *The Biology of Belief*, 2005. p, 108.

5  Lipton, Bruce, PhD. Presentation to Chiropractors. Video recording. April 2003.

6  Abraham, Carolyn. "Study finds Vioxx took deadly toll." Jan 25, 2005. www.theglobe andmail.com/servlet/story/RTGAM.20050125.wvioxx25/BNStory/specialScienceand Health.

7  Dr. Barbara Starfield, "Doctors Are the Third Leading Cause of Death in the US, Causing 250,000 Deaths Every Year." *Journal of the American Medical Association*. Vol. 284. July 26, 2000.

8  Null, Gary PhD; Dean, Carolyn, MD, ND; Feldman, Martin, MD; Rasio, Debora, MD. *Death by Medicine*. October 2003. Abstract.

9  Philp, Margaret. "Canadians Enjoy Long and Healthy Lives." *Globe and Mail*. Jun. 5, 2000.

10  Berens, Michael J. "Dirty Hospitals Kill 75,000 Patients a Year Unnecessarily." *Reader's Digest*. Feb. 2003.

11  Baker, Ross and Associates. "The Canadian Adverse Events Study." Canadian Medical Association Journal. May 25, 2004. http://www.cmaj.ca/cgi/content/full/170/11/1678.

12  Robbins, Joel, DC, ND, MD. *College of Natural Health Extension Course*. 1995. Lecture note.

13  Sapp, Amy; McDonald, Shannon. "Production and Consumption of Meat: Implications for Global Environment and Human Health." *Harvard School of Public Health*. Dec. 13, 2001.

14  Goodall, Jane. *Harvest for Hope*. 2005. pp. 117–133.

15  Miller, Neil Z. *Vaccines: Are They Really Safe and Effective?* 1996. p. 17.

16  Scheibner, Viera, Ph.D. *Vaccination: 100 Years of Orthodox Research Shows That Vaccines Represent a Medical Assault on the Immune System*. 1993. p. xv.

17  Miller, Neil Z. Op. cit. pp. 19–38.

18  Scheibner, Viera. Op. cit. p. xvii.

19  Lanctôt, Guylaine, MD. *The Medical Mafia*, 1995. pp. 117–118.

20  http://www.informedchoice.info/cocktail.html; http://www.rense.com/general59/vvac.htm; http://www.tetrahedron.org/articles/vaccine_awareness/ingredients.html.

21  Woodruff, Croft. "The Flu Vaccine Myth." *Alive Magazine*. Apr. 2000.

22  Ibid.

23  Robbins, Joel, DC, ND, MD. *Health Through Nutrition*. 1992. p. 55; Griffin, G. Edward. *World Without Cancer*, "Cartels: The Escape from Competition." 1980. pp. 241–268.

24  http://www.dr-rath-foundation.org/open_letters/interview4.

## CHAPTER 7

1   Robbins, Joel, DC, ND, MD. *College of Natural Health Extension Course*. 1995. Lecture note.

2   Owen, Bob L., PhD, DSc. *You Don't Have to Die Sick*. 1994. p. 64.

3   Weindruch, Richard, PhD. "Caloric Restriction and Aging." *Scientific American*. Jan. 1996.

4   Robbins. Op. cit. Sec. 4, p. 49.

5   Appleton, Nancy, PhD. "Lick the Sugar Habit." *Health Freedom News*. 1994.

6   Hiestand, Denie and Shelley. *Electrical Nutrition*. 2001. p. 81.

7   Zovluck, Bernarr, DC, DD. "Why All Should Eat Only Raw Foods Always." http://www.living-foods.com/articles/eatonlyraw.html.

8   Basey, Marleeta F. *Mother Earth News*. Dec. 2004.

9   Campbell, T. Colin, PhD; Campbell, Tomas M., II. *The China Study*. 2004.

10  Morter, M. T., Jr., BS, MA, DC. *Correlative Urinalysis*. 1987. pp. 79, 84.

11  Robbins. Op. cit. Sec. 8, pp. 3, 4.

12  Fallon, Sally; Enig, Mary G. http://www.westonaprice.org. Permission to reproduce facts and quotes originally published by them is gratefully acknowledged.

13  http://www.ratical.org/ratville/soydangers.html#p1.

14  Ibid.

15  Fallon, Sally and Enig, Mary. Third International Soy Symposium Report. *Nexus Magazine*. Vol. 7.3. Apr/May 2000. pp. 4, 7, 8.

16  Ibid. p. 5.

17  Ibid. p. 6.

18  Jensen, Bernard, DC, *Doctor-Patient Handbook*. 1980. p. 8.

19  Jensen, Bernard, DC, *Doctor-Patient Handbook*. 1980. Walker, Norman, DSc, PhD. *Colon Health*. 1995. Anderson, Richard, ND, NMD. *Cleanse & Purify Thyself*. 1994.

20  "What's Wrong With Food Irradiation?" Feb. 2002. http://www.organicconsumers.org/Irrad/Irrad/irradfact.rtf/

## CHAPTER 8

1   Wentz, Myron, Dr. *A Mouth Full of Poison.* Sanoviv. 2004. p. 14.
2   "The Mercury Menace." *http://pressherald.mainetoday.com/specialrpts/mercury.*
3   http://www.un.org/earthwatch/toxicchem/heavymetals.html.
4   Vimy, Murray J, DDS. *Toxic Teeth: A Guide to Mercury Exposure from "Silver" Fillings.* 1992. pp. 7–13.
5   http://www.whale.to/b/huggins_h.html.
6   Lee, John R., MD; with Virginia Hopkins. *What Your Doctor May Not Tell You About Menopause: The Breakthrough Book on Natural Progesterone.* 1996. p. 51.
7   *Clinical Toxicology of Commercial Products.* 5th Edition. 1984. p. ll4.
8   "Fluoride May Not Prevent Cavities, and Can Cause Health Problems." http://thyroid.about.com/cs/toxicchemicalsan/a/fluoridepr.htm.
9   http://www.aerias.org/kview.asp?DocId=133&spaceid=1&subid=7.
10  *US Environmental Protection Agency Report.* 1999.
11  http://www.garynull.com/Documents/erf/need_for_civic_action.htm.
12  Dako, Pete. "Constituents of Tobacco Smoke." http://www.swen.uwaterloo.ca/~as3/archive/science.html#Smoke.
13  http://www.holisticvetpet ceteraare.com.
14  http://www.energytools.biz/mag_field_therapy.htm.
15  Gamble, Steve. "The Dangers of EMF Radiation and What We Can Do to Improve our Health in Today's Polluted World." http://www.equilibra.uk.com/emfsbio.shtml.


## CHAPTER 9

1   Robbins, Joel, DC, ND, MD. *College of Natural Health Extension Course.* 1995. Sec. 12. p. 5.
2   Smith, Marshall. "SARS: The Mystery Disease." Brother Jonathan Gazette. Mar. 31, 2003. http://www.brojon.org/frontpage/SARSFEVER.html.
3   Robbins. Op. cit.
4   Smith. Op. cit.
5   Ibid.
6   Robbins. Op. cit. p. 9.
7   Jensen, Bernard, DC; Anderson, Mark. *Empty Harvest.* 117.
8   Henderson, Doug, *Diet and Exercise is a Crock.* 2000.
9   Shippen, Eugene, MD; Fryer, William. *The Testosterone Syndrome.* 1998. p. 81.
10  Ibid. p. 83.
11  Goldhamer, Alan, DC, http://www.healthpromoting.com.
12  Ruff, Howard J. *Famine and Survival in America.* 1974. pp. 83–86.
13  http://womenshealth.about.com/cs/hysterectomy/l/aahysteralternt.htm.
14  http://www.mayoclinic.com/health/uterine-fibroids/UF99999/PAGE=UF00010&.

15  http://www.healingdaily.com/conditions/hormone-replacement-therapy.htm.

16  Johnston, Laurance, PhD. "Natural Prostate Health." http://www.healingtherapies. info/natural_prostate_health.htm.

17  Sieber, Paul, MD. "Overview of Prostate Problems." http://www.seekwellness.com/ prostate.

18  Shippen. Op. cit. p. 98.

19  Lee, John R., MD. *Hormone Balance for Men.* 2003. pp. 15, 16.

20  Ibid. p. 23.

21  Ibid. p. 20.

22  Ibid. p. 15.

23  Shippen. Op. cit. pp. 23–26.

24  Ibid. pp. 79–95.

25  Ibid. pp. 115–133.

26  Ibid. p. 106.

27  Fair and Heston. 1977; Pfeiffer, 1978. http://www.doctoryourself.com/prostate.html.

28  Lee. Op. cit. p9.

29  Shippen. Op. cit. p. viii.

30  Lee, John R., MD; Virginia Hopkins. *What Your Doctor May Not Tell You About Menopause: The Breakthrough Book on Natural Progesterone.* 1996.

31  Fallon, Sally; Enig, Mary G., PhD. "Teens Before Their Time." http://www.weston aprice.org/soy/teensbeforetime.html.

32  Wright, Jonathan V., MD; Lenard, Lane, PhD. *Why Stomach Acid is Good for You.* 2001. p. 59.

33  Ibid. p. 20.

34  *Metabolic Syndrome.* http://www.americanheart.org/presenter.jhtml?identifier=4756.

35  Brown, Michael. *The Presence Process.* 2005. p. 280.

36  Perricone, Nicholas, MD. *The Wrinkle Cure.* 2000.

37  Connolly, Robert, Dr. "Psoriasis Can Be Cured." http:// www.psoriasiscured.com.

38  For a discussion of this, see: http://www.geocities.com/HotSprings/4966/fm.htm.

39  http://www.imbris.net/~bblinzler/candida.html.

40  Huggins, Hal E, DDS, MS; Levy, Thomas E, MD, JD. *Uninformed Consent: The hidden Dangers in Dental Care.* 1999. pp. 80, 81.

**CHAPTER 10**

1  Morter, M. T. Jr. BS, MA, DC. *pH: Your Potential for Health.* 2000.

2  Robbins, Joel, DC, ND, MD. *College of Natural Health Extension Course.* 1995. Lecture note.

3  Whang, Sang. *Reverse Aging.* 1994. p. 67.

4  Cochran, Mark, BS, DC, ND. *The Secrets of pH Concerning Health and Disease.* 2003. p. 4.

5  Bartlett, Peter. "Using pH as a Measure of Digestive Physiology." *Positive Health.* Issue

13. July/Aug 1996. http://www.positivehealth.com.

6 Baroody, Theodore A., ND, DC, PhD. *Alkalize or Die,* 2002; Cochran, Mark, BS, DC, ND. *The Secrets of Health and Disease.* 2003; Morter, M. T., Jr., BS, MA, DC. *Correlative Urinalysis, The Body Knows Best.* 1987.

7 Morter, M. T., Jr., BS, MA, DC. *Correlative Urinalysis.* 1987. pp. 33–38.

8 Ibid. p. 51.

9 Ibid. p. 83.

10 Guyton, Arthur C., MD. *Textbook of Medical Physiology.* 2nd. ed. Philadelphia, PA, and London, Eng.: W. B. Saunders. 1961. pp. 125–126.

11 Morter, M. T., Jr., BS, MA, DC. *Correlative Urinalysis.* 1987. p. 115.

12 http://www.ztherapy.org/oxygen.html.

13 *The Wellness Revolution for Organizations.* Issue 3. October 21, 2003.

14 Naesens, Gaston. http://www.euroamericanhealth.com/gaston.html.

15 Cousens, Gabriel, MD. *Rainbow Green: Live-Food Cuisine.* 2003. pp. 6, 13.

16 Gdanski, Ron. *Cancer: Cause, Cure and Cover-up.* 2000. p. 60.

## CHAPTER 11

1 http://www.beyondveg.com/novick-j/nutrition-education/physicians-2.shtml.

2 CBS News. May 26, 2005.

3 Campbell, Colin T, PhD. *The China Study.* 2005.

4 Robbins, Joel, DC, ND, MD. *College of Natural Health Extension Course.* 1995. Sec. 3. p. 65.

5 Postawski, Kacper, M. "Powerful Sleep." http://www.powerfulsleep.com.

## CHAPTER 12

1 Ray, Timothy, OMD Lac. "The "Low Battery" Focus." *Explore Magazine.* Vol. 10.4.

2 Davis, Adelle. *Let's Eat Right To Keep Fit.* 1970. p. 63.

3 Gordon, Richard. *Quantum-Touch, The Power to Heal.* 2002.

4 Werner, Dr. *Pulsating Electromagnetic Resonance Therapy.* http://www.naturalhealth-web.com/articles/Werner.html.

5 DeloRey, Herbert, NMD. Edmonton General Hospital. hdelorey@yahoo.ca.

6 Nelson, William, MD. Author of *The Pomorpheus,* 1982. Inventor of the Quantum Xrroid system.

7 Nelson, William, MD. *Manual for the Quantum Xrroid (Medical) Unconscious Interface, QXCI–QMCI.*

8 DeloRey. Op. cit.

9 http://www.google.ca/search?hl=en&lr=&oi=defmore&defl=en&q=define: Biophoton.

10  http://www.oirf.com/recinstr/photon2.html.

11  http://community-2.webtv.net/essentialhealth/aromatherapy.


## CHAPTER 13

1  Stockton, Susan. *The Terrain is Everything*. 2000.

2  Irons, V. E., Dr. *Reactions*. Vol. IV, Number 5.2. Company Manual. n.d.

3  Ibid. pp. 3, 4.

4  Robbins, Joel, DC, ND, MD. *Health Through Nutrition*. 1992. p. 42.

5  Robbins, Joel, DC, ND, MD. *College of Natural Health Extension Course*. 1995. Lecture note.

6  O'Brien, Michael, MD. Avena Originals Health Seminar. Red Deer, AB. 2001. Lecture note.

7  Walker, Norman W., DSc, PhD. *Colon Health: The Key to a Vibrant Life*. 1995. p. 9.

8  http://www.meridianinstitute.com/newslet/Vol6-4/6-4.html.

9  http://www.thecolonet.com.

10  Walker, Norman W. Op. cit. p. 27.

11  Clark, Hulda Regehr, Ph.D, ND. *The Cure for all Diseases*. 1995. p. 558.

12  Cochran, Mark, BS, DC, ND. *The Secrets of pH Concerning Health and Disease*. 2003.

13  http://www.homecraft.bc.ca/sauna.htm.

14  Wilson, Lawrence. *Townsend Letter for Doctors and Patients*. Nov. 2000. http://find articles.com/p/articles/mi_m0ISW/is_2002_Nov/ai_93736414.

15  Ibid.

16  http://www.infaredhealth.com/fir_energy.html.

17  http://www.tohealth.com.au/hpress.htm. "Hypothermic Detoxification Therapy Using the Far Infrared Sauna."

18  Multiple Chemical Sensitivity. http://www.infaredhealth.com/article_pages/fir_sauna_detox.html.

19  Rogers, Sherry, Dr. "The Ultimate Solution to Disease." *Total Wellness*. May 2000. http://www.physiotherm.net/medicalStudies/48/Rogers_InfraredSaunas.html.


## CHAPTER 14

1  http://www.natural-health.co.uk/cell.html.

2  Jhon, Mu Shik, Dr. *The Water Puzzle and the Hexagonal Key*. 2004. pp. 67–85.

3  Ibid. p. 16

4  Ibid. pp. 35, 39, 78.

5  Ibid. p. 73.

6  Ibid. pp. 45, 46.

7   http://www.harmonikireland.com/living_water.htm.

8   Morter, M. T., Jr., BS, MA, DC. *Correlative Urinalysis*. 1987. p. 156.

9   Popp, Fritz, Dr. http://www.implosionresearch.com/water.html.

10  http://www.wateralive.excelexgold.com.

11  Emoto, Masaru. *The Hidden Messages in Water*. 2004. pp. 5, 129, 130.

## CHAPTER 15

1   DeVries, Arnold. *The Elixir of Life*. 1958. p. 4.

2   Robbins, Joel, DC, ND, MD. *Health Through Nutrition*. 1992. p. 4.

3   Ibid.

4   Ibid.

5   O'Brien, Michael, MD. Avena Originals Health Seminar. Red Deer, AB. 2001. Lecture note.

6   Boutenko, Victoria. *Green for Life*. 2005. p. 9.

7   Wildman,Derek. E. et al. *Implications of Natural Selection in Shaping 99.4% Nonsynonymous DNA Identity Between Humans and Chimpanzees: enlarging Genus Homo*. National Academy of Sciences. May 19, 2003 (#2172).

8   Blood Type Facts. http://www.bloodbook.com/type-facts.html.

9   Boutenko. Op. cit. p. 17.

10  Ibid. pp.31–36.

11  Ibid. pp. 41–47.

12  Ibid.

13  Ibid. pp. 69–77.

14  Robbins, Joel, DC, ND, MD. *Pregnancy, Childbirth & Children's Diet*. p. 17. n.d.

15  http://www.drdonnavice.com/drrobbins/index.php.

16  Dorland's Illustrated Medical Dictionary.

17  Bateson-Koch, Carolee, DC, ND. *Allergies: Disease in Disguise*. 1994. pp. 91, 92. http://www.alive.com.

18  Howell, Edward, Dr. *Enzyme Nutrition*. 1985. p. xv.

19  Roy, Leo, MD, ND. *Enzymes: Weavers of Life*. 1994. p. 12.

20  Howell. Op. cit. p. 26.

21  Ibid. p. 27.

22  Howell, Dr. Edward. "Enzymes and Longevity." Interview. http://www.dreddyclinic.com/online_recources/articles/aging/enzymes-and-longevity.htm.

23  Howell, Edward, Dr. *Enzyme Nutrition*. 1985. p. 26.

24  Miller, Jonathon. "Enzymes, Essential for Life." 2004. http://www.reallywell.com/enzymes.htm.

25  Ruff, Howard J. *Famine and Survival in America*. 1974. p. 82.

26  Ibid. p. 83.

27  Ibid. p. 85.

28  Harris, Robert S. Ph.D; Loesecke, S. B. *Nutritional Evaluation of Food Processing.* 1971. p. 233. (Quoted in *Famine and Survival in America* by Howard J. Ruff. 1974. p. 87.)

29  O'Brien, Michael, MD. Avena Originals Health Seminar. Red Deer, AB. 2001. Lecture note.

30  Ruff. Op. cit. p. 82.

31  http://www.avenaoriginals.com/library/article_display.asp?a=Probiotics.

32  Robbins, Joel, DC, ND, MD. *College of Natural Health Extension Course.* 1995. Sec. 3. p. 30.

33  Erasmus, Udo, *Fats that Heal, Fats that Kill.* 1994. pp. 3. http://www.alive.com.

34  Ibid. p. 9.

35  Ibid. p. 236.

36  Erasmus, Udo. *Choosing the Right Fats.* 2001. pp. 10, 11. http://www.alive.com.

37  http://www.bantransfats.com/abouttransfat.html.

38  Erasmus. Op. Cit. pp. 93–98.

39  Erasmus, Udo. *Fats that Heal, Fats that Kill.* 1994. p. 64. http://www.alive.com.

40  http://www.hps-online.com/food.

41  Erasmus. Op. Cit. p. 70.

42  http://proliberty.com/observer/20011010.htm.

43  Enig, Mary PhD. Presentation at AVOC Oils Symposium. Ho Chi Min City, Vietnam. Apr. 25, 1996.

44  Erasmus. Op. Cit. p. 30.

45  Thampan, P.K. "Facts and Fallacies About Coconut Oil." *Asian and Pacific Coconut Community.* 1994. p. 8.

46  http://www.mercola.com.

47  http://www.cancerchoices.com/guide/colostrum.htm.

48  http://www.firstmilking.com/when_you_should_expect_results.htm.

49  Erasmus, Udo. *Fats that Heal, Fats that Kill.* 1994. p. 279.

50  Hemp Facts. http://www.geocities.com/capitolhill/2343/hemp.html.

51  Bennett, Chris. "Hemp Seed, the Royal Grain." http://www.votehemp.com/produc-tion/faq_1.html.

52  Osburn, Lynn. "Hemp Seed: The Most Nutritionally complete Food Source in the World." *Hemp Line Journal.* July–Aug 1992.

53  http://www.newtreatments.org/reams.

54  Ibid.

55  de Langre, Jacques PhD. *Seasalt's Hidden Powers.* 1994. p. 2.

56  de Langre. Op, cit. p. 11.

57  Ibid. p. 21.

58  http://www.mnwelldir.org/docs/nutrition/salt.htm.

59  de Langre. Op. cit. p. 57.

60  McCauley, Bob. *Confessions of a Body Builder.* 2000. p. 82.

**CHAPTER 16**

1 Murray, Richard P., DC, PA. "Natural vs Synthetic." *Biomedical Nitty-Gritty Newsletter*, Vol. 3.1. Jan 1982.

2 Ibid.

3 http://liquid-vitamins.info/.

4 Tennant, Jerry, MD. "Phytoplankton, Making History for Mankind." *Tennant Institute of Integrative Medicine.* n.d. p. 1.

5 "The Mathematical Ocean." Feb. 9, 2005. http://www.nasa.gov/vision/earth/lookingat earth/plankton.html.

6 Williams, Ron. *Another Day*, ForeverGreen. DVD. 2005.

7 Ibid.

8 Rowe, Bob, DC. "Optimum Health and UMAC CORE." 2005.

9 Williams. Op. cit.

10 "Stevia, Sweetener of the Future." *Christine's Cleanse Corner.* http://www.transformy-ourlife.com/miscprods/stevia.htm.

11 Butler, Graham, BSc, CNPA. "Stevia: A Sweet Tradition." http://www.alive.com/1475 a4a2.php.

12 http://www.health2us.com/csapps.htm.

13 "Government Reports on Colloidal Silver." http://www.happyherbalist.com/fda_report.htm.

14 Ibid.

15 "A Few Unique plus Traditional Uses for Colloidal Silver." http://www.silvergen.com/colloidal_silver_uses.htm.

16 "Colloidal Silver: The Rediscovery of a Super Antibiotic?" http://www.all-natural.com/silver-1.html.

17 "Great Info About Colloidal Silver." http://www.infobasset.com/colloidal-silver.

18 Harris, Larry C. Interview by *The Wednesday Report.* http://www.thewednesdayre-port.com/articles/research/weapons_of_mass_destruction-threat_scenario.htm.

19 http://www.the7thfire.com/health_and_nutrition/Colloidal_Silver.htm.

20 *The Colloidal Silver Handbook.* http://www.cerebrex.com/archives.htm.

21 Becker, Robert O., MD. *The Body Electric.* 1985. p 167.

22 "Colloidal Silver: The Rediscovery of a Super Antibiotic?" Op. cit.

23 Baranowski, Zane, CN. "Colloidal Silver: The Natural Antibiotic." http://www.elixa.com/silver/zaneuse.htm.

24 Two sources: http://shesacancersurvivor.com/silver/index.htm; and, http://www.sota instruments.com.

25 http://www.chisuk.org.uk/articles/result.php?key=37.

26 "Grapefruit Seed Extract—A natural antibiotic." *The Grisanti Report.* No. 1231. http://www.drgrisanti.com/grapefruit.htm.

27  Privitera, James R, MD. "Olive Leaf Extract." http://curezone.com/foods/oliveleaf. asp#priv.
28  Klatz, Ronald, Dr.; Kahn, Carol. *Grow Young with HGH*. 1997. pp. 43, 44.

## CHAPTER 17

1  Lipton, Bruce, PhD. *The Biology of Belief*. 2005. p. 134.
2  Ibid. p. 166.
3  Brown, Michael. *The Presence Process*. 2005. p. 35.
4  Tolle, Eckhart. *The Power of Now*. 1997. p. 18.
5  Ibid. p. 29.
6  Ibid. p. 24.
7  Ibid. p. 16.

## CHAPTER 18

1  Lipton, Bruce, PhD. *The Biology of Belief*. 2005.
2  Ibid. p. 136.
3  Ibid. p. 148.
4  Ibid. p. 150.
5  Childre, Doc; Martin, Howard. *The HeartMath Solution*. 2000. p. 37.
6  Zukav, Gary; Francis, Linda. *The Heart of the Soul: Emotional Awareness*. 2001.
7  Loyd, Alexander, ND, MS; Johnson, Ben, MD, DO, NMD. *The Healing Codes*. 2005. p.11.
8  Hawkins, David R., MD, PhD. *The Eye of the I*. 2001. p. 142.
9  Green, Glenda. *Love Without End: Jesus Speaks*. 1999. p. 124.
10  Childre, Doc; Martin, Howard. Op. cit. p. 27.
11  Walsch, Neale Donald. *Questions and Answers on Conversations with God*. 1999. p. 121.

## CHAPTER 19

1  Hawkins, David R., MD, PhD. *Power vs Force: The Hidden Determinants of Human Behavior*. 2001. p. 185.
2  Lipton, Bruce, Ph.D. *The Biology of Belief*. 2005. pp. 135, 136.
3  Ibid. p. 138.
4  Ruiz, Don Miguel. *The Four Agreements*. 1997. p. 5.
5  Lipton. Op. cit. p. 163.
6  Ruiz. Op. cit. p. 13.
7  *Bible, King James Version*. Luke 17: 21.

8   Berg, Yehuda. *The Power of Kaballah.* p. 107.

9   Ibid. p. 14, 19.

10  Ibid. p. 123.

11  Hargis, David M. *The Constantine Conspiracy.* 1994. pp. 25–30.

12  Braden, Gregg. *The Isaiah Effect: Decoding the Lost Science of Prayer and Prophecy.* 2000. p. 35.

13  *Bible.* Op. cit. Matthew 21: 22.

14  Horowitz, Leonard, DMD, MA, MPH. *Healing Celebrations.* 2000. pp. 160, 161.

15  Cho, David Yonggi, Dr. *The Fourth Dimension.* 2001. pp. 51–53.

16  Mains, Karen Burton. *You Are What You Say: Cure for the Troublesome Tongue.* 1988.

17  Losier, Michael. *Law of Attraction.* 2003.

18  Walsch, Neale Donald. *Conversations with God, Book 1.* 1995. p. 180.

19  Lipton, Bruce PhD. *The Biology of Belief.* Video. 2001.

20  Dyer, Wayne, W., PhD. *The Power of Intention.* 2004. p. 4.

21  Ibid. p. 10.

## CHAPTER 20

1   *Bible, New King James Version.* Luke 23: 34.

2   Ibid. John 8: 32.

3   Ibid. Matt 9: 22.

4   Ruiz, Don Miguel. *The Four Agreements.* 1997. p. 50.

5   Maté, Gabor, MD. *When the Body Says No: The Cost of Hidden Stress.* 2003. pp. 197, 198.

6   Maté, Gabor, MD. *Scattered Minds,* 1999. p. 32.

7   Tracy, Brian. "Activating Your Success Mechanism." http://www.wcool.com/religion/goals.html.

8   Kuskoff, Vladimir. "Self-discovery by Observation." http://members.surfeu.fi/wpk/articles.

## CHAPTER 21

1   Arlin, Stephen; Dini, Fouad; Wolfe, David. *Nature's First Law: The Raw Food Diet.* 2000. p. 62.

2   Ibid.

3   Morter, M. T., Jr. *pH: Your Potential For Health.* 2000. p. 7.

4   Morter, M. T., Jr. *Correlative Urinalysis.* 1987. p. 138.

5   Ibid. p. 137.

6   Ibid. pp. 134, 135.

7   Ibid. pp. 46, 135.

8    Wright, Jonathan, V., MD; Lenard, Lane, PhD. *Why Stomach Acid is Good for You*, 2001. p. 157.

9    Cousens, Gabriel, MD. Author of *Conscious Eating*. http://www.living-foods.com/ articles/vinegartruth.html.

10   Lee, John R., MD; Hopkins, Virginia. *What Your Doctor May Not Tell You About Menopause*. 1996. p. 71.

11   Examples are: *Juicing for Health*, by Dr. Joel Robbins; *Fresh Vegetable and Fruit Juices* by Dr. N. W. Walker; and *Juice Fasting & Detoxification*, by Steve Meyerowitz.

12   O'Brien, Michael, MD. Avena Originals Health Seminar. Red Deer, AB. 2001. Lecture note.

13   http://www.foodmarketexchange.com/datacenter/product/organic/details/dc_pi_ organic_05.htm.

14   http://www.mercola.com/2003/dec/27/toxic_metals.htm.

15   *Aluminum.* www.luminet.net/~wenonah/hydro/al.htm.

16   Wagenheim, Brooke. "Common Parasites Threaten Everyone." Feb. 2003. http://www. southsidepride.com/2003/February/Articles/parasites.html.

17   Robbins, Joel, DC, ND, MD. *College of Natural Health Extension Course*. 1995. Sec. 3, p. 3.

**CHAPTER 22**

1    O'Brien, Michael, MD. Interview by author. December 9, 2000.

2    http://www.avenaoriginals.com.

3    *Memoirs of Dr. John R. Christopher.* http://www.healthyherbalist.com.

4    Robbins, Joel, DC, ND, MD. *Attitudes and Health*. 1992. p. 37.

**CHAPTER 23**

1    O'Brien, Michael, MD. Interview by the author. December 9, 2000.

**APPENDIX 1**

1    Robbins, Joel, DC, ND, MD, *Health Through Nutrition*. 1992. p. 15.

2    Baroody, Theodore A., ND, DC, PhD. *Alkalize or Die*, 2002.

The following books and booklets are ones I have found to be very informative and helpful for understanding the truth of natural health for the body. The titles in **bold-face type** are particularly recommended. Please keep in mind that no single book has all the answers, nor do all books agree on every point. Read with a discerning mind, and in time, the picture of what contributes to true health will come clearer for you.

Arlin, Stephen; Dini, Fouad; Wolfe, David. *Nature's First Law: The Raw Food Diet.* San Diego, CA: Maul Brothers Publishing. 2000.

Baroody, Theodore A., ND, DC, PhD. *Alkalize or Die.* Waynesville, NC: Holographic Health Press. 2002.

Bateson-Koch, Carolee, DC, ND. *Allergies: Disease in Disguise.* Burnaby, BC: Alive Books. 1994.

Berg, Yehuda. *The Power of Kabbalah.* Los Angeles, CA: Kabbalah Center International. 2004

Bieler, Henry G., MD. *Food is Your Best Medicine.* New York: Ballantine Books. 1982.

Blaylock, Russell L., MD. *Excitotoxins: The Taste that Kills.* Santa Fe, NM: Health Press. 1997.

Boutenko, Victoria. *Green For Life.* Raw Family Publishing. Ashland, OR: Raw Family Publishing. 2005.

Braden, Gregg. *The God Code.* Carlsbad, CA: Hay House. 2004.

Braden, Gregg. *The Isaiah Effect: Decoding the Lost Science of Prayer and Prophecy.* Nevada City, CA: Harmony Books. 2000.

Bragg, Paul C., ND; Bragg, Patricia ND, PhD. *Apple Cider Vinegar: Miracle Health System.* Santa Barbara, CA: Health Science. n.d.

Bragg, Paul C., ND; Bragg, Patricia ND, PhD. *The Miracle of Fasting.* Santa Barbara, CA: Health Science. n.d.

Brotman, Juliano. *Raw: The Uncook Book.* New York: HarperCollins. 1999.

Brown, Michael. *The Presence Process.* Vancouver, BC: Namaste Publishing. 2005.

Burroughs, Stanley. *The Master Cleanser.* Newcastle, CA: Burrough Books. 1976.

Campbell, T. Colin, PhD; Campbell, Tomas M II. *The China Study.* Dallas, TX: BenBella Books. 2004.

Carter, Albert, E. *The Miracles of Rebound Exercise.* Edmonds, WA: National Institute of Reboundology & Health. 1979.

Childre, Doc; Martin, Howard. *The HeartMath Solution*, New York: HarperCollins. 1999.

Clark, Hulda Regehr, PhD, ND. *The Cure for all Diseases*. San Diego, CA: ProMotion Publishing. 1995.

Cochran, Mark, BS, DC, ND. *The Secrets of pH Concerning Health and Disease: The Short Version*. 2003.

Cousens, Gabriel, MD. **Rainbow Green Live-Food Cuisine**. Berkeley, CA: North Atlantic Books. 2003.

Dahl, Lila. **Change Your Mind, Change Your Life.** Victoria, BC: Mind Revision. 2002.

Davis, Adelle. *Let's Eat Right To Keep Fit*. New York: Signet Books. 1970.

DeVries, Arnold. *The Elixir of Life*. Chicago: Chandler Book Company. 1952.

de Langre, Jacques, PhD. **Seasalt's Hidden Powers**. North Carolina: Happiness Press. 1994.

Dyer, Wayne W., PhD. *The Power of Intention*. Carlsbad, CA: Hay House. 2004.

Ehret, Arnold, Prof. *Mucusless Diet Healing System*. Beaumont, CA: Ehret Literature Publishing Co. 1972.

Elliot, David A. **The Electric Universe.** Burnaby, BC: Inklination Press. 1996.

Emoto, Masaru. **The Hidden Messages in Water.** Hillsboro, Oregon: Beyond Words Publishing Inc. 2004.

Erasmus, Udo. **Choosing the Right Fats.** Burnaby BC: Alive Books. 2001.

Erasmus, Udo. **Fats that Heal, Fats that Kill.** Burnaby BC: Alive Books. 1994.

Gdanski, Ron. *Cancer: Cause, Cure and Cover-up*. Grimsby, ON: Nadex Publishing. 2000.

Gordon, Richard. *Quantum-Touch: The Power to Heal*. Berkeley, CA: North Atlantic Books. 2002.

Gray, Robert. *The Colon Health Handbook*. Oakland, CA: Rockridge Publishing Company. 1983.

Green, Glenda. *Love Without End: Jesus Speaks*. Fort Worth, TX: Heartwing Publishing. 1999.

Griffin, G. Edward. **World without Cancer**. Westlake Village, CA: American Media. 1980.

Hawkins, David R., MD, PhD. **Power vs. Force: The Hidden Determinants of Human Behavior.** Sedona, AZ: Veritas Publishing. 2001.

Hay, Louise L. *Heal Your Body*. Carlsbad, CA: Hay House. 1988.

Hiestand, Denie and Shelley. **Electrical Nutrition.** Vancouver, BC: ShellDen Corp. 1999.

Horowitz, Leonard, DMD, MA, MPH. *Healing Celebrations*. Sandpoint, ID: Tetrahedron Publishing Group. 2000.

Horowitz, Leonard, DMD, MA, MPH. **Emerging Viruses—AIDS & Ebola—Nature: Accident or Intentional.** Rockport, MA: Tetrahedron Inc. 1997.

Howell, Edward, Dr. *Enzyme Nutrition*. Wayne, NJ: Avery Publishing Group. 1985.

Huggins, Hal E., DDS, MS; Levy, Thomas E, MD, JD. **Uninformed Consent: The Hidden Dangers in Dental Care.** Charlottesville, VA: Hampton Roads Publishing. 1999.

Hume, E. Douglas. *Bechamp or Pasteur: A Lost Chapter in the History of Biology.* Mokelumne Hill, CA: Health Research. 1996.

Jarvis, D. C., MD. *Folk Medicine: A New England Almanac of Natural Health Care from a noted Vermont Country Doctor.* New York: Ballantine Books. 1985.

Jensen, Bernard, DC. *Doctor-Patient Handbook.* Provo, UT: BiWorld Publishers. 1976.

Jensen, Bernard, DC. *Breathe Again Naturally.* Escondido, CA: Bernard Jensen Enterprises. 1983.

Jensen, Bernard, DC; Anderson, Mark. *Empty Harvest.* Garden City Park, NY: Avery Publishing Group. 2002.

Jensen, Bernard, DC. **Tissue Cleansing Through Bowel Management.** Escondido, CA: Bernard Jensen Enterprises. 1981.

Klatz, Ronald, Dr. *Grow Young with HGH.* New York: Harper Collins Publishers. 1997.

Jhon, Mu Shik, Dr. *The Water Puzzle and the Hexagonal Key.* Uplifting Press, Inc. 2004.

Lanctôt, Guylaine, MD. **The Medical Mafia.** Miami, FL: Here's The Key. 1995.

Lee, John R., MD; Virginia Hopkins. **What Your Doctor May Not Tell You About Menopause.** New York: Warner Books. 1996.

Lipton, Bruce, PhD. **The Biology of Belief.** Santa Rosa, CA: Mountain of Love/Elite Books. 2005.

Lopez, D. A., MD; Williams, R. M., MD, PhD; Miehlke, M., MD. **Enzymes: The Fountain of Life.** Charleston, SC: Neville Press. 1994.

Losier, Michael. *Law of Attraction.* Victoria, BC: Michael J. Losier. 2003.

McCauley, Bob. *Confessions of a Body Builder.* Lansing, MI: Spartan Enterprises. 2000.

Maté, Gabor, MD. *When the Body Says No: The Cost of Hidden Stress.* Toronto, ON: Random House. 2003

Maté, Gabor, MD. *Scattered Minds.* Toronto, ON: Alfred A. Knopf. 1999.

Meinig, George E., DDS, FACD. **Root Canal Cover-Up.** Ojai, CA: Bion Publishing. 1993.

Mendelsohn, Robert S., MD. **Confessions of a Medical Heretic.** New York: Warner Books. 1980.

Meyerowitz, Steve. **Juice Fasting & Detoxification.** Great Barrington, MA: The Sprout House. 1996.

Meyerowitz, Steve. **Sproutman's Kitchen Garden Cookbook.** Great Barrington, MA: The Sprout House. 1994.

Miller, Neil Z. **Vaccines: Are They Really Safe and Effective? A Parent's Guide To Childhood Shots.** Santa Fe, NM: New Atlantean Press. 1996.

Morter, M. T., Jr., BS, MA, DC. **pH: Your Potential For Health.** Rogers, AR: Morter Health System. 2000.

Morter, M. T., Jr., BS, MA, DC. **Correlative Urinalysis: The Body Knows Best.** Rogers, AR: B.E.S.T. Research. 1987.

Owen, Bob L., PhD, DSc. *You Don't Have to Die Sick.* Cannon Beach, OR: Health/Hope Publishing House. 1994.

Page, Linda, ND, PhD. **Healthy Healing: A Guide to Self-Healing for Everyone.** http://healthyhealing.com: Healthy Healing Publications. 1998.

Perricone, Nicholas, MD. *The Wrinkle Cure.* New York: Warner Books. 2000.

Pottenger, Francis M., Jr. **Pottenger's Cats: A Study in Nutrition.** San Diego, CA: Price-Pottenger Nutrition Foundation, Inc. 1995.

Robbins, Joel, DC, ND, MD. **Attitudes and Health,** Colonia, NJ: Vitality Unlimited. 1992.

Robbins, Joel, DC, ND, MD. **Health Through Nutrition.** Colonia, NJ: Vitality Unlimited, 1992.

Robbins, Joel, DC, ND, MD. **College of Natural Health Extension Course.** Lindstrom, MN: College of Natural Health. 1995.

Robbins, Joel, DC, ND, MD. **Pregnancy, Childbirth & Children's Diet.** Tulsa, OK: Health Dynamics Corp. n.d.

Robbins, Joel, DC, ND, MD. **Juicing for Health.** Tulsa, OK: Health Dynamics Corp. 1994.

Roy, Leo, MD, ND. *GI Detox.* Westbank, BC: Datic Health Resources. 1994.

Roy, Leo, MD, ND. *Oils, Fats, Cholesterol.* Westbank, BC: Datic Health Resources. 1994.

Roy, Leo, MD, ND. *Your Liver: The Laboratory of Living.* Westbank, BC: Datic Health Resources. 1994.

Ruiz, Don Miguel. *The Four Agreements*. San Rafael, CA: Amber-Allen Publishing. 1997.

Scheibner, Viera, PhD. **Vaccination: 100 Years of Orthodox Research Shows That Vaccines Represent a Medical Assault on the Immune System.** Victoria, Australia: Australian Print Group. 1993.

Shannon, Nomi. **The Raw Gourmet**. Burnaby, BC: Alive Books. 1999.

Tolle, Eckhart. **The Power of Now: A Guide to Spiritual Enlightenment.** Vancouver, BC: Namaste Publishing. 1997.

Vimy, Murray J., DDS. **Toxic Teeth.** Calgary, AB: Murray J. Vimy. 1993.

Whang, Sang. *Reverse Aging*. Englewood Cliffs, NJ: Siloam Enterprise. 1994.

Walker, N. W., DSc, PhD. **Fresh Fruit and Vegetable Juices.** Prescott, AR: Norwalk Press. 1978.

Walker, N. W., DSc, PhD. *Colon Health: The Key to a Vibrant Life.* Prescott, AR: Norwalk Press. 1995.

Walsch, Neale Donald. **Conversations with God, Book 1.** Charlottesville, VA: Hampton Roads Publishing. 1995.

Walsch, Neale Donald. *Questions and Answers on Conversations with God.* Charlottesville, VA: Hampton Roads Publishing. 1999.

Weimar Institute. **Recipes from the Weimar Kitchen**. Weimar, CA: Weimar Institute. 1983.

Wentz, Myron Dr. *A Mouth Full of Poison.* Medicis, SC: Sanoviv. 2004

Wigmore, Ann, ND, DD. *Recipes for Longer Life.* Boston, MA: Rising Sun Publications. 1978.

Wright, Jonathan V., MD; Lenard, Lane, PhD. ***Why Stomach Acid is Good for You.*** New York: M Evans and Company. 2001.

Zukav, Gary; Francis, Linda. *The Heart of the Soul.* New York

# ILLUSTRATION CREDITS

Table 2.1 and Figs. 3.1, 3.2, 3.3, 3.4, 9.1 from Robbins, Joel, DC, ND, MD. *College of Natural Health Extension Course*. Lindstrom, MN: College of Natural Health. 1995.

Tables 5.1, 5.2 and Fig. 4.1 from Robbins, Joel, DC, ND, MD. *Health Through Nutrition*. Colonia, NJ: Vitality Unlimited. 1992.

Fig. 4.2. from Meinig, George E. DDS, FACD. *Root Canal Cover-Up*. Ojai, CA: Bion Publishing. 1993.

Tables 7.1, 12.1 and Figs. 7.1, 7.2 adapted from various sources by Ron Garner.

Figs. 10.1, 10.2, 20.1 by Ron Garner.

Figs. 13.1, 13.2 from Irons, V. E. *Reactions*. Cottonwood, CA: Distributor Manual. Vol. IV, Number 5. 1996.

Table 14.1 and Figs. 14.1 14.2, 14.3 photographs by Mr. and Mrs. Excelex. 2001.

Figs. 14.4, 14.5 from research (2006) of Mr. and Mrs. Excelex and somatoscope images courtesy of C.E.R.B.E. Inc., Quebec, Canada.

Fig. 16.1. from Roy, Leo, MD, ND. *Deception by Vitamins*. Kelowna, BC: Datic Health Resources. 1994.

# INDEX

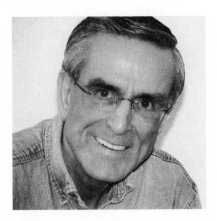

RON GARNER, BEd, MSc, Diploma in Natural Health, is a health researcher, educator, author, and speaker. For a major part of his life, he worked in the public school system in Canada, where he held positions as a teacher, Principal, Deputy Superintendent in British Columbia, and also served as Regional Superintendent of Schools in the Yukon Territory.

Marrying his teaching and writing skills, he presents complex subjects in an organized, easy-to-understand manner. Underneath the content of his writing, the reader finds evidence of his passion for truth and desire to help others.

His own search for health solutions has convinced him that the human body is a miraculous self-healer—if it is given the support it requires to build and maintain health.

He currently resides in British Columbia, Canada.

# n Namaste Publishing

OUR PUBLISHING MISSION
To make available publications that acknowledge, celebrate,
and encourage others to express their true essence and
thereby come to remember
*Who They Really Are.*

NAMASTE PUBLISHING
P.O. Box 62084
Vancouver, British Columbia  v6j 4a3
Canada
www.namastepublishing.com

EMAIL
namaste@telus.net

PHONE
604-224-3179

FAX
604-224-3354

TO PLACE AN ORDER
www.namastepublishing.com
or, email: namasteproductions@shaw.ca

To schedule Ron Garner for a teaching or speaking event,
email: namasteteachings@telus.net

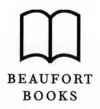

**BEAUFORT
BOOKS**

Beaufort Books is dedicated to publishing the highest quality fiction and non-fiction books and making them available to the general public.

For more information about Beaufort Books
and our other publications, contact:

Beaufort Books
27 West 20th Street
Suite 1102
New York, NY 10011

PHONE
212-727-0190

FAX
212- 727-0195

EMAIL
service@beaufortbooks.com
www.beaufortbooks.com